Aranzio's Seahorse and the Search for Memory and Consciousness

Aranzio's Seahorse and the Search for Memory and Consciousness

ALAN J. McCOMAS

Neuroscientist and Emeritus Professor of Medicine,
McMaster University, Hamilton, Canada

(Drawings by Marie Levesque)

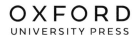
OXFORD
UNIVERSITY PRESS

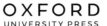

Great Clarendon Street, Oxford, OX2 6DP,
United Kingdom

Oxford University Press is a department of the University of Oxford.
It furthers the University's objective of excellence in research, scholarship,
and education by publishing worldwide. Oxford is a registered trade mark of
Oxford University Press in the UK and in certain other countries

First Edition published in 2023

Impression: 1

Published in the United States of America by Oxford University Press
198 Madison Avenue, New York, NY 10016, United States of America

British Library Cataloguing in Publication Data

Data available

Library of Congress Control Number: 2022938815

ISBN 978–0–19–286824–4

DOI: 10.1093/oso/9780192868244.001.0001

Printed in the UK by
Bell & Bain Ltd., Glasgow

Memory, guiding us through the day, is who we are.

To my wife, Marie Ambruz, who made this book possible

Prologue

Even as late as the middle of the 20th century, little was known of the ways by which the human brain was able to create, store, and retrieve memories. Over the course of the next 70 years explanations would gradually emerge. In some cases the new knowledge would come from chance while in others it would be the result of careful experiment. Though many people would be involved, there were some whose contributions would prove especially important. At the time this story begins, in 1944, they included established clinicians at the height of their fame as well as students on the thresholds of their careers. And then, just as important as the investigators, there would be a small number of patients with very striking and unusual symptoms.

Curiously, most of the new knowledge about memory would concern a part of the brain that had been largely overlooked in the past, even though its structure had been well described. Because its curved shape resembled that of a seahorse, this part of the brain had been given the Greek name for that marine creature—*hippocampus*.

It was Giulio Cesare Aranzio[1] who, in the 16th century, had thought of the name. A native of Bologna, a thriving medieval city in what is now northern Italy, he had been a renowned teacher of anatomy and surgery in the university. And the University of Bologna, like the hippocampus, was unique, though in a different way—founded by scholars in 1088, it had been the world's first university.

When Aranzio had discovered the unusually shaped structure in the brain, he could hardly have imagined what purpose it might have served. But for those who, in the centuries to come, were preoccupied with that greatest of mysteries, the nature of consciousness, it was this structure, the hippocampus, with its ability to store memories, that offered a solution.

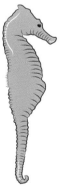

Note

1. S.C. Bir, S. Ambekar, S. Kukreja, and A. Nanda, 'Julius Caesar Arantius (Giulio Cesare Aranzi, 1530–1589) and the Hippocampus of the Human Brain: History behind the Discovery' (2015) 122 *Journal of Neurosurgery* 971–5.

Aranzio (also Aranzi, Arantius) was born in Bologna and received a medical doctorate from the University of Bologna, having been taught the practice of surgery by his uncle, a highly regarded and influential practitioner. Appointed to a university position himself, Aranzio continued to lecture in both anatomy and surgery until his death. In addition to discovering the hippocampus, he made a number of other important contributions to anatomical knowledge; these included the attachments of the external ocular muscles, the path of the optic nerve, and various structures in the heart (including the nodules in the semilunar valve that now bear his name). Aranzio was a contemporary of, and would have been familiar with, the better-known medical scholar, Andreas Vesalius (1514–1564) who spent part of his career at the University of Padua, some 100 kilometres to the north of Bologna.

Contents

II. THE EVOLUTION OF CONSCIOUSNESS

A. GENERAL ISSUES

B. LIMBIC SYSTEM AS LOCATION OF CONSCIOUSNESS

C. SHORT-TERM MEMORY AS THE MECHANISM OF CONSCIOUSNESS

D. NEURAL MECHANISMS INVOLVED

E. RECAPITULATION, SYNTHESIS, AND EPILOGUE

Note to Reader

Against the convention in journal articles but in the interests of readability, first names have been used rather than surnames as in the description of a young or future neuro-scientist, or of one of two neuroscientist spouses. First names have sometimes been used to emphasize gender as well, in recognition of the more difficult paths that many female neuroscientists have been obliged to follow. Had Brenda Milner not accompanied her husband to Canada she could have taken up her scholarship to continue studying at Cambridge University. Denise Albe-Fessard had started her scientific career in France as a lowly laboratory assistant before rising to become the pre-eminent authority on deep brain structures. At the present time Sheena Josselyn combines her outstanding optogenetic research with the many demands of motherhood. And who but a woman could have shown the same compassion and interest in her subject as Suzanne Corkin did for Patient H.M?

Also against convention but with the aim of making the text flow better, birth (and death) dates have been omitted for those who form part of the modern story (post-1944) while being provided for long-deceased persons.

The illustrations are an important feature of the book not only as further sources of information but as momentary relief in places where the text is detailed. Many have been supplied by Wikimedia Commons, Creative Commons, or the Wellcome Gallery of Images, to all of whom the author is greatly indebted.

Introduction

Galvani's Spark, the first book in what is now a trilogy, was intended as homage to a remarkable group of individuals who, through the last two centuries particularly, had devoted themselves to exploring the nature of nerve impulses—the brief electrical signals that enable information to be transmitted from one part of the nervous system to another and that are ultimately responsible for movements, sensations, thoughts, and dreams. The adjective 'remarkable' is fitting. They were persons, mostly men, who had had original ideas and who had set about testing them, usually with apparatus they had built themselves. The expenses had often come out of their own pockets for there were no research grants as there are now, nor had they been part of any international consortium of neuroscientists, as is the custom today. As pioneers, they had been obliged to find their own ways of exploring the nervous system. In the context of the history of neuroscience, theirs was the 'heroic age'.

Sherrington's Loom, the second book, was different. It was intended for a graduate student or lay person who wished to know more about the science relevant to consciousness. It did not aim to describe how consciousness came about—how nerve impulses were somehow translated into thoughts and sensations—but instead identified some of the key experiments that would have to be taken into account in any explanation of the basis of consciousness.

The present study was perhaps inevitable, though I would never have contemplated tackling the neural underpinnings of consciousness before. How the attempt arose, and the realization of the importance of memory in addressing the mystery of consciousness, are described in the next section. It is a rather long account and a very personal one, but I hope it will be seen as relevant to what follows.

The new book has been divided into two parts, the second of which deals with the evolutionary origin of consciousness, the role of memory, and the identification of the brain structures that are especially involved. The evidence for the various propositions is considerable and for this reason much of it is presented for an initial inspection in a historical account of research into the neural basis of memory. It is this account that forms the first part of the book. As a history it is complete in itself, while drawing attention to neuroscientists of the heroic age other than those already considered in *Galvani's Spark* and *Sherrington's Loom*.

Central to both parts of the book is a structure buried deeply at the base of each of the two hemispheres that make up most of the human brain. For a long time it was overlooked by neuroscientists more interested in studying how the brain enabled objects to be seen, sounds heard, and touch felt—or how muscles were called into action for

Aranzio's Seahorse and the Search for Memory and Consciousness. Alan J. McComas, Oxford University Press.
© Oxford University Press 2023. DOI: 10.1093/oso/9780192868244.003.0001

movement. But, through accident and experiment, it turned out that the small deep part, the hippocampus, was every bit as important as the two hemispheres. In fact, it was more important, for it served to keep a record of events, places, people, and objects. It was where memory was created, stored, and retrieved.

The first part of the present book, then, deals with memory and the emerging recognition of the importance of the hippocampus—a part of the brain's limbic system. The history begins with the observations of the psychologist Brenda Milner on her famous subject, the patient Henry Molaison. I have tried to describe something of the setting in which a study has been carried out, not just that of Brenda Milner but those of the many who followed her—the anatomists, neurophysiologists, molecular biologists, and neurologists. This is not simply for the sake of writing a fuller account. There are stories to be told. Why, for instance, did a particular scientist decide to pursue a certain line of work? Why was another one obliged to stop his or her research? Was luck involved in a major discovery—perhaps in the form of a chance observation during an experiment? Why was an important clue not recognized or followed up? I have cast my net widely in order to include work that, although not directly related to the memory–consciousness story, was important at the time for an understanding of the working of the nervous system and for the future direction of neuroscience. Melzack and Wall's gate theory of pain and Hagbarth's introduction of single fibre recordings in human peripheral nerves are two examples. Though the present book and its two predecessors are largely concerned with the history of neuroscience, the content and cast of characters differ; in a number of respects, however, the three books complement each other.

The second part of the book begins by gathering evidence from a variety of sources pointing to the hippocampus and related parts of the limbic system as the conscious-generating part of the human brain. Since these structures had been shown (in Part I) to be responsible for the formation, storage, and retrieval of memory, their involvement in seizures and other disturbances of consciousness constitutes evidence for a link between memory and consciousness. A second argument for the relationship comes from evolution. Memory, and with it an elemental consciousness, must have developed as primitive creatures became increasingly successful in their search for food, sexual partners, and safety. A third argument is provided by the necessity of memory, no matter how brief, for perceptions and thoughts. Also included in Part II is consideration of the numerical issues involved in the operations of the hippocampal neurons.

In summary, the second part of the book draws heavily on the first, but whereas the first deals with historical fact, the purpose of the second is to put forward and to justify an idea. It proposes that the hippocampus and its neighbouring structures are where consciousness is generated.

And that memory, ever-changing short-term memory, is what consciousness is.

I have endeavoured to set out the evidence for this conclusion, and the historical narrative that preceded it, in a manner that will be understood by laypersons as well as by those working on the brain. For the latter, and especially for young neuroscientists embarking on brain studies, there should be interest in learning the historical background to the present concepts of memory and consciousness. For established psychologists used to theoretical models of working memory and attention the book may prove more of a challenge. Nevertheless, while accepting a role for such models in the past, there should be no hesitation in abandoning them as contradictory evidence comes from the experimental laboratories. I am thinking especially of the exciting results of recording from single neurons in the brains of conscious human beings and of the ingenious experiments using optogenetics in rodents, both of which are discussed in this book.[1]

To those interested in the philosophy of scientific investigation (epistemology), the approach adopted in the book is reductionist—one that attempts to solve a problem by breaking it into parts, finding a solution to each part, and then assembling the various answers into a coherent explanation for the whole. It is a tried and trusted way, one that a neuroscientist employs whenever he or she stimulates the brain, or sticks recording electrodes into single cells or small groups of cells. The opposite of this 'outside in' approach is an 'inside out' one, that attempts to interpret the incessant rhythmic electric activity going on inside the brain in terms of function. Just as in the patient on the neurology ward, whose abnormal electroencephalogram (EEG) discharges herald a change in consciousness, it is the brain itself that controls the study.[2]

Now for the personal story.

Notes

1. Not surprisingly, there is much that could be added concerning models of brain function. **Working memory** is a term introduced to replace 'short-term memory'; it is conceived to have two brain compartments handling visual and auditory information respectively, both under the control of a third area, the 'central executive'. All three regions are assigned to the cerebral cortex, to the exclusion to the hippocampus (the one area of the brain shown convincingly to have a memory function!) A review of 'working memory' by one of its originators is: A. Baddeley, 'Working Memory: Looking Back and Looking Forward' (2003) 4 *Nature Reviews Neuroscience* 829–39. Similarly, for **attention** there is, among others, the multi-layered model of Shallice and Burgess (T. Shallice and P. Burgess, 'The Domain of Supervisory Processes and Temporal Organization of Behaviour' (1996) 351(1346) *Philosophical Transactions of the Royal Society, B* 1405–12). As described in the present book (Chapter 45), such models are inconsistent with the results of experiments involving the timing of 'willed' actions and of observations on patients with 'split brains'.
2. The ingenious 'inside-out' approach to studying the brain is one pursued by Györgi Buzsáki (G. Buzsáki, *The Brain from Inside Out* (New York, NY: Oxford University Press, 2019)).

The Journey that Led to the Book

Regardless of topic, it is natural to question an author's credentials. One is reassured if the author of a gardening book has spent hours on his or her knees, trowel in hand, attending to a herbaceous border. Or, in the case of a cookery book, a reader would have more confidence in an author with kitchen experience than in a food dilettante.

In my own case, though I cannot claim to have worked on the hippocampus, I have studied various aspects of brain function both as a neurophysiologist and as a neurologist. This is not an apology. Sometimes a broad view, coming from a wide practical experience, is as valuable as a more specialized one. After all, the brain is a complex system of many parts and interconnections. But as to how my experience was gained, and how the present book came to be written, is a long story.

It began sixty years ago when I pushed open the door to a laboratory in London.

The room had been darkened, the blinds pulled down over the large windows overlooking the street. The small amount of light that still crept in was enough to make out the figures grouped around the table to the far end of the laboratory. To one side of the table were two racks of electronic equipment, the contents linked by loops of black cable. Occupying the top of one rack was an oscilloscope with a green spot that slowly and repeatedly made its way across the screen. As it did so, its otherwise smooth journey was interrupted by sudden brief spikes; at the same time there would be a popping sound from a loudspeaker. Each spike on the screen and each pop from the loudspeaker signalled the firing of an impulse by a neuron in the spinal cord of a sleeping cat.

It was my introduction to high-level neurophysiology at University College London (UCL) and the wonder of that experience would determine my career. How extraordinary, how exciting it was, to be able to listen in to the workings of the nervous system of another creature and to do so in 'real' time. That was the beauty of classical neurophysiology—what you saw and what you heard was happening there and then.

As a recently qualified medical graduate, still in my mid-20s, I could not hope to compete with those who had been longer in that kind of research, and for a while I was uncertain whether to make the attempt. Back in my own laboratory, a smaller room down the corridor, I tried and after days and weeks of frustration had good luck. Rather than deplete the cat population of London any further, I had chosen to experiment on rats. And rather than search for signs of impulse activity in the spinal cord I had directed my attention to one of the nuclei at the bottom of the brain stem. There the nerve cells of interest were clustered together and proved easy to find with an exploring glass microelectrode. Each one encountered would have its 'receptive field' mapped out—that is, the part of the rat hindpaw projecting to that nerve cell. Then, by repeatedly

Aranzio's Seahorse and the Search for Memory and Consciousness. Alan J. McComas, Oxford University Press.
© Oxford University Press 2023. DOI: 10.1093/oso/9780192868244.003.0002

applying a fine glass probe attached to a piezoelectric device (a Rochelle salt crystal) it was possible to measure the thresholds to touch at different points on the skin precisely.

I loved doing the experiments. Long after the physiology staff and technicians had left, the rat and I would still be together in our own darkened room. I felt that there was a communion between us, as if the creature wished to reveal the secrets of its brain. It reached the point, one that other neurophysiologists have surely experienced, when I could sense what would be seen and heard before the electrode was gently moved to a new position. They were long experiments, the discharges of each cell photographed on 35-millimetre film that would be developed before leaving the laboratory. Sometimes, near the end of the experiment, my wife[1] would appear, having caught the 134 bus from Muswell Hill, and would heat up a can of soup over the Bunsen burner for us to have together before setting off for home.

The experimental results and the discussion as to their meaning had the makings of a paper. With two fingers tapping away on the keys of a rented typewriter, my wonderful wife, a nurse without any secretarial training, typed out the manuscript with its carbon copies and off it went to the *Journal of Physiology* — and was accepted![2]

Although the publication was barely noticed by those working on touch sensation there had been great enjoyment in the work and, importantly, John (later, Sir John) Gray, my professor at UCL, had been generous with his red pen in demonstrating how to write science.[3]

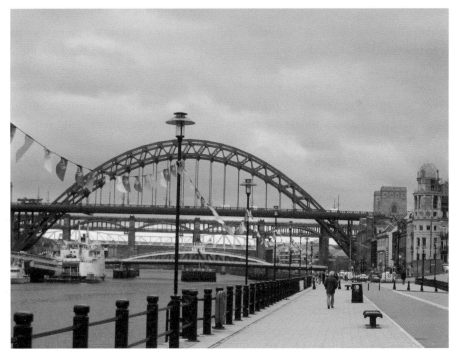

The bridges of Newcastle upon Tyne, surely one of the best city river scenes in the United Kingdom. Photograph by author.

Back in the north of England, in Newcastle-upon-Tyne, I was employed as a research neurophysiologist by another fine person, a neurologist who, by virtue of his organizational skills and commitment to his specialty, would become the Lord Walton of Detchant.[4] That was far into the future, however. My immediate charge was to establish a laboratory for research on skeletal muscle and its nerve supply, in the hope of making discoveries about the nature and possible treatment of diseases such as muscular dystrophy, myasthenia gravis, and amyotrophic lateral sclerosis (ALS).

Not having worked on muscle at UCL, it was a formidable challenge. However, I started making glass microelectrodes, just as in London, but this time using them to stimulate and record from inside single muscle fibres of patients with muscle problems. Then, a few years later and following a chance observation, it became possible to devise an electrophysiological method for estimating the numbers of motor nerve cells in the spinal cord and brain stem.[5] These were the neurons that, by sending impulses down their axons (nerve fibres), could excite the muscle fibres and cause them to contract. The estimates could be done within a few minutes on live human beings, those who were healthy and those with neuromuscular disorders. With other young neurologists as colleagues, the results flowed and the papers appeared.[6]

But there was something missing—there was little or no opportunity for brain research.

And then the opportunity came, but not in a way that could have been foreseen. A newly appointed neurosurgeon to the university hospital began to operate on patients with parkinsonism and on others suffering from intractable pain.[7] The operations were stereotaxic, which meant that, rather than removing a large flap of bone to obtain access to the brain, a thin probe was inserted through a small opening in the skull and then carefully advanced towards the target neurons deep in the brain. It was an ordeal for the patients undergoing the procedure since they were not only conscious throughout but, as a preliminary step, were obliged to have a metal frame attached to their skulls. Once the frame was in place the neurosurgeon could consult the X-rays and calculate where, deep inside the brain, lay the thalamic neurons that had to be destroyed. The problem was that human brains and skulls differed from one individual to another, and an atlas of brain structure was of only limited assistance. And, fifty years ago, the computed tomography (CT) and magnetic resonance imaging (MRI) scanners had yet to be invented.

Enter the neurophysiologist with a recording electrode! Each of the many nuclei in the thalamus has its own function and the cells making up the nuclei have their own distinctive discharges. The neurophysiologist's task was to locate those neurons responding to touching the skin on the opposite side of the body, or perhaps to bending and straightening the fingers. The neurosurgeon would then know exactly where to make the small lesion that would interrupt the neural circuits responsible for the uncontrollable tremor of the parkinsonian patient or the distress of the patient with unbearable pain.

A glass microelectrode would have been impractical for recording and so we employed a stiff tungsten wire, insulated almost to its pointed tip. And, once we had isolated the impulse activity of a joint or touch cell, we would spend a few minutes to do a little brain research. We thought we might be able to alter the pattern of the nerve impulses by asking the patient to attend to the part of the body from which we were recording or, alternatively, by diverting his or her attention elsewhere. The brief experiments should have confirmed what we and others were thinking, namely that the brain could modulate incoming sensory information according to the need of the moment. It was difficult to envisage any other function for the bundles of nerve fibres that were known to run from the cerebral cortex to the various sensory nuclei in the spinal cord and brain stem.[8]

To our disappointment there were no discernible effects of attention or distraction. Nevertheless, how remarkable it was to be recording from deep inside the brain of a human being, one who was not only fully conscious but able to report what he or she was thinking or feeling! As others would show later, there was another part of the brain—the hippocampus, the subject of this book—where it mattered very much what one was thinking or feeling.

Other than sensation, I was interested in consciousness. Indeed, one does not have to be a neurophysiologist to wonder how the brain gives us an awareness of ourselves and our surroundings, enables us to think and plan ahead, and, in the most gifted of our species, makes possible the creation of beautiful art and science.

But how does one go about investigating consciousness? If a philosopher, the approach might be an attempt to understand the nature of reality, the place of the individual in the universe. Or perhaps he or she might ascribe to the view that consciousness, or at least its forerunner, is a feature of all matter (panpsychism). A psychologist would be more direct, seeking clues as to the workings of the conscious brain from observations of human behaviour. The specialist in artificial intelligence or robotics would look at the challenge differently, perhaps arguing that any system that is capable of mimicking, or even surpassing, human cognition must therefore be conscious. All of these approaches are valid, raising and occasionally answering questions of supreme interest, but they still leave consciousness as a seemingly inexplicable phenomenon.

What of the neuroscientist? Though destined to be thwarted by the so-called hard problem (the feeling of self, the redness of a rose, etc.), he or she can get closer to an understanding of consciousness through a reductionist approach, and for reasons that would seem obvious to most of us, including philosophers such as John Searle. Thus, clinical and scientific evidence identifies consciousness as a function of the brain; the brain, like other parts of the nervous system, operates by transmitting and receiving brief electric signals (the nerve impulses); therefore it should ultimately be possible, by studying impulse activity in different parts of a conscious brain, to detect the 'neural correlates of consciousness' (a term invented by Francis Crick and Christof Koch). If the conscious brain happens to be a human one, one that can report directly to an observer manipulating an electrode, so much the better. To promote such an approach is not to deny the validity of others, but caution is required. Functional magnetic resonance imaging (fMRI), so often the basis of a research paper, certainly has a place in the investigation of consciousness but has potential flaws.[9] Similarly, it remains to be seen whether the outcome of mapping every nerve fibre and synaptic connection in all or part of a brain (a 'connectome' project) will justify the enormous effort and expense involved.

In *Sherrington's Loom. An Introduction to the Science of Consciousness*,[10] an attempt was made to review the history of neuroscientific research into consciousness, identifying some of the important meetings devoted to that topic, as well as the most significant experimental observations and the scientists responsible for making them. The book included several speculations as to how various brain systems functioned, drawing heavily on the concept of 'gnostic' units—a concept developed by the late Polish neuroscientist and psychologist, Jerzy Konorski. In contrast to these speculations, *Sherrington's Loom* offered little as to how and in which part(s) of the brain consciousness developed, other than suggesting involvement of the limbic system (a part of the brain that includes the hippocampus). One of the reasons for not pursuing the location issue was that Antonio Damasio had covered this topic extensively in *Self Comes to Mind. Constructing the Conscious Brain*, which had appeared in 2010.[11] I was content to leave it at that, and then an event took place that caused me to change my mind.

What happened was this. As an emeritus professor no longer engaged in laboratory research, I volunteered to organize a symposium on consciousness. It was not difficult to identify local speakers, some of them neurologists, others experimental psychologists, and one a philosopher-neuroscientist. Our external speaker was an expert in artificial intelligence from an American university.

And so, in mid-October 2019, the appointed day for the '*Exploring Consciousness Symposium*' arrived. It had been a beautiful Fall with day after day of sunshine to set off the colours of the trees around the campus. Early in the morning on the day of the symposium the weather abruptly changed. But despite the peals of thunder and the torrential rain, there was a respectable audience. And so, with an excellent introductory talk by the philosopher-neuroscientist, the meeting began. Everything was going well and by lunchtime even the weather had improved. It was after one of the talks in the afternoon that the first doubt came.

Sue, an experimental psychologist who had been an enormous help in organizing the meeting, had just finished her talk ('*Self-consciousness, the mind's theatre and the default network*'). It had been a fascinating lecture, well-delivered with good slides, but there was something that had bothered me. Raising my hand during the question period, I pointed out that a particular interpretation of the data could not be correct because backward masking experiments clearly showed that the brain operated in 'chunks' of time, each chunk lasting some 50–100 ms (one 'ms' is a thousandth of a second, a millisecond). I knew this for a fact because I had done such experiments myself many years previously.[12] Sue, quite unperturbed, replied that time-chunking could not apply to such conscious activities as talking and thinking. And, of course, she was right—but the experimental evidence for time-chunking was incontrovertible. How could this apparent contradiction occur?

That was the first reason for disquiet. The second had come after the symposium while reviewing the PowerPoint slides used in my own talk. The intended highlight of the presentation had been some very exciting work from Los Angeles featuring recordings from single neurons in the human hippocampus.[13] I had tried to attract one of the authors of the published study to come and speak, but without success. To compensate for presenting this work 'second-hand' I had ended my talk by showing a rather dramatic video of a patient in whom both hippocampi had been largely destroyed by a viral infection of the brain. Again, it was not my own work and, 35 years after it had been made, it was possible that the video was no longer in the public domain. But, through the wonder of the Internet, I had found the video and had used it.[14] And then, after the symposium, watched it again. And again. And as I watched the patient, Clive Wearing, struggling through each day with a total inability to remember anything beyond a few seconds, it became obvious that here was information of inestimable value for an understanding of consciousness.

In the weeks following the symposium I continued to think about the apparent contradiction in Sue's talk and about Clive's astonishing video and what they might tell us about consciousness. As anyone who has tackled a difficult conceptual problem knows, it is easy to so completely immerse oneself in it that there is little awareness of the outside world. And then one day, while walking through the neighbourhood park, I thought of a way of reconciling the two items with an understanding of consciousness. It required a different approach, one that was logical and potentially powerful—evolution.

It was not a new approach. Charles Darwin had spent the latter part of his life puzzling over when, in the course of animal evolution, consciousness had appeared.[15] That monkeys, chimpanzees and domestic animals such as cats, dogs and horses, were conscious, he had no doubt. But what about those 'simpler' creatures that had emerged on their own branches of the evolutionary tree? Did they have some sort of consciousness? The situation had changed dramatically since Darwin's time such that we now had a huge mass of information about the fine structure, development, and function of various parts of the brain. Might not this data enable a solution to be found for Darwin's dilemma, at the same time bringing us closer to an understanding of the nature of consciousness?

I believe it does. The key is the evolutionary acquisition of memory, for with memory came consciousness.

With one small exception, a clinical one, I cannot take credit for any of these observations nor, as stated earlier, did I ever perform any laboratory experiments on memory or the hippocampus. It is understandable therefore that those working in the field might question the appropriateness of an outsider writing a book such as this. I also appreciate that, in place of the efforts of solitary hippocampal neuroscientists of 50 years ago, there is now a small army at work, one that has its own journal. Indeed, some workers have now retired after devoting their entire careers to investigating just one aspect of hippocampal structure or function. As someone commented recently, hippocampal research is being conducted on an industrial scale.

There is, of course, an inherent danger in all this specialized activity, one that recalls the old Indian parable of the six blind men encountering an elephant for the first time. (For one, feeling the tusk, it was a spear while for another, feeling the trunk, it was a snake; similarly an ear was mistaken for a fan, a leg for a tree-trunk, the flank for a wall, and the tail for a rope). In the case of the hippocampus, its function has been assigned by different neuroscientists to memory, movement, and olfaction (smell) respectively, with a reluctance to accept that the same structure may actually serve all three. And, were that not enough, there is a strong argument, one made in this book, for the hippocampus being largely responsible for consciousness.

I would add something else to this apologia. Though exploration of the nature and whereabouts of consciousness in the brain is an endeavour logically justified, any attempt carries risk. As the book relates, Wilder Penfield—an internationally renowned neurosurgeon—suffered academic humiliation at the hands of Francis Walshe for having proposed a 'centrencephalic' locus for consciousness. And, as I discovered when writing the final sections of the book, a few years before the Penfield-Walshe debacle there had been Russell Meyers' demolition of Walter Dandy's proposal for consciousness in the basal ganglia.[16] Like Penfield, Dandy had been a giant in neurosurgery and in both instances professional reputations had offered no haven from the withering attacks.

There is also this to consider. The great problem that confronts anyone attempting to find a 'centre' for consciousness within the brain, or, indeed, attempting to explain any aspects of consciousness, is that final proof is elusive, if not impossible. The situation is very different to those in mathematics and the physical sciences in which solutions are to be found in equations and particles. The best that can be done for consciousness is to assemble the pertinent evidence and put forward the most plausible explanation(s). In tackling this challenge the neuroscientist confronts a situation which is potentially favourable—there is an enormous, indeed staggering, amount of information at his or her disposal. Given the evidence to be presented, it will be for the reader to decide the strength or weakness of the case for the hippocampus and the limbic system, through the generation of memory, as the keys to consciousness.

A last note. The writing of this book began well before the appearance of COVID-19 and was completed in the darkest days of the pandemic. As reports appeared of patients losing their senses of smell and taste, it was natural to wonder about the likely involvement of the hippocampus by the virus. After all, the human hippocampus evolved from the 'smell brains' of our evolutionary ancestors and remains only two synapses apart from the olfactory receptors in the nose. Does the hippocampus, then, hold the key to an understanding of the memory loss and brain 'fog' of 'long-COVID'? If so, the more we can learn about the hippocampus, the better.

It is now time to begin the story of the research that revealed memory as a function of the hippocampus.

Notes

1. My late wife, Kate (née Welsh) was a superb nurse, both on the neurological ward and in the neurosurgical operating theatre. In late life she had the misfortune to suffer from an especially malignant, and ultimately fatal, form of migraine.
2. A.J. McComas, 'Responses of the Rat Dorsal Column System to Mechanical Stimulation of the Hindpaw' (1963) 166 *Journal of Physiology* 435–48.
3. Simultaneously with a group in Mexico, John Gray (1918–2011) had been the first to record a 'generator potential' in a specialized touch receptor, the Pacinian corpuscle. Later Gray served as Secretary to the Medical Research Council (United Kingdom), during which time he was knighted. He subsequently returned to neurophysiology, studying sensory systems in fish.
4. John Nicholas Walton (1922–2016) was born in County Durham (United Kingdom), studied at the Newcastle-upon-Tyne Medical School, and became a neurologist with special interest and expertise in muscle disorders. His hugely successful career included presidencies of several medical organizations, among them the World Federation of Neurology. He was an active member of the House of Lords, contributing to debates on medical ethics and new genetic treatments. His autobiography *The Spice of Life: From Northumbria to World Neurology* was published in 1993 (London: Royal Society of Medicine).
5. A.J. McComas, P.R.W. Fawcett, M.J. Campbell, and R.E.P. Sica, 'Electrophysiological Estimation of the Number of Motor Units within a Human Muscle' (1971) 34 *Journal of Neurology, Neurosurgery and Psychiatry* 121–31.
6. A.J. McComas, 'Invited Review: Motor Unit Estimation: Methods, Results and Present Status' (1991) 14 *Muscle & Nerve* 1123–30.
7. Mr John Hankinson, FRCS.
8. Perhaps the most likely explanation is that the descending fibres from the cortex are already working, and doing so continuously. By exerting inhibition on the neurons in the sensory pathways they are compensating for the overgrowth of synaptic connections during the foetal and postnatal development of the nervous system. The descending inhibition makes touch and joint sensation more precise.
9. Regarding fMRI, there has been an unfortunate tendency both to overinterpret its results and to regard them as infallible. Impressive though it undoubtedly is, the methodology remains a very indirect one for localizing brain function (it measures oxygen uptake from the blood rather than impulse activity in neurons). Further, the mathematics used in creating the multitude of 'voxels' that make up the final pictures has been called into question (A. Eklund, T.E. Nichols, and H. Knutsson, 'Cluster Failure: Why fMRI Inferences for Spatial Extent Have Inflated False-Positive Results' (2016) 113(28) *Proceedings of the National Academy of Sciences of the USA* 7900–5). Nor can experts agree on the interpretation of the same scan data (R. Botvinnik-Nezer, F. Holzmeister, C.F. Camerer, A. Dreber, J. Huber. …. .[T. Schonberg]. Variability in the Analysis of a Single Neuroimaging Data Set by Many Teams' (2020) 582 *Nature* 84–8). To emphasize its potential for errors, fMRI was once used to 'show' that the brain of a dead salmon could respond to human facial expressions! (C.M. Bennett, A.A. Baird, M.B. Miller, and G.L. Wolford, 'Neural Correlates of Interspecies Perspective Taking in the Post-Mortem Atlantic Salmon: An Argument for Proper Multiple Comparisons Correction' 1(1) *Journal of Serendipitous and Unexpected Results* 1–5).
10. A.J. McComas, *Sherrington's Loom. An Introduction to the Science of Consciousness* (New York: Oxford University Press, 2019).
11. Damasio A. *Self Comes to Mind. Constructing the Conscious Brain*. New York: Random House, 2010.
12. N.J. MacIntyre and A.J. McComas, 'Non-Conscious Choice in Cutaneous Backward Masking' (1996) 7 *NeuroReport* 1513–16.

13. R.Q. Quiroga, L. Reddy, G. Kreiman, C. Koch and I. Fried, 'Invariant Visual Representation by Single Neurons in the Human Brain' (2005) 435 *Nature* 1102–7.

14. The video concerns patient Clive Wearing. See Chapter 20.

15. See: C.U. Smith, 'Darwin's Unsolved Problem: The Place of Consciousness in an Evolutionary World' (2010) 19(2) *Journal of the History of the Neurosciences* 105–20.

16. Walter Dandy (1886–1946), twice nominated for a Nobel Prize, had been the head of neurosurgery at Johns Hopkins Hospital. A quick and brilliant surgeon, he had also been an innovator. Long before CT or MRI scans, he had invented imaging of the brain by taking X-rays after air had been injected into the ventricles or lumbar subarachnoid space (pneumoencephalography). Dandy had been the first to treat cerebral aneurysms by occluding their necks with silver clips, and he had also worked out the generation, flow and absorption of cerebrospinal fluid (CSF) in the brain and spinal cord. Ironically, Dandy died of a sudden heart attack on the very day that his basal ganglia hypothesis of consciousness appeared in the prestigious *Bulletin of the Johns Hopkins Hospital* and he thereby avoided Russell Meyers' subsequent attack. See: W.E. Dandy, 'The Location of the Conscious Center in the Brain: The Corpus Striatum' (1946) 79 *Bulletin of the Johns Hopkins Hospital* 34–57. Also: R. Meyers, 'Dandy's Striatal Theory of 'the Center of Consciousness.' Surgical Evidence and Logical Analysis Indicating its Improbability' (1951) 65(6) *AMA Archives of Neurology and Psychiatry* 659–71.

PART I
MEMORY

1

The Undisturbed Seahorse

(Western Europe, 16th–20th centuries)

Following Aranzio's discovery, the hippocampus continued to be regarded as a distinct anatomical feature of the brain, one that medical students would be required to identify in the course of their dissections of the human body. But that was all. In the latter part of the 19th century, however, the situation started to change. Anatomists now had powerful light microscopes, among them the beautiful instruments manufactured by the German firm of Carl Zeiss in Jena. In Pavia, in what would become northern Italy, Camillo Golgi (1843–1926; Figure 1.1)[1] had discovered a silver staining method that enabled the fine structure of neurons to be distinguished. Detailed drawings of cells and fibres in various parts of the brain and spinal cord were produced, published, and discussed at meetings of anatomists. The great Spanish neuroscientist, Santiago Ramon y Cajal (1852–1934),[2] was one of those to recognize and describe the unusual architecture of the hippocampus.

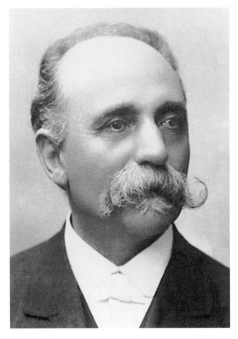

Figure 1.1 Camillo Golgi (1843–1926), photographed prior to 1906, the year in which he shared the Nobel Prize in Physiology or Medicine with his scientific rival Ramon y Cajal.

Aranzio's Seahorse and the Search for Memory and Consciousness. Alan J. McComas, Oxford University Press.
© Oxford University Press 2023. DOI: 10.1093/oso/9780192868244.003.0003

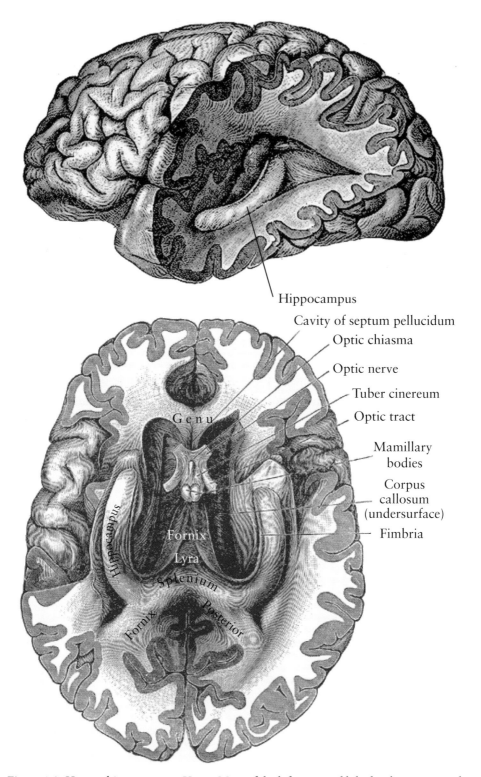

Hippocampus
Cavity of septum pellucidum
Optic chiasma
Optic nerve
Tuber cinereum
Optic tract
Mamillary bodies
Corpus callosum (undersurface)
Fimbria

Genu

Hippocampus

Fornix

Lyra

Splenium

Posterior

Fornix

Figure 1.2 Human hippocampus. *Upper.* Most of the left temporal lobe has been removed to show the deeply lying left hippocampus from above. *Lower.* The lower (inferior) parts of both cerebral hemispheres are absent so as to provide a view of the interiors of the upper parts, including the two hippocampi. Originals prepared by Henry Carter (1831–1897) for inclusion in Gray's classic *Anatomy of the Human Body* (Wikimedia Commons).

It was then, towards the end of the 19th century, that certain regions of the brain became identified as those concerned with vision, hearing, and touch or with the production of movement. Other regions of the cerebral cortex were simply labelled 'association areas' and viewed by many as being of lesser importance; indeed, neurosurgeons were prepared to remove large parts, or to sever their connecting fibres, in attempts to improve psychiatric patients. In this quest they had had some guidance from those who had performed similar surgeries on primates—neurophysiologists and adventurous clinicians such as John Fulton (1899–1960), Heinrich Klüver (1897–1979), and Paul Bucy (1904–1992) in the United States and, much earlier, Sanger Brown (1852–1928) and Victor Horsley (1857–1916)[3] in Britain.

The hippocampus, in comparison, remained uncharted territory. Part of the reason for its neglect may have been its inaccessibility, its position deep within the temporal lobe (Figure 1.2). Another reason may have been the challenge of its multitude of nerve fibre connections. And finally, there was its 'primitive' histological structure and the fact that it was a part of the brain that had evolved early—'old brain' (archepallium). Surely the new brain ('neocortex') that, comprising the bulk of the cerebral hemispheres, would be more important and therefore more interesting to investigate!

And then, in 1957, had come the publication of a study of patients who had undergone surgery involving the hippocampus and the first indication of its great importance for memory. How that study had come to be made is the starting point of the modern story, one that had its origin during the final stages of the Second World War (Figure 1.3).

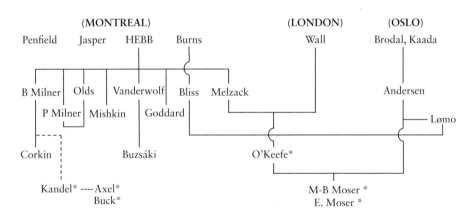

Figure 1.3 Scientific family tree. Many, though far from all, of the neuroscientists investigating memory either trained under, or worked with, others at one period. The strong influence of Montreal is evident. (Note that though Kandel never collaborated with Brenda Milner, it was the latter's work that inspired him to study memory—hence the interrupted line.) Asterisk indicates Nobel Prize.

Notes

1. A brief account of Camillo Golgi's life is given in my earlier book Alan J. McComas, *Galvani's Spark. The Story of the Nerve Impulse* (New York: Oxford University Press, 2011).

2. Santiago Ramon y Cajal is regarded by many as the greatest neuroscientist of all, renowned not only for the beautiful illustrations accompanying his descriptions of the nervous system but also for his insights as to how those parts might function. Though sharing the 1905 Nobel Prize for Physiology or Medicine, Cajal and Golgi had opposing views as to whether or not the nervous system was one vast syncytium of protoplasm (Golgi) or a multitude of nerve cells (neurons) closely apposed but nevertheless separate from each other (Cajal's conclusion, the correct one). Cajal's own story of his improbable life is recounted in S.R. Cajal, *Recuerdos de mi Vida* (*Recollections of my Life*) published in two volumes (Madrid:1901–1917). The autobiography was subsequently translated into English by E.H. Craigie and J Cano (1966) published by MIT Press. Other accounts of Cajal's life include that in *Galvani's Spark* (see note 1) and there is more about Cajal in Chapter 32.

3. Victor (later, Sir Victor) Horsley not only had a strong claim to be considered the pioneer of modern neurosurgery but was a neuroanatomist and early neurophysiologist. Among his achievements, while at University College London and the National Hospital for Nervous Diseases, were the introduction of beeswax to stop bleeding from cranial bones, the first use of electrical stimulation of the brain during surgery for epilepsy, the earliest recording of a nerve compound action potential, and the invention (with Clark) of a stereotaxic apparatus for exploring deep brain structures.

2

A Portentous Crossing

(Montreal, 1944–1948: Donald Hebb, Peter and Brenda Milner)

There was the war and there was the book.

It was the Second World War that had brought them together but it was Donald Hebb's book that would determine their futures.

Peter Milner[1] and Brenda Langford[2] had met at a research establishment on the south coast of England. It was in 1942, a year in which the war with Hitler's Germany was going badly for Britain and its allies. Both Peter and Brenda were involved with Britain's top-secret radar; though colleagues, their backgrounds were very different. Peter, having graduated in electrical engineering at Leeds University, was responsible for designing a training system for future radar operators while Brenda's function was to devise the optimal layout of information on the radar screen. She had been given this task because of her familiarity with experimental psychology, a subject in which she had excelled while a student at Cambridge University.

Whereas Brenda had only developed an interest in psychology after entering university, Peter had been fascinated by electric gadgetry from an early age. As a boy he had learned much from his father, a research chemist, who enjoyed building radios in their Yorkshire home; at the age of ten the boy had already built his first transmitter. Slim and dark-haired, Peter would later be recognized, even by his university colleagues, as having exceptional intelligence. His electrical engineering expertise in the development of one war-time secret, radar, was noted and made him an obvious choice for another secret undertaking—atomic energy research. For several reasons, including the presence of a supply of uranium isotope (in 'heavy' water), it had been decided that the nuclear programme would be started in Canada rather than in the United Kingdom. Before setting off across the Atlantic in a troopship, however, Peter had an additional project in mind—the clever and attractive young psychologist, Brenda Langford.

Newly married, the Milners disembarked in Boston and then, two days later, took the train across the border to Montreal; it was early November 1944 and the Canadian winter was already under way. Though the Milners could not have known it, they had arrived in the city that would be their home for three-quarters of a century.

In 1944, Montreal was like other Canadian cities in feeling the effects of war. While its men, recruited into the armed forces from all walks of life (including the universities), were playing a major part in the final push to end the European conflict, the Montreal women were working long hours for little pay in the factories. Yet, despite these and other changes brought about by the war, Montreal had retained its grandeur. Built on

Aranzio's Seahorse and the Search for Memory and Consciousness. Alan J. McComas, Oxford University Press.
© Oxford University Press 2023. DOI: 10.1093/oso/9780192868244.003.0004

a large island at the confluence of the St Lawrence and Ottawa rivers, it had taken its name from the small mountain at its centre. With roughly one million inhabitants, it was not only the largest city in Canada but the most cosmopolitan; one indication of its importance and attractiveness was the express train service to and from New York City. Though the majority of Montreal's inhabitants were descendants of the original French settlers, there were substantial populations with English, Scots, and Irish backgrounds, and even larger numbers with Italian roots. There was a strong and active Jewish community too, one that Mordecai Richler would describe in his novels.[3]

Yet, as the Milners soon discovered, the social structure of Montreal was a fractured one. Although most of its citizens had been brought up and educated as francophones, it was the anglophone minority that controlled the banks, the legal system, the insurance firms, and the largest businesses. In addition, the anglophones had their own schools, their own hospitals (Montreal General and the Royal Victoria), and their own university––McGill, the most prestigious university in the country, had been started in 1810 following the gift of a Scottish immigrant fur-trader. Even the homes were separate. While the francophones lived on the northern part of the island, the mansions of Westmount, nestling on the southwest foot of Mount Royal, formed an exclusive enclave for the wealthiest anglophones. Though they lived in the same island-city, there was little contact between the francophones and anglophones; in the writer Hugh MacLennan's description, they existed as two solitudes.[4]

Montreal was religious. The Catholic Church had come to Canada in the form of the missionaries who had accompanied the first French explorers in the early 1600s. Over the following three centuries the influence of the Church had spread. Every small town in Quebec had come to have its silver-spired church with its neighbouring presbytery and school, while the larger towns and cities had Catholic hospitals too. In Montreal the Milners would have been aware of the heavy Catholic presence, reflected in the many nuns and black-robed priests mingling with other passers-by on the city streets.

In 1944, however, Brenda's preoccupation was finding employment while her husband was working on the atomic energy project. Ideally, it would be a job that would further her academic career for, though it had made use of her training in experimental psychology, her war-time work had not been intellectually satisfying. Rather boldly, given her English upbringing, she looked not to McGill, where the Psychology Department was understaffed and mostly dormant, but to the Université de Montréal, a Catholic university on the north side of Mount Royal where all tuition was given in French. It was there that the atomic energy project had been started and where Peter was working. The head of the university's new Institut de Psychologie, a Dominican priest, on learning of Brenda's Cambridge background, promptly engaged her to lecture and organize practical classes. The attraction for Father Mailloux was that, at the time Brenda had been an undergraduate, the head of the Psychological Laboratory at Cambridge had been Frederic Bartlett (1886–1969), author of the influential book *Remembering*.[5] One of Bartlett's scientific contributions had been to argue that there was often a reconstructive element in the recall of a memory, such that details were influenced by the social background of the individual. At the time it had been proposed, Bartlett's idea had caused a major change in thinking about memory since to many, psychologist and layperson alike, memories had been regarded as potentially infallible. Today, however, it is widely accepted that false memories can be readily created in response to suggestion or by the brain's own tendency to fill any gaps in its recollections of the past.

The Psychology Laboratory at Cambridge had had its origins in the work of William Rivers (1864–1922), famous for his studies of Melanesian native societies and for being one of the first to recognize and treat soldiers from the First World War for what is now termed post-traumatic stress disorder (PTSD).[6] In addition, Rivers had carried out the meticulous testing of his friend and colleague, Henry Head (1861–1940), when the latter had had the nerves on the back of his forearm surgically divided as part of a study on sensation in skin and deeper tissues. Despite Rivers' death in 1922, the Laboratory had gradually strengthened and included Kenneth Craik and Oliver Zangwill in addition to Bartlett, its first appointed Professor.[7] It was Zangwill, with his deep husky voice, who had supervised Brenda's studies and it was he who had pointed out that patients with brain damage offered unique opportunities for studying how the brain normally functioned. It was an observation that the young student would exploit to the full years later.

Transplanted to Montreal and now with the prospect of teaching psychology (including the work of Bartlett) entirely in French, Brenda not only rose to the challenge but became eligible for a tenured position in the university. Despite the security that the latter would afford, the young Englishwoman wanted more. Accordingly she began to attend and participate in seminars in the psychology department at McGill. In 1947 the seminars would be given by a recently appointed professorial recruit to the department, Donald Hebb (see Figure 2.1).[8]

Donald Hebb, author of the book.

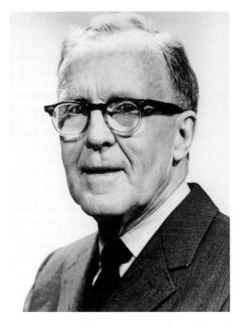

Figure 2.1 Donald Hebb. Courtesy of the University of British Columbia Archives (41.1/2039-1).

A pleasant man with a ready smile and eyes that twinkled behind his spectacles, Donald Olding Hebb (1904–1985) had been born in Chester, Nova Scotia, a breathtakingly picturesque small town on the Atlantic coast of Canada. The son of doctors, Hebb had shown indecision in his early career. Intending to become a novelist, he had gained an arts degree at the nearest university, Dalhousie in Halifax. Hebb had then briefly become a schoolmaster before giving that profession up and working his way across Canada as an itinerant labourer. Next, he had taken up school-teaching again, this time in Montreal, where he simultaneously became a graduate student at McGill University. It was then that he had become interested in the physiological background of psychology, prompting him to study for a PhD with the eminent US psychologist, Karl Lashley (1890–1958).[9] The thesis work, completed at Harvard University, was carried out on the visual systems of rats that had been raised in the dark. A year later, in 1937, Hebb was back in Canada, this time to work at the Montreal Neurological Institute. The attraction was the presence of Wilder Penfield, the renowned neurosurgeon, and the opportunity of studying, in Penfield's patients, the possible effects of frontal lobe surgery on intelligence.

After two scientifically productive years in Montreal, Hebb had moved again, this time to the eastern end of Lake Ontario, where he had accepted a teaching position at Queen's University in Kingston. Again, good experimental work was accomplished, part of which involved the design and construction of a special maze for testing rats. Hebb remained restless, however, and after only three years at Queen's was off again, this time to work in Florida with Karl Lashley, his former PhD supervisor. Though the change gave Hebb the opportunity to study chimpanzees rather than rats, the experiments did not go well, largely because of the difficulty in training the animals. After five years Hebb made his final move and once again, it was to Montreal that he turned; this time, however, he came as Professor of Psychology at McGill University.

At this stage in his career, Hebb was well positioned to influence the future direction of psychology. Both as a student and then as a teacher, he was familiar with the classical psychological studies of human subjects––studies that had to do with attention, perception, memory, and so on. His association with Lashley, first as a graduate student and then as a junior colleague, had introduced him to animal experimentation. And then there had been his time with Penfield, when he had been able to observe the behavioural consequences of removing parts of the human brain as treatment for tumours or seizures.

There was, however, something missing. Thus, although it was possible to make measurements in psychology, such as the minimum time taken to respond to a stimulus ('reaction time'), or the relationship between the size of a stimulus and its perception (the Fechner Law),[10] what did these values represent? In particular, what was going on in the neurons (nerve cells) and in the connections (synapses) that they formed with one another? It was the lack of information about underlying neural mechanisms that had so frustrated the great Harvard psychologist, William James (1842–1910), a half-century earlier. For want of this knowledge James had been dependent on his own introspection to gain insights into the workings of the brain. Time and again, as one reads his *Principles of Psychology*, published in 1890,[11] one comes across his frustration in not being able to suggest the neural basis of behaviour.

In addition to his own observations, Hebb had kept abreast of the advances in neuroscience since James' time, most of which had come from neuropsychologists' experiments in stimulating and recording the brain. Hebb was able to draw on this new information to suggest possible explanations for different aspects of behaviour and to put his ideas into the manuscript for a textbook. Before committing himself to a final version, however, Hebb tried his ideas out on an audience that was both discriminating and close at hand––the departmental graduate students. It was a mutually beneficial arrangement. As they considered one of the chapters during their weekly seminar with the professor, the students would learn some psychology and, just as important, hear suggestions as to the neuroscience underlying the various behaviours. Hebb's experience as a schoolmaster had made him an effective teacher and he had little difficulty in holding the attention of the students. Very often the discussions would continue into the late evening and, in the following days, there would be original publications for the students to consult in the library. Hebb, in turn, profited from the seminars since they enabled him to discover aspects of the book that needed clarification or expansion.[12]

Among Hebb's students, several of whom went on to make fine academic careers, was one a little older and more mature than the others––Brenda Milner. An early photograph shows Brenda as a slender young woman with thick brown hair and pleasant features. Hebb would, in addition, have noted that she was well spoken and neatly dressed. However, it was her wide and generous smile that people remembered––that, and the intelligent eyes below the broad forehead (Figure 2.2). Also, unlike her shy husband,

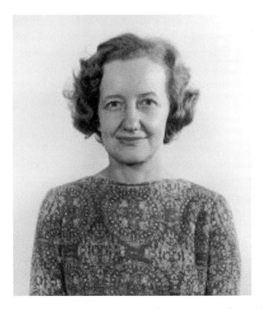

Figure 2.2 A youthful Brenda Milner. Courtesy of Dr Milner. A later photograph of the subject is provided in the Epilogue.

Brenda was vivacious and always at ease in talking, whether to large groups or in private conversation.

Enthused by the seminars with Donald Hebb, Brenda applied and was accepted into the psychology graduate programme at McGill. Her excitement was conveyed in the letters to husband Peter, by now at a new atomic energy establishment at Chalk River. And then a remarkable thing happened. Peter, whose training and entire professional life up to that point had been in engineering, found Brenda's recounting of Hebb's ideas so intriguing that he resolved to enter the field of experimental psychology himself. Leaving Chalk River, then a small and desolate community north of Ottawa,[13] he became, briefly, an undergraduate student and then, like his wife, a graduate student in the McGill psychology programme.

And it was Peter, the former electrical engineer, who struck gold first.

Notes

1. P.M. Milner, *The History of Neuroscience in Autobiography*, L.R. Squire (ed.) (San Diego, CA: Academic Press, 2014) 8: 290–323..

2. B. Milner, *The History of Neuroscience in Autobiography*, L.R. Squire (ed.) (San Diego, CA: Academic Press, 1998) 2: 276–305..

3. For example: M. Richler, *The Apprenticeship of Duddy Kravitz* (London: Andre Deutsch, 1959) and *Barney's Version* (Toronto: Knopf Canada, 1997).

4. H. MacLennan, *Two Solitudes* (Toronto: Macmillan of Canada, 1945).

5. F.C. Bartlett, *Remembering. A Study in Experimental and Social Psychology* (Cambridge: Cambridge University Press, 1932).

6. Rivers' psychiatric work in the First World War, particularly that involving the treatment of the poets, Siegfried Sassoon and Wilfred Owen, was brilliantly imagined in Pat Barker's novel: P. Barker, *Regeneration* (London: Viking Press, 1991).

7. After the Second Word War, the Laboratory, now Department, included Richard Gregory (1923–2010), an inventor, experimental psychologist, and author famous for his original insights into visual mechanisms. The well-known contemporary neuroscientist, V.S. Ramachandran, is one of those who had studied with him. One of the later recruits to the Department was the American, Lawrence Weiskrantz, probably best known for his discovery of 'blindsight'.

8. P.M. Milner and B.A. Milner. 'Donald Olding Hebb. 22 July 1904–20 August 1985' (1996) 42 *Biographical Memoirs of Fellows of the Royal Society* 192–204.

9. For more on Lashley, see Chapter 4.

10. The Fechner Law states that the perception of a stimulus is proportional to the logarithm of its intensity.

11. W. James, *Principles of Psychology* (Cambridge, MA: Harvard University Press, 1890).

12. D.O. Hebb, *The Organization of Behavior. A Neuropsychological Theory* (New York, NY: Wiley & Sons, 1949).

13. Chalk River continues as a research centre in nuclear physics. It was where the CANDU nuclear reactors were developed and, until 2018, was an important world source of nuclear isotopes for medical treatment and research. While at Chalk River, Bertram Brockhouse performed neutron bombardment studies for which he was awarded a Nobel Prize in Physics in 1994 (by then he was a professor at McMaster University).

3

Graduate Studies at Montreal Neurological Institute

(Montreal, 1948–1954: Peter and Brenda Milner, James Olds, Wilder Penfield, Herbert Jasper)

As part of their graduate work, doctoral students in the sciences are required to undertake original research and to present their findings, together with the relevant historical background, in a printed thesis. Most often the topic for the thesis will be some aspect of their supervisor's research and this makes good sense. Not only will the supervisor, as an expert in the field, be able to give the student appropriate guidance but it is likely that all the equipment required for the student's experiments will already be available in the laboratory.

It was not like that for Peter Milner, who had to start from scratch. Intrigued by some of the speculations in Hebb's book, he had set out to discover the effect on behaviour of stimulating the reticular formation in the brain stem. The reticular formation had recently come into prominence through the work of Horace Magoun and Guiseppe Moruzzi in Chicago,[1] though it was also being studied, as a part of the brain stem, by Herbert Jasper and his young colleagues at the Montreal Neurological Institute (MNI), only a short walk from the university. The two groups had shown that stimulating the reticular formation could arouse a sleeping animal, altering the electrical activity of the brain at the same time. Because of this awakening effect, the neurons in the reticular formation were said to comprise 'the reticular activating system'. But, Milner wondered, what would be the effect of stimulating this system in an animal that was already awake? Would it tend to repeat a behaviour that had been associated with stimulation? To Milner's disappointment, rather than favouring a behaviour, the effect of prior stimulation was to make the rat avoid it. Milner abandoned the experiments—perhaps unwisely, since stimulated avoidance would have been an interesting subject for exploration, offering a number of further experimental approaches. Instead Peter Milner chose another topic for his thesis, the possibility that the perception of time could be altered in a brain made hyperactive by stimulation of the reticular formation—in the same way, perhaps, that thoughts flash through the human mind at times of crisis or, in the other direction, that 'a watched pot never boils'.

Magoun and Moruzzi's experiments, as well as Jasper's, had been carried out in cats, which until then, had been the favoured species for neurophysiologists. Compared with dogs, cats have much less variety in the shapes and sizes of their cerebral cortex,

Aranzio's Seahorse and the Search for Memory and Consciousness. Alan J. McComas, Oxford University Press.
© Oxford University Press 2023. DOI: 10.1093/oso/9780192868244.003.0005

and there were good atlases available for locating deeper structures in the cat brain. On the other hand, many neuroscientists were reluctant to use domestic animals for their research and rats were a good alternative. Rats are intelligent enough to learn their way through mazes and, as Skinner and Lashley had shown, they can solve other suitably designed cognitive problems provided they are given food rewards. And rats are cheap and, unlike rabbits, survive experiments well. It was rats that Hebb had seen Lashley use in his unsuccessful attempts to locate memory in the brain.

The general nature of the experiments would have appealed to Peter Milner because of his training and experience in electrical engineering—though there was a delicacy involved that had been missing in his work on nuclear reactors. The stimulating system that he had devised used two fine insulated silver wires, cemented together to form a stiff 'needle' for penetrating the brain. With a rat brain atlas for guidance, the wires were inserted into the reticular formation and held in place by being cemented to the skull.

As Milner was nearing the end of his doctoral work, he was joined by a younger man, a graduate student from Harvard. James Olds, too, had been strongly influenced by Hebb's book and wished to test some of the new thinking by animal experiments in the author's department. Like Peter Milner, Olds was also interested to see if the behaviour of rats could be altered by brain stimulation. To this end he adopted Milner's technique for inserting and maintaining electrodes in position and found, in his first rat, that stimulation caused the animal to advance, explore, and sniff. Surprisingly, the rat would repeatedly return to the place where it had been stimulated, as if it was seeking more of something it liked. Olds and Milner decided to test this idea by seeing if the rat would stimulate itself, rather than be stimulated by an observer. Accordingly Milner made a box with a lever mounted on one of the sides; pressing on the lever would allow current to flow through the implanted electrodes in the brain (via a light cable suspended from the ceiling and thence through a step-down transformer to the mains supply).

And so the experiments began (Figure 3.1). The two graduate students observed that the rat, during the inspection of its new surroundings, pressed the lever. Rats being curious creatures, this was to be expected. What was novel, however, was that the rat returned to press the lever again and again, finally stopping when the stimulating current was switched off. The only possible interpretation of this behaviour was that the rat had been enjoying the effect of stimulating its own brain. Indeed, James Olds and Peter Milner had discovered that there was a 'pleasure centre' (or 'reward centre') in the mammalian brain. What they did not know, at least until they had seen an X-ray of the rat's head, was that the stimulating electrodes had not been in the reticular formation, as Olds had intended, but further forward in the midbrain.[2] Later work would identify a small collection of nerve cells (the nucleus accumbens, a part of the 'limbic system') as the pleasure centre. The incorrect placement of the electrodes by the students was forgiveable—the brain stem of the rat is so slender that it is easy to miss the reticular formation when approaching it blindly from above. Alternatively, the stimulating needle might have moved slightly if the cement had not fully hardened when the wires on the outside of the rat's head were being bent.

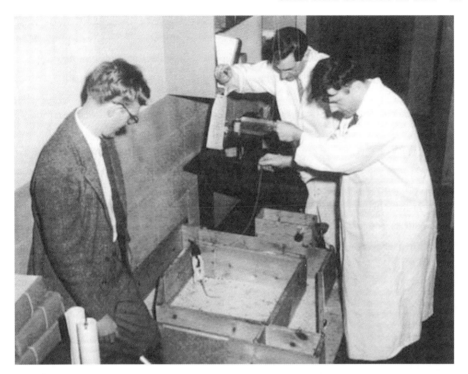

Figure 3.1 Rat self-stimulation experiment in 1954 by Peter Milner (furthest from camera) and James Olds; Seth Sharpless, another young member of the McGill Psychology Department, is in the foreground. The rat is being placed in a box with a runway to test its tendency to return to the place where it had previously received stimulation. The event was a re-enactment for an article in the *Montreal Star* reporting the discovery of a pleasure centre in the brain. (Archival material reproduced courtesy of The Woodbridge Company Ltd.)

The finding of a pleasure centre in the brain was a huge discovery, leading to a much better understanding of certain behaviours, and of addiction in particular. Olds pursued this line of enquiry, first for his doctoral thesis and then, after leaving Montreal, for the remainder of his career.[3] Peter Milner, having been a partner in the discovery and initial report, completed his own doctoral thesis (on time estimation). He then turned his attention to evaluating some of Hebb's ideas, for example, by emphasizing the need for inhibition to control the hypothetical neural assemblies. A supremely intelligent man, and one of the founders of artificial intelligence, Peter Milner's distinguished career would include a period as Head of the McGill Psychology Department.[4]

In 1948, however, it was Donald Hebb who had become the Head of the Department at McGill. The appointment had meant him giving up any experimental work of his own and he could do no more than make suggestions regarding the experiments and other types of study undertaken by the departmental graduate students. What he did do, and do very well, was lecture to the undergraduate students[5]—and they, the students, had Hebb's new book to help them.

Entitled *The Organization of Behavior. A Neuropsychological Theory*,[6] the book was an instant success, attracting the attention not only of students but of established psychologists and neuroscientists as well. Two of Hebb's propositions were especially noteworthy. One was that an infant's learning depended on neurons working in groups ('cell assemblies'), each of which was responsive to a particular stimulus, such as something heard or something seen. The respective assemblies would then form synaptic connections with each other, if the stimuli occurred at the same time (e.g. the sight of a mother and the sound of her voice). The second proposition was related to the first, namely:

> When an axon of cell A is near enough to excite cell B and repeatedly or persistently takes part in firing it, some growth process or metabolic change takes place in one or both cells such that A's efficiency, as one of the cells firing B, is increased.

Much later, neuroscientists would express Hebb's dictum more simply as

> Cells that fire together wire together

and it would not be Hebb but a later neuroscientist who would win a Nobel Prize for showing how this came about.

While her husband was making a ground-breaking discovery in the animal laboratory, Brenda Milner was engaged in a very different type of research. Hebb had approached Penfield at the MNI and asked if one of his own graduate students could examine those patients who had had parts of their temporal lobes removed as treatment for severe epilepsy. Unlike the excitement of being able to see results of various interventions immediately, as Peter and James Olds had been able to do, Brenda would be obliged to pursue a slower, more laborious, and less clear path.

At the time of this request, Penfield was in the prime of his career and was the best-known neurosurgeon in North America and probably in the world (Figure 3.2).[7] His fame had come from his practice of stimulating the exposed cortex in conscious patients and noting their responses before deciding which damaged or diseased tissue could be safely removed. As a graduate student studying patients, Brenda would sometimes stand in the gallery of the operating theatre with the interns and residents and watch Penfield at work. It would have been difficult not to be impressed both by the nature of the procedures—the exposure and then the stimulation of the cortex—and by the intellectual stature of the person undertaking them.

Though Penfield was famous as a neurosurgeon, there was much more to him than that. Not only was he the Director of the MNI, but he had been the Institute's founder. He was also an accomplished neurohistologist and someone who saw, in his work as a neurosurgeon, the opportunity to explore the relationship between brain and mind. His success and his eminence had not been easily won, however.

Born in the United States, Penfield had been an athlete at college and had won a Rhodes scholarship to study medicine at Oxford immediately prior to the First World War. After the war had broken out, but prior to the entry of the United States into the

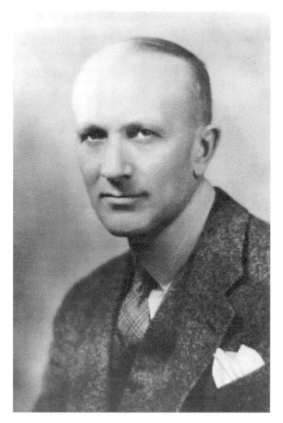

Figure 3.2 Wilder Penfield. The photograph was taken in 1934, the year that the Montreal Neurological Institute was completed (Wikimedia Commons).

conflict, he had volunteered as a medical orderly. Almost immediately he had had a near-death experience, being flung high into the air and breaking his leg after a torpedo struck the ship in which he was crossing to France from England. After the war he had resumed his medical studies in Oxford, coming into contact with both Sir William Osler (1849–1919) and Charles Sherrington (1856–1952). Sherrington, a senior figure shortly to be knighted, was regarded as the greatest neurophysiologist of his time.[8] Included among his many achievements had been his mapping of the motor cortex in a variety of primates, work that had obvious relevance to Penfield's own research later. Sherrington was more than a neurophysiologist, however, as Penfield and other young men in the Oxford laboratory would discover. Sherrington was also a philosopher, historian, poet, and bibliophile who delighted in far-reaching discussions with his students. Penfield had absorbed and adopted this wide view of life, and it would continue to be reflected in his own writings. Later, at the National Hospital for Nervous Diseases in London's Queen Square, Penfield had been taught by some of the Britain's most distinguished neurologists and had also assisted at neurosurgical operations.

It was while he was at Queen Square that Penfield had become interested in the microscopic nature of the scar tissue that formed when the brain was injured. He continued this work after resuming his neurosurgical practice in New York. Dissatisfied with his own attempts at histology, he then decided to study in Madrid with Pio del Rio Hortega, one of Ramon y Cajal's former protégés. This undertaking, associated with a loss of income, involved Penfield sitting at a desk and learning histology in the company of much younger students. Using the beautiful staining methods pioneered by Golgi and Cajal but then modified by del Rio Hortega, Penfield was able to replicate a discovery made by his new master—the existence of a special type of glial (auxiliary) cell in the nervous system, the oligodendrocyte. Others would subsequently confirm del Rio Hortega's suggestion that these cells were able to form the fatty (myelin) sheaths surrounding nerve fibres, enabling the fibres to transmit impulses rapidly and economically down their lengths.[9] Penfield's was a fine piece of original work and the experience encouraged him, after returning to New York, to bring neuropathology closer to neurosurgery and neurology—if possible, in the same part of the hospital.

Penfield's growing reputation had attracted attention in Montreal and had resulted in him moving to that city as head of the new specialty of neurosurgery at the Royal Victoria Hospital. It was in Montreal that Penfield began to operate on cortical scars, thinking them likely to have triggered epileptic seizures in his patients. Before resecting the damaged tissue, however, he would explore the brain with electrical stimulation so as to determine what could be safely removed. An operation of this kind involved incising and retracting the scalp under local anaesthesia so as to expose the skull, and then using a drill and flexible saw to remove a large flap of bone over part of the brain. Penfield would then stimulate different points on the exposed cortex, noting the response in each instance and marking the location with a small numbered 'ticket'. In this way he had been able to show that stimulating the strip of cortex immediately in front of the main fissure (the central sulcus) resulted in muscles twitching on the opposite side of the body; this, then, was the 'motor cortex'. Stimulating behind the main fissure elicited sensations from the body surface; this was the 'somatosensory cortex'. As with the motor cortex, there was much more brain surface given over to the hand and mouth than to the trunk and legs, and in both types of cortex the body was represented upside down (Figure 3.3).

Penfield had not been the first to stimulate the human brain during surgery. Even in Canada, in the small settlement of St Anthony's at the tip of the northern peninsula of Newfoundland, there had been a teenaged girl with epilepsy who had been investigated in this way in 1909.[10] However, the most thorough of the early pioneers of cortical stimulation had been Fedor Krause (1857–1937)[11] in Berlin who had investigated a considerable number of patients and published a detailed map of the movements evoked by stimulation of the motor strip. His former junior, Otfrid Foerster,[12] had carried on with this work in his own clinic in Breslau. At that time Foerster was both a neurosurgeon and a neurologist, a brilliant pioneer who had made several original contributions to both fields. Such was his fame that it was Foerster who had been invited by the Russian government to treat Lenin after a stroke. Penfield had visited Foerster in 1928 and had stayed long enough to have witnessed Foerster's technique for operating on the human brain under local anaesthesia and for stimulating the exposed surface.

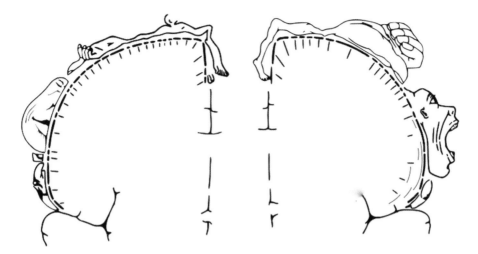

Figure 3.3 Homonculi representing body surface (*left*) and of movements (*right*) in the postcentral and precentral gyri respectively, as determined by Penfield and his collaborators using electrical stimuli to the cortical surface. (By mailto:ralf@arc.in-berlin. de [public domain], via Wikimedia Commons).

Penfield had only been in Montreal for a very few years when he brought off a major coup—funding from the Rockefeller Foundation to establish a neurological institute. It was the fulfilment of a dream, a place not only for neurologists and neurosurgeons to see and treat patients but for those specialists on the periphery whose reports were often crucial—the radiologists, pathologists, and chemists. At the top of the new building (Figure 3.4) there was an animal house, for research was to be closely allied to clinical practice. After the Institute's opening in 1934, Montreal could boast of having the premier facility of its kind in the world, one superior in several respects to Britain's National Hospital for Nervous Diseases in London's Queen Square or to any of the well-known hospitals and clinics in the United States. The Institute had been Penfield's creation and now, 15 years later, it was in this imposing stone building, attached to the Royal Victoria Hospital by a bridge, that Brenda Milner had come to watch Penfield operate and to examine some of his patients.[13]

Penfield had become attracted to the idea of removing part of a temporal lobe as a treatment for epilepsy. While with Foerster in Breslau he had watched the famous neurologist-surgeon resect scar tissue from the temporal lobe of a young man whose seizures had followed a serious head injury. The operation had been a success and had raised the possibility that the temporal lobe might, in some patients, be the source of seizures perhaps unrelated to injury but to some other type of malfunction—an abnormal blood supply, for instance. In evaluating his patients for surgery he was helped by a man whose growing reputation would parallel Penfield's. Brenda Milner would have seen him during her visits to the surgical theatre, standing at the front of the gallery and operating his electronic equipment: Herbert Jasper (Figure 3.5).

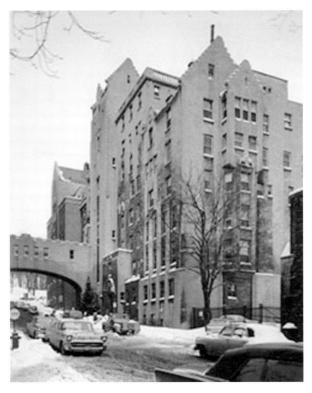

Figure 3.4 The Montreal Neurological Institute in 2011. Original photo in colour by Jeangagnon (Wikimedia Commons).

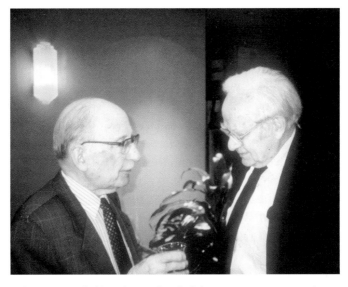

Figure 3.5 Herbert Jasper (left) and David Hubel during an international symposium celebrating Jasper's 90th birthday (photograph by author).

Jasper, like Penfield, had been born in the western United States, though in Oregon.[14] The son of a minister, he had been attracted to the study of the mind early on and had carried out some experiments on peripheral nerve and muscle at the University of Iowa and then, in greater depth, at the Sorbonne in Paris.

The two men were physical opposites. Penfield was a big man—he had played football for the Princeton football team and had captained the college wrestling team—and had an undeniable presence. Jasper, bespectacled and sporting a moustache, was slight and could easily have been overlooked in any gathering. In other respects, however, the two were very similar. Both were good organizers. Penfield had demonstrated this by creating and running the MNI, while Jasper had built up a first-class neurophysiology department, one that combined clinical and basic research. Both were ambitious and both were drawn to the mind-brain problem. And both excelled in what they did.

One of Jasper's successes had been in electroencephalography (EEG). The first published account of spontaneous slow electrical waves in the human brain had been by Hans Berger in Germany in 1929.[15] What had seemed an unlikely discovery was subsequently verified by Adrian and Matthews at Cambridge a few years later and then pursued in a handful of laboratories, one of them being Jasper's at Brown University on Rhode Island.

Jasper had been the first to show that an epileptic focus could be localized with the EEG, a result that had captured Penfield's interest and had led to Jasper being recruited to the staff of the newly founded neurological institute in Montreal. Jasper's research interests were many; other than demonstrating the clinical usefulness of the EEG and devising the standard 10–20-electrode recording system he had introduced monopolar needle recording into EMG (electromyography). At the time of Brenda Milner's arrival at the Institute Jasper was investigating the interactions between the cortex and the thalamus; among other achievements he would, with Allan Elliott, identify gamma-amino butyric acid (GABA) as an inhibitory neurotransmitter in the mammalian brain.[16]

Jasper was an accomplished organizer, as already noted. In August 1953 he had brought together many of the senior figures in clinical and basic neuroscience for a symposium entitled *Brain Mechanisms and Consciousness*.[17] The date of the symposium had been chosen so as to immediately precede the XIX International Physiological Congress in Montreal, which most of the symposium participants would also be attending. The Congress, a three-yearly event, had not been held in North America since the Boston meeting in 1929 and the Montreal Congress had brought together eminent physiologists from both sides of the Atlantic, most of the Europeans arriving by boat. For his own meeting Jasper had kept the number of invitees small and, as venue, had chosen a resort hotel in the Laurentian Mountains north of Montreal.[18] A photograph of the symposium faculty (Figure 3.6) shows the most illustrious neuroscientist of the time, the Nobel Laureate Lord Adrian, in the front row with Wilder Penfield, sporting a bow tie, next to him. On the other side of Lord Adrian, in the centre of the group, stands the organizer of the meeting, Herbert Jasper. There is a third representative from Montreal for near the end of the second row, and smiling broadly, is Donald Hebb.

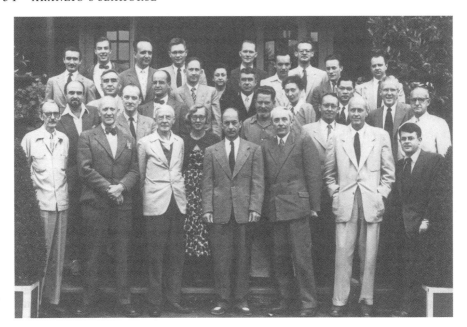

Figure 3.6 Participants in the Laurentian Conference on Brain Mechanisms and Consciousness held at the Alpine Inn, Ste Marguerite, Quebec, in August 1953. Front row, from left: Lashely, Penfield, Adrian, Brazier, Jasper, Bremer, Magoun, Greene. Second row: Gastaut, Rioch, Fessard, Morison, Hess, Olszewski, Grey Walter, Mahut, Jung, Li, Hebb, Kubie. Third row: Ajmone-Marsan, Whitlock, Moruzzi, Nauta, Courtois, Ingvar, Buser.

(Reproduced with permission from: Jasper HH. Historical perspective. In: Consciousness: at the frontiers of neuroscience, ed HH Jasper et al. *Advances in Neurology*, 1998; 77: 1–6).

The temporary presence of prominent international neuroscientists in Montreal, before and after the symposium, would have caused great interest and excitement among the staff and students at the Institute and in the university. Indeed, it is very likely that some of the visitors would have given lectures and visited the local laboratories. Peter Milner would certainly have been interested in anything that Horace Magoun or Giuseppe Moruzzi might have said about the reticular activating system, the topic of Peter's research. And then there had been the son of a second Nobel Laureate, Walter Hess, reporting on the results obtained by his father of stimulating structures in and around the hypothalamus. It was in the vicinity of the hypothalamus that Peter Milner and James Olds had discovered the 'pleasure centre' in the rat brain.

Jasper's symposium had been a great success, in no small part due to the intimacy developed by the small number of participants. There had been opportunities to continue discussions of their work around the dinner table in the evenings or while walking through the extensive grounds of the Alpine Inn. Interestingly, though the presentations at the symposium had covered both human and animal studies, there had been no mention of memory.

Brenda Milner had not been particularly interested in memory, however, when she had embarked on her research with Penfield's patients, possibly because, at that stage of her career, she had absorbed virtually all that was known about it. Indeed, she had lectured on the subject to her francophone students at the Université de Montréal while pursuing her own graduate studies at McGill. Her research on the effects of temporal lobe ablation had been completed the year before the Laurentian symposium on consciousness and had gone as well as she might have expected, given that there were a number of problems inherent in a study of that type. One such problem was that all of the patients referred by Penfield had abnormal brains—responsible for their seizures— prior to surgery. The surgery itself might have added to their dysfunction but the site and extent of the surgery varied from one patient to the next. In some it was just the anterior pole of one temporal lobe that had been removed while in others the resection had been more extensive and included much of the hippocampus and adjacent structures. In a few patients, those who had failed to respond and who required a second operation, the entire temporal lobe had been removed on one side Another problem confronting Brenda was that some brain activities normally involve both hemispheres; an intact hemisphere can then compensate for partial removal of the other one, thereby obscuring its normal function.

Brenda submitted her thesis and was awarded her PhD in 1952. Two years later an account of her work appeared in the *Psychological Bulletin*.[19] Most of the lengthy paper was devoted to a comprehensive review of the literature concerning temporal lobe ablations in animals (especially monkeys); the most important of these studies had been conducted by another of Hebb's graduate students, Mortimer Mishkin, during his doctoral research at Yale. In her 1954 paper Brenda's own findings occupied a scant two pages at the end. She had investigated 25 patients with partial or total removal of their left or right temporal lobes and, for controls, had compared them with 13 patients in whom Penfield had resected parts of the frontal or parietal lobes. Using a battery of tests, Brenda had found that the temporal lobe patients had difficulty in the interpretation of complex pictures. In addition, the right temporal lobe seemed to be especially concerned with spatial relationships. It was already well established that in a right-handed person, the left temporal lobe was important for speech and, intriguingly, a few of the patients with left-sided resections had difficulty remembering words or short stories that had been read to them.

Overall, the human studies had not added much to what had already been known from the animal work. The literature review had been masterly, however, and there was an elegance and authority in the writing, with phrases such as 'The argument does not seem convincing', 'The deficit is admittedly hard to define', and 'The evidence at present is not sufficient to settle the question finally one way or the other'.

By the time her publication appeared Brenda was working full-time as a researcher at the MNI and had been given an office of her own by Penfield, together with a small stipend. She had taken to the clinically related work and had not been dissuaded by Hebb's cautionary advice. Hebb had no doubt been mindful of the difficulties he had experienced at the Institute prior to the Second World War. In a hospital or an institute such as the MNI, there is—or was—a well-established hierarchy with the consulting specialists at the top, the residents and interns below, and the technical staff and nurses lower still. A non-clinical research worker such as Brenda would have been at the very bottom. Among other frustrations she would sometimes find that her patient had been taken from his or her room for an X-ray or for treatment, or even discharged, and so not available to her. In deciding to pursue postdoctoral research full time, Brenda had been obliged to resign her tenured position at the Université de Montréal. The decision must have involved some heart-searching because of the financial security the former position would have provided throughout her academic career and there would have been a pension on retirement. However, the sacrifice would shortly bring its reward—a reward in the form of three unusual patients.

One of the patients was destined to become well known throughout the neurological world and to be the subject of two books and numerous scientific papers. He would also help to make Brenda famous.

Notes

1. F. Moruzzi and H.W. Magoun, 'Brain Stem Reticular Formation and Activation of the EEG' (1949) 1 *Electroencephalography and Clinical Neurophysiology* 455–73.
2. J. Olds and P. Milner, 'Positive Reinforcement Produced by Electrical Stimulation of the Septal Area and Other Regions of the Rat Brain' (1954) 47 *Journal of Comparative and Physiological Psychology* 419–27. The description of how the discovery was made is given in Peter Milner's autobiographical essay: P.M. Milner, *The History of Neuroscience in Autobiography*, L.R. Squire (ed.) (Washington, DC: Society for Neuroscience, 2014) 8: 290–323.
3. R.F. Thompson, 'James Olds. May 30 1922–August 21 1976' (1999) 77 *Biographical Memoirs of the National Academy of Sciences* 246–63.
4. Entry for P.M. Milner in *The History of Neuroscience in Autobiography* (see note 2).
5. As related by Peter Milner, Hebb would continue to give a course of undergraduate lectures throughout all his years at McGill, with as many as a thousand students attending. He also continued to give lectures to graduate students.
6. D.O. Hebb, *The Organization of Behavior. A Neuropsychological Theory* (New York, NY: Wiley & Sons, 1949).
7. The information about Penfield's life and career as a neurosurgeon is taken from his autobiography: W. Penfield, *No Man Alone. A Neurosurgeon's Life* (Boston, MA: Little Brown, 1977).
8. There are several biographies of Sherrington and an account of his life and work is included in: A.J. McComas, *Galvani's Spark. The Story of the Nerve Impulse* (New York, NY: Oxford University Press, 2011).
9. The life and work of Pio del Rio Hortega (1882–1945), including his discovery of oligodendroglia and microglia, is given in: F. Pérez-Cerdá, M.V. Sánchez-Gómez, and C. Matute, 'Pio del Rio Hortega and the Discovery of the Oligodendrocytes' (2015) 9 *Frontiers in Neuroanatomy*: article 92 (doi:103389/fnana.2015.00092). Because of the Spanish Civil War, del Rio Hortega was obliged to abandon his laboratory in Madrid and to continue his career in Argentina.
10. G.W.N. Fitzgerald, The making of a rural general surgeon. Chapter 5.2.5 in *WONCA Rural Medical Education Guidebook*. Bangkok: WONCA, 2014. Dr John Mason Little, who had trained

in Boston, performed the intraoperative electrical stimulation in the course of his ten years' surgical experience in Newfoundland.

11. Fedor Krause. <en.wikipedia.org/wiki/Fedor_Krause> accessed 25 April 2022.

12. Otrid Foerster, 1873–1941 <http://www.en.wikipedia.org/wiki/Otfird_Foerster> accessed 25 April 2022. Foerster, a German, had trained in neurology but later combined his neurological practice with neurosurgery. In addition to his cortical surgery for epilepsy, he devised spinal operations for the relief of spasticity and intractable pain, and he was able to map some of the human dermatomes (skin areas supplied by the sensory nerve fibres of individual nerve roots).

13. When Penfield had worked with the architects in the design of the Montreal Neurological Institute he had asked that the ceiling of the entrance to the building be decorated with oligodendroglia cells together with the names of the Greek fathers of medicine.

14. H.H. Jasper, *The History of Neuroscience in Autobiography*, L.R. Squire (ed.) (Washington, DC: Society for Neuroscience, 1996) 318–46.

15. For a recent account of the discovery and verification of EEG, see: A.J. McComas, *Sherrington's Loom. An Introduction to the Science of Consciousness* (New York: Oxford University Press, 2019) 122–40.

16. K.A.C. Elliott and H.H. Jasper, 'Gamma-Amino Butyric Acid' (1959) 39(2) *Physiological Reviews* 383–406. Note: gamma-amino butyric acid (GABA) was first shown to be an inhibitory transmitter at the crayfish neuromuscular junction, before its role in the mammalian central nervous system was determined.

17. The proceedings of the symposium were published in the following year: J.F. Delafresnaye (ed.), *Brain Mechanisms and Consciousness* (Springfield, IL: Charles Thomas, 1954).

18. In Ste Marguerite-du-lac-Masson, Quebec. The Alpine Inn, the venue for the symposium, continues to operate seventy years later, though now in competition with more modern (and possibly more comfortable) local hotels and spas.

19. B. Milner, 'Intellectual Function of the Temporal Lobes' (1954) 50(1) *Psychological Bulletin* 42–62.

4

Bold Surgeon and Compliant Patient

(Hartford, Connecticut, 1953: William Scoville, Brenda Milner, Henry Molaison)

The first of the three patients was a civil engineer who had required a second operation by Penfield on his left temporal lobe. The later surgery had been restricted to the medial part of the lobe and had resulted in pronounced difficulty in remembering. The patient could recall nothing of the months immediately before his operation, nor could he retain any new information once his attention had shifted. This perplexing case was followed by a similar one. The patient, a 28-year-old glove cutter, had also undergone resection of much of the left medial temporal lobe. In this instance the inability to remember events that had taken place prior to surgery; that is, the retrograde amnesia extended back four years.

Penfield and Brenda Milner had been puzzled. Why should memory have been impaired in these two patients and not in any of the others that had undergone unilateral temporal lobe surgery? What had made them different? In the end, the surgeon and the psychologist could only postulate that there must have been some abnormality on the unoperated (right) side, such that it could not compensate for the removal of tissue on the left. And so it proved, for when the first patient died from a pulmonary embolus nine9 years later, the autopsy revealed a long-standing degeneration of the right hippocampus.

These results, though unexpected, were nevertheless in line with Penfield's earlier suspicion that the temporal lobes, whatever other functions they might have, were concerned with memory. The first hint had come when he had been stimulating the lobe prior to surgery. In a small number of patients the stimuli had evoked sights or sounds that appeared to be from the past.[1] In some instances it was overheard conversations or a person calling, in one it was people approaching, while in another it was the noise and vision of circus wagons. Sometimes the people were familiar and sometimes not. In some cases the location of the hallucination could be described. Results such as these had led Penfield to suppose that, rather like a continuously running video-camera, the temporal lobes were creating an unbroken record of life experiences.

But which parts of the temporal lobes were involved in memory? The division of the human cerebral cortex into lobes is based entirely on the pattern of the surface folds and this varies, not only between one individual and another but often between the two hemispheres in the same person. Further, there is no *a priori* reason why different functions of the brain should correspond precisely to the folding pattern, for

Aranzio's Seahorse and the Search for Memory and Consciousness. Alan J. McComas, Oxford University Press.
© Oxford University Press 2023. DOI: 10.1093/oso/9780192868244.003.0006

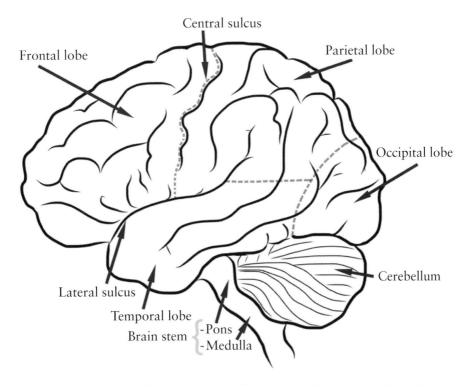

Central sulcus

Frontal lobe

Parietal lobe

Occipital lobe

Cerebellum

Lateral sulcus

Temporal lobe

Brain stem { -Pons
              -Medulla

Figure 4.1 Outer surface of left hemisphere of human brain showing the lobes, sulci (fissures), and gyri (convolutions). The gyri immediately in front of, and behind, the central sulcus house the motor and body surface maps respectively (see Figure 3.3) while the temporal lobe gyri are important for memory; the hippocampus is on the inner (medial) side of the hemisphere and therefore not visible.

the latter evolved as the means of maximizing the area of cortex within the confines of the skull. Despite this caveat the temporal lobe, like the other lobes, continues to be divided anatomically on the basis of its folds—the 'gyri' separated from each other by the 'sulci'. Thus, there is a superior gyrus, most of which forms the bottom of the prominent lateral sulcus (Figure 4.1). The middle gyrus is on the outside (lateral) surface of the lobe, while the inferior and fusiform gyri are on the bottom (inferior) surface. The inner (medial or 'mesial') surface is more complicated. The front (anterior) part is the uncus and, a little further back, lie the amygdala and adjacent hippocampus. In the few patients who had reported 'memories', Penfield's stimulating probe had been on the superior surface of the temporal lobe, deep within the lateral sulcus; in these original experiments he had not stimulated the hippocampus or the neural structures immediately adjacent to it. In Penfield's operations on the temporal lobe, the further back from the anterior pole that he removed tissue, the less that would be left of the hippocampus on that side.

There is another uncertainty about Penfield's observations. Were the patients really recalling events from the past, or were the reported experiences fabricated by the brain, as happens in dreaming or in the hallucinations associated with temporal lobe epilepsy?

Penfield's conclusion that the temporal lobes were the seat of memory did not go unchallenged, especially by the professor and head of psychology at Harvard University.

Karl Lashley (1890–1958)[2] was a skilful and original investigator with a penetrating mind who had carried out extensive research on primates and other species. For the experiments on memory he had used rats; they were cheap, easy to handle, and smart enough to be trained and tested. Rather to his surprise, Lashley had observed that the animals could still remember how to work their way through mazes after varying amounts of brain had been removed, though their proficiency in the task was proportional to the amount of cortex remaining. From this he had deduced that memory—the 'engram'—was distributed widely in the brain (the principle of 'mass action') rather than in a single location, as Penfield was proposing. Further, from his rat experiments, it seemed to Lashley that one part of the brain could take on the functions of another ('equipotentiality').

An exciting if unconventional speaker, Lashley was well known to psychologists and even to the public. Donald Hebb had twice worked under his direction, first at Harvard and then in Florida at the Yerkes Primate Center, and there were other future leaders in psychology and neurophysiology who had also started their careers with Lashley. Unsurprisingly, in view of his eminence, Lashley had been one of the small group Jasper had invited to the Laurentian symposium on consciousness in 1953; on that occasion Lashley had chosen to talk about perception rather than memory. The group photo shows him standing at the end of the front row—a slim professorial figure with glasses. There is a look of ill-health, however, and within six months Lashey would collapse in front of his students from the effects of a severe haemolytic anaemia. In four years he would be dead.

Understandably, Brenda Milner's study of Penfield's two patients with memory loss following unilateral temporal lobectomy had attracted the attention not only of experimental psychologists like Lashley but of a wider audience as well. Penfield had decided to present the work at the 1955 annual meeting of the American Neurological Association in Chicago.[3] In making Brenda his co-author, Penfield did more than acknowledge her careful work; he had come to appreciate her intelligence and abilities as an investigator, coupled with her maturity of thought and expression. He was also aware of her excellent undergraduate record at Cambridge, one that had won her a two-year research scholarship immediately before the war. Notwithstanding the great difference in professional seniority between the head of the Institute and the new post-doctoral fellow, the two were closer when it came to understanding the workings of the brain.

The next development involved another surgeon and a third patient—as it turned out, by far the most important patient of the three.

William Scoville had been one of those to receive a booklet containing the programme and abstracts of the talks for the Chicago meeting, including the précis of the presentations to be given by Penfield and Brenda Milner. The Connecticut neurosurgeon had previously met Penfield at a neurosurgical conference in Santa Fe, New Mexico and, on that occasion, had told the older man of his own experience with medial temporal lobe surgery in psychiatric patients. In 1955, the year of the presentation in

Chicago, Penfield had written to Scoville, reminding him of their earlier discussion, and asking if Brenda Milner could examine some of his, Scoville's, operated patients. Scoville, in turn, replied that he would be delighted to have Brenda visit. There was only one patient who had not been psychotic, however, and he had undergone surgery for epilepsy. Scoville went on: 'his memory is absolutely no good: cannot even be sent to the store alone for purchases'.

William Beecher Scoville (1906–1984; Figure 4.2)[4] had been an undergraduate at Yale before starting medical school in Philadelphia. His middle name was the legacy of a grandfather who had achieved national prominence by preaching against slavery prior to the Civil War. Following his graduation from the University of Pennsylvania Scoville had been an intern in psychiatry in his hometown of Hartford, Connecticut. Then had come a move to New York, first to study psychiatry and then to learn neurology. It was only then that he had found his true calling—neurosurgery. After completing his training in that specialty under leading neurosurgeons in Boston and Baltimore (at Johns Hopkins Hospital), Scoville had returned to Connecticut. Though Hartford was a small city in comparison with those in which he had studied, it was important, nonetheless. Situated on the Connecticut River, it had been settled early, first by the Dutch and then by the British. In the 19th century it had become an important

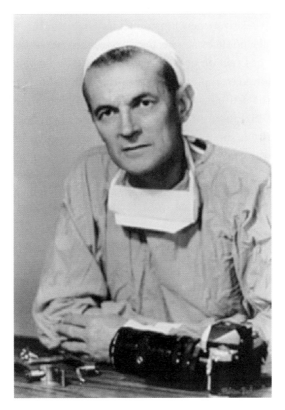

Figure 4.2 William Beecher Scoville, Henry Molaison's neurosurgeon. Photograph courtesy of Luke Dittrich.

manufacturing centre while also serving as the State capital. Included among its medical facilities was a large mental asylum that provided work for neurologists and psychiatrists, and sometimes for neurosurgeons too. The asylum had become a showpiece following its opening in 1822, both for the quality of care for its patients and for the impressive building and grounds.[5] Charles Dickens, in 1842, had been one of those to have visited the asylum. A century later the asylum had been renamed 'The Institute of Living' at the instigation of its ambitious superintendent. It was he, Dr Burlingame, who had not only encouraged Scoville to operate on some of the Institute's patients but had had a psychosurgery operating theatre built for him. Remarkably, there had also been a research laboratory constructed, together with a monkey-house.[6]

However, it was not only at the Institute of Living that Scoville had found work or, rather, had been invited to work; the huge State Hospital in nearby Middletown had also had need of his services. The request had come at a time when public mental hospitals in the United States were hopelessly overcrowded and the patients, for the most part, poorly looked after. Further, there was little that could be offered in the way of treatment. In Connecticut a state committee had proposed neurosurgery as a partial solution to the wretched situation; operations would be performed in both the public hospitals and the private Institute for the Living. The particular procedure that the committee had in mind was frontal lobotomy and William Scoville, already familiar with it, would become one of its foremost practitioners.

The operation was relatively new. It had had its origins in the observation, in John Fulton's physiological laboratory at Yale, that two belligerent chimpanzees had become more tractable after destruction of their frontal lobes. This finding, reported in 1935, had been swiftly followed by application of the principle to human patients in Portugal, a move directed by the neuroanatomist, Egas Moniz, and one for which he would later be awarded a Nobel Prize.[7]

Rather than remove tissue, Moniz had devised a novel and seemingly elegant procedure. The key instrument was an adjustable wire loop that, with the loop closed, was inserted into the brain through a small incision in the forehead and a hole in the underlying skull. Once in position, the loop was opened and rotated through 360 degrees, thereby severing the fibres connecting the neurons in the frontal lobes from the rest of the brain. Four such procedures were carried out on each frontal lobe. In view of the encouraging reports on patients treated by Moniz's group, the procedure was adopted elsewhere and especially in the United States by Walter Freeman and James Watts. Rather than use a collapsible wire loop to cut the nerve fibres, Freeman and Watts, together with their many followers, preferred a fine scalpel blade; subsequently Freeman devised an instrument resembling an ice-pick that could be driven into the frontal lobe through the thin bone at the back of the eye socket. The various types of operation were referred to as 'frontal lobotomies'.

It is surprising that the lobotomies were performed so readily. The operation would eventually fall into disrepute but not before an estimated 40,000 patients had been treated in the United States, together with 17,000 or so in Britain. In most instances there had been no proper controls, no further trials in primates, no careful assessments of mental abilities and mood, no separation of patients by diagnosis, and no systematic search for possible side effects. Indeed, the *laissez-faire* attitude was in sharp contrast to the situation today, where any experiment on human subjects, even one involving the slightest needle prick or the administration of a harmless (placebo) pill, still requires the consent of a hospital or university ethics committee as well as that of the patient.

To William Scoville and the other neurosurgeons practicing lobotomy in the 1940s and 1950s the frontal lobes presented something of an enigma, however. Their large sizes suggested that their evolution from smaller primate brains must have been responsible for the enormous intelligence of the human species and perhaps for human consciousness. Years later, Francis Crick and Christof Koch would go so far as to suggest, erroneously, that the final stage of visual processing, the act of seeing, took place in the prefrontal area.[8] And yet there were some observations suggesting that the massive frontal lobes did relatively little, especially in comparison with more posterior parts of the brain in which even a small lesion could have devastating consequences. Penfield had been aware of this conundrum when he had been obliged to operate on his older sister soon after his appointment as neurosurgeon in Montreal. In attempting to excise her malignant glioma, he had removed the greater part of her right frontal lobe (while preserving the motor strip) and had been astonished at the preservation of her personality and mental faculties.[9] And in 1848 there had been the remarkable case of Phineas Gage.

Gage had been the young foreman of a gang of workers engaged in constructing a railway line through the mountains of Vermont and was an expert in demolishing rock. However, on this occasion there was an accident—while Gage was still working his tamping rod ignited the blasting powder in the hole that had been drilled in the rock. The force of the explosion drove the iron rod through Gage's left cheek, and thence behind the left eye, up through the base of the skull and the left frontal lobe, and out of the top of the head (Figure 4.3). The tapered rod, one metre long, three centimetres in diameter, and smeared with blood and brain, had landed some twenty-five metres away. Gage, who had been knocked to the ground, was able to get up and walk. On being taken to the nearest doctor, he remarked: 'Doctor, here's business enough for you.' Despite the destruction of his left frontal lobe (though evidently sparing the motor strip) and the subsequent development of a large cerebral abscess, Gage recovered physically. And though his personality had deteriorated in the immediate aftermath of the accident, that recovered too, such that he was eventually able to operate a stage-coach business successfully in Chile for seven years.[10]

Gage's history, the relatively benign consequences of frontal lobe injury or disease in other patients, and observations on patients following prefrontal leucotomy, led to a puzzling conclusion. Other than effecting movements (including those of the eyes and vocal cords) and having some influence on behaviour, the massive frontal lobes appeared to have little function. And despite considerable recent research, including brain scans in humans and single neuron recordings in animals, there is not much to add. In view of their size and their evolutionary development, it is tempting to suppose that the frontal lobes are concerned with 'higher mental reasoning', and there are some

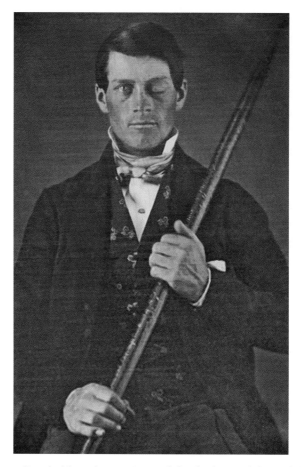

Figure 4.3 Phineas Gage holding the tamping rod that had passed through his left orbit and frontal lobe. Prepared from a daguerrotype, this photograph is originally from the collection of Jack and Beverly Wilgus, and now in the Warren Anatomical Museum, Harvard Medical School. (Creative Commons Attribution-Share Alike 3.0 unported license.)

observations that would support that view. Perhaps, too, the frontal lobes have a role in 'working' memory—holding and manipulating information for a few seconds—but the evidence is conflicting. Brenda Milner, who had long been interested in the frontal lobes, would herself suggest that patients with frontal lobe damage or ablations had difficulty in adapting to change. But even if these various functions were present, they still seemed meagre when matched against the billions of neurons contained within the lobes.

As already noted, William Scoville would have been well aware of the frontal lobe enigma during the time that he was performing leucotomies on patients in the Connecticut mental asylums in the late 1940s. He had carried out a large number and had pioneered orbital undercutting as a means of minimizing the amount of tissue destruction. In this new procedure he had approached the brain from the front, removing a disc of bone above each eye before gently raising the frontal lobes and cutting their nerve fibres from below. Even with this modification, however, the results had not been as impressive as he would have liked and this, allied to uncertainty about the normal function of the frontal lobes, was sufficient reason for him to consider the temporal lobes as alternative targets.

Scoville had some information to guide him, for the effects of removing both temporal lobes in monkeys had been examined by Heinrich Klüver and Paul Bucy in Chicago in the late 1930s. They had observed marked changes in behaviour, the animals becoming more docile and less given to rage and fear; in addition, the monkeys appeared not to recognize objects with which they had previously been familiar and would repeatedly explore them with their mouths and nostrils.[11] Unknown to the Chicago investigators and to Scoville, very similar findings had been published fifty years previously, by Sanger Brown and Victor Horsley in London's University College.[12]

In 1950 Scoville had performed bilateral temporal lobe surgery for the first time; this had been on a young woman with a ten-year history of schizophrenic symptoms. Using the same frontal approach as before, Scoville had removed the uncus on each side with a suction catheter, leaving the hippocampus intact; he had then performed similar surgery on another three patients in the same afternoon. The results in these and other patients were inconclusive, leading Scoville to remove more of the medial temporal lobe, including varying amounts of the hippocampus, in additional cases. He was encouraged by the fact that, in some cases, the patients appeared to have forgotten the delusions that had caused their original hospitalization—though it was not appreciated at the time, it was a strong hint that the temporal lobes were concerned with memory.

In August 1953 Scoville would operate on a young man, a patient who differed from all the previous ones in that he was not psychotic (Figure 4.4). Rather, Henry Molaison's problem was that he was severely epileptic. It is possible that his seizures were the sequel to a head injury in childhood; according to his mother, they had started the year following an accident in which he had been knocked down by a bicycle on one of Hartford's streets and rendered unconscious for several minutes. It is equally likely that the seizures were the result of a genetic predisposition, since there was a history of epilepsy on his father's side of the family.[13] Initially the attacks were minor, lasting less than a minute and consisting of unawareness and detachment from his surroundings; generalized seizures, with loss of consciousness, jerking of the limbs, and urinary incontinence, had appeared several years later. Like other neurosurgeons, Scoville was familiar with Penfield's use of temporal lobe surgery for cases of intractable epilepsy and he was also familiar with the use of EEG as a means of localizing the site of the seizures—an investigation that Herbert Jasper had pioneered before his move to Montreal. To help him determine the side of the brain generating Henry Molaison's seizures, Scoville had engaged his own electroencephalographer, the gifted Russian emigré Wladimir Liberson. Having accessed his patient's medial temporal lobes, Scoville placed a recording electrode on each in turn but neither revealed the locus of the seizures to Liberson. Uncertain of the side of the problem but ever bold, Scoville proceeded to suck out both medial temporal lobes, including much of their most prominent structures, the hippocampi (Box 4.1).

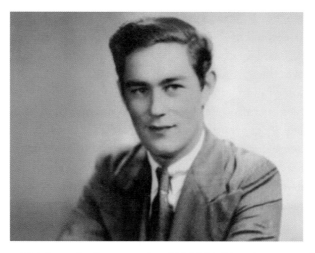

Figure 4.4 Henry Molaison, the former patient H.M. This historic image, taken shortly before the temporal lobe surgery that would destroy his long-term memory is included as a 'fair use' reproduction in that it is essential to this narrative, appears to be unique, and there is no known copyright holder. (Wikipedia file: Henry Gustav 1.jpg.)

Box 4.1. Human hippocampus.

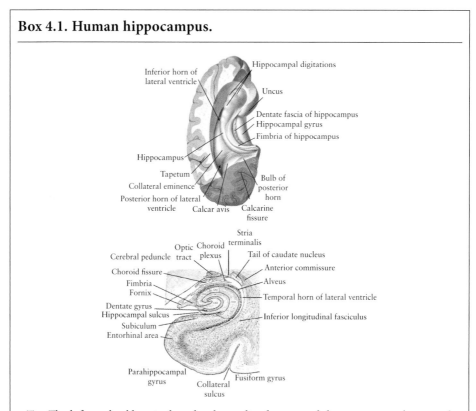

Top. The left cerebral hemisphere has been sliced open and the top removed to reveal the hippocampus lying in the floor of the lateral ventricle. The resemblance to a seahorse is obvious. (Wikimedia Commons. Author, Johannes Sobotta, 1908.

Bottom Transverse cut through the medial temporal lobe showing the structures bordering the hippocampus and linked to it. (Wikimedia Commons. J.A. Kieman, modified from Edinger, 1899 (L. Edinger, *The Anatomy of the Central Nervous System of Man and of Vertebrates in General*. F.A. Davis: Philadelphia, PA. 5th edition, 1899).

When Giulio Cesare Aranzio was dissecting a human brain and identified a structure that had not been previously described, it is probable that he had been systematically cutting out and removing tissue from the temporal lobe. If so, he would have seen the hippocampus from above. It would have appeared as a white strip which curved upwards and then ran forwards in an arc approaching the midline, becoming thinner as it did so. If the human subject had died within a day or so, the structure would have glistened with moisture, for it lay in the floor of one of the fluid-filled cavities in the brain, the lateral ventricle. It was the nerve fibres leaving the structure and lying on its surface that gave the latter its striking whiteness. When the structure was dissected away from its neighbouring parts, it did indeed have the appearance of a seahorse, one that was lying down in the brain, its tail formed by the curved arc (Figure).

The hippocampus is not, of course, a separate structure but rather one with several parts and a host of connections. At the front (anterior) end it abuts a large collection of nuclei which together form the *amygdala* and to which it has reciprocal connections. Running along the medial aspect of the hippocampus is a bulge of cortex—the *dentate gyrus*. A transverse cut through this part of the temporal lobe shows that the hippocampus lies atop the curvature of the *parahippocampal gyrus* (Figure, *bottom*); this last structure contains the entorhinal cortex, the lateral part of which sends fibres into the hippocampus (the *perforant path*). The parahippocampal gyrus also houses the *subiculum*, which is an important source of fibres leaving the hippocampal region. Many of these efferent fibres enter and run in the *fornix*—the prominent curved arc that forms the tail of the seahorse. At the end of its arc fornix splits up to connect with a number of structures (amongst them the *thalamus*, *mammillary bodies*, and *brainstem nuclei*).

When William Scoville carried out his more extensive medial temporal lobe resections, as in Henry Molaison, he would have removed not only much of the hippocampus but also the amygdala and the part of the parahippocampal gyrus as well.

Although he had, by then, performed bilateral temporal lobotomy on many occasions, Henry Molaison had been the first patient who, apart from his seizures, had been mentally normal. The choice of tense is important for, as he recovered from the operation, Henry Molaison had made an alarming discovery about himself—*he could no longer remember*.

Henry Molaison was the non-psychotic patient that Scoville had singled out for mention in his correspondence with Penfield. He would become Brenda Milner's third subject with memory loss and there would be many scientific papers written about him. During his lifetime he would be known as Patient H.M.

On the evening of 25 April 1955, with Penfield's encouragement, Brenda Milner travelled from Montreal to Hartford, Connecticut, to examine Henry Molaison as well as several other patients that Scoville had operated upon. By day it would have been a beautiful journey, especially the first part as the train made its way south through the eastern townships of Quebec before entering the mountains of Vermont and running alongside Lake Champlain.

At the Hartford Hospital[14] Brenda was met by Scoville and it was the neurosurgeon who introduced Henry Molaison to her. It had been twenty months since his operation and Henry was now twenty-nine. Brenda found the young man to be pleasant and polite, and willing to participate in the various tests that she had brought with her. She began by asking him to remember the number, 584. On returning twenty minutes later, having had a cup of coffee elsewhere, Brenda was surprised to discover that Henry had retained the number. 'How did you do it?', she enquired. It transpired that Henry had added the three digits and then divided the sum in such a way as to give the three digits back again. It had been a simple arithmetic trick for keeping the digits in his mind.

'Do you remember my name?', Brenda then asked.
'I'm having difficulty with my memory,' the young man replied.
'Do you still remember the number?' Brenda went on. Henry looked blank.
'Number? Was there a number?'[15]

It was an exciting introduction to a study that would transform the science of memory.

Over the next few days, Brenda took Henry through a series of formal memory tests. The first of these was the Wechsler Memory Scale and consisted of a standard series of general questions beginning with the patient's age, the present year and month, and the name of the President of the United States. After this came a test of visual memory, the ability to recall simple geometric shapes that had been shown to him. Brenda then examined Henry's verbal memory by asking him to repeat unusual pairings of words. Finally, she told him a short story and asked him to repeat it. The tests were arranged so that Henry would have the opportunity to give his answer immediately after the presentation and then after an interval of twenty minutes.

Next came an intelligence test, again one that had been devised a few years previously by David Weschler at New York's Bellvue Hospital. Some of the questions tested general knowledge, such as the names of countries, cities, or persons, while others were philosophical. Mental arithmetic was also tested, as was the ability to arrange visual shapes. The results of the two examinations were surprising because while Henry's intelligence, as tested, was well above average, his memory was not—in fact, his memory score was the lowest Brenda Milner had ever encountered. Even so, it was not a total loss of memory because Henry could still recall events that had taken place in childhood and up to a few years of his surgery. But new information, whether it was something said or seen, a place visited, or someone he had recently met, none of this could be retained for longer than half a minute. While Henry's short-term memory was still present, his long-term memory was mostly absent.[16]

Over the next few days Brenda would examine eight more Connecticut patients who had also undergone bilateral medial temporal lobectomy, in all but two cases for treatment of their schizophrenia. It had not been easy since, for a variety of reasons that included their mental illness, none had been able to cooperate as readily as Henry Molaison.

There was one more patient to be studied, someone else that Scoville had operated upon, but in order to see him Brenda would have to travel to a large mental hospital just south of Chicago. Though it involved another long journey, the results would be as striking and as important as those found in Hartford.

Patient D.C. was a forty-seven-year old doctor with paranoid schizophrenia, who had undergone surgery on both medial temporal lobes together with orbital undercutting. In the days following the surgery he had been unable to find his way back to his hospital bed or to recognize the hospital staff. When examined by Brenda Milner one year later in a different hospital he attributed his unfamiliarity with his surroundings to his arrival on the previous day—in fact, he had been transferred six weeks previously. Like Henry Molaison, D.C. was found to have a high IQ and like Henry Molaison his memory score was strikingly low.

With ten patients having undergone thorough psychological testing, William Scoville and Brenda Milner had enough material to begin writing their paper.

Notes

1. W. Penfield and P. Perot, 'The Brain's Record of Auditory and Visual Experience: A Final Summary and Discussion' (1963) 86 *Brain* 595–696.
2. Among the biographies of Lashley that by Sir Frederic Bartlett (Brenda Milner's former departmental head in Cambridge) is especially well written, capturing the essence of a captivating but highly unusual person. See: F.C. Bartlett, 'Karl Spencer Lashley 1890–1958' (1960) 5 *Biographical Memoirs of Fellows of the Royal Society* 106–18.
3. A full account of the study of the two patients did not appear until three years later: W. Penfield and B. Milner, 'Memory Defect Produced by Bilateral Lesions in the Hippocampal Zone' (1958) 79(May) *AMA Archives of Neurology and Psychiatry* 475–97.
4. A detailed account of Scoville's early life, family relationships, professional training, and, ultimately, surgery on psychiatric patients is given by his grandson, Luke Dittrich, in the *New York Times* bestseller: L. Dittrich, *Patient H.M. A Story of Memory, Madness and Family Secrets* (New York, NY: Random House, 2016).
5. The information about the Institute of Living also comes from Luke Dittrich (see note 4). An interesting fact to have emerged from Dittrich's research was that Scoville's wife was at one time a patient at the Institute and it is even possible that she may have been operated upon by her husband.
6. Mortimer Mishkin, a fellow graduate student with Brenda Milner at McGill, was one of those who would come to work there. Karl Pribram, a noted neuroscientist, had been the head of the Institute's laboratory at that time.
7. An excellent comprehensive account of the history of prefrontal lobotomy (leucotomy) is given in Wikipedia (<http://www.en.wikipedia.org/wiki/lobotomy> accessed 20 April 2022). It appears that Moniz may have had the idea of his surgery prior to the conference during which he heard Fulton speak. Several years before that, however, Walter Dandy had performed a bilateral

prefrontal lobectomy on a patient with a tumour (meningioma) at Johns Hopkins Hospital without any significant mental consequences.

8. F.H.C. Crick and C. Koch, 'Are We Aware of Neuronal Activity in Primary Visual Cortex?' (1995) 375 *Nature* 121–4.

9. W. Penfield, *No Man Alone. A Neurosurgeon's Life* (Boston, MA: Little Brown, 1977) 207–21.

10. A full account of Gage's injury, treatment, recovery, and subsequent life is provided by Wikipedia (<http://www.en.wikipedia.org/wiki/Phineas Gage> accessed 20 April 2022). The article includes the debate as to what extent Gage's personality changed following the accident and subsequent brain infection. Gage's brain injury, and its relevance for an understanding of brain function, is the main topic of a book by Antonio Damasio (A.R. Damasio, *Descarte's Error. Emotion, Reason and the Human Brain* (New York, NY: GP Putnam, 1994).

11. H. Klüver and P.C Bucy, 'An Analysis of Certain Effects of Bilateral Temporal Lobectomy in the Rhesus Monkey, with Special Reference to "Psychic Blindness"' (1938) 5 *Journal of Psychology* 33–54.

12. P.S.S.V. Pannemreddy and J.L. Stone, 'Sanger Brown and Edward Schäfer before Heinrich Klüver and Paul Bucy: Their Observations on Bilateral Temporal Lobe Ablations' (2017) 43(3) *Neurosurgical Focus* 1–7.

13. S. Corkin, *Permanent Present Tense. The Unforgettable Life of the Amnesic Patient, H.M.* (New York, NY: Basic Books, 2013).

14. The Hartford Hospital was where the surgery had been performed. The hospital was adjacent to the Institute for Living.

15. As recounted during an interview for the Canadian National Film Board, 17 July 2018 <https://www.youtube.com/watch?v=ChuCQn6MwLw> .

16. William James may have been the first to distinguish between short-term and long-term memories. See: W. James, *Principles of Psychology* (Cambridge, MA: Harvard University Press, 1890).

5

Triumph and an Unprovoked Attack

(Montreal, London, 1957; Wilder Penfield, Francis Walshe)

The paper by William Scoville and Brenda Milner, entitled 'Loss of Memory after Bilateral Hippocampal Lesions' appeared in the February 1957 issue of *The Journal of Neurology, Neurosurgery and Psychiatry*.[1] The latter had been a good choice of journal for, while lacking the prestige of the much older *Brain*, it tended to attract articles with greater scientific content. Further, as the title of the journal implied, the published material came not only from neurology but from a variety of disciplines, and it was to this wide field that the Scoville and Milner paper instantly appealed. The article contained diagrams showing exactly what had been attempted by the surgeon, together with summaries of the psychological test results in each of the ten patients. The importance of the work was evident in the penultimate sentence: 'It is concluded that the anterior hippocampus and hippocampal gyrus, either separately or together, are critically involved in the retention of current experience.'

The publication must have given the first author considerable satisfaction. William Scoville had had a strong academic leaning earlier in his career and had since kept himself up to date with the primate research in John Fulton's laboratory at Yale. More than that, Scoville had, through his innovative surgery—first the orbital undercutting and now the bilateral medial temporal lobectomies—contributed to knowledge of brain function himself. Already the author of several surgical papers, he would continue to publish and teach neurosurgery for the remainder of his career. And he had invented and patented a retractor as well as a special clip for closing veins during aneurysm surgery.

The new contribution, the study with Brenda Milner, was a major one. For the first time, memory had been clearly linked to a specific region of the brain and the Scoville and Milner paper would become a classic citation. But the study had also left a large question mark, one that could have set memory research back in the years to come. Fortunately it would be largely disregarded even by those who took the trouble to read the paper rather than simply cite it. The uncertainty concerned the amygdala.

This complex structure, composed of several nuclei, lay in front and alongside the head of the hippocampus and there were fibre connections between the two, indicative of a shared function. Yet in a patient in whom Scoville had performed a limited resection, allegedly removing both amygdala but sparing the hippocampi, there had been no disturbance of memory. Scoville and Milner had written: 'Removing only the uncus and amygdala bilaterally does not appear to cause memory impairment.' But the

Aranzio's Seahorse and the Search for Memory and Consciousness. Alan J. McComas, Oxford University Press.
© Oxford University Press 2023. DOI: 10.1093/oso/9780192868244.003.0007

authors seemed reluctant to accept the absence of a role for the amygdala for they had added elsewhere: 'It is not known whether the amygdala plays any part in this mechanism (retention of current experience) since the hippocampal complex has not been removed alone but always together with the uncus and amygdala.'

The key role of the amygdala in memory would only become apparent much later. Before then, however, Henry's memory would be studied again and again, and in more and more detail. It would become clear that his memory for the present was limited to a mere 30 seconds or so. Though it was not stated in the original paper, the presence of this short-term memory implied that a part of the brain other than the hippocampus must be responsible for it. Such an interpretation was justified given the information provided in Scoville and Milner's paper. But had Scoville's resections of Henry's two hippocampi been as extensive as he had claimed? Half a century would elapse before there was a definitive answer—and it would be a surprise.

In 1957, however, Brenda Milner's role in identifying the hippocampus as a brain region essential for memory was a triumph for the Department of Psychology at McGill University, but it was only one of several successes for the revitalized department.

Donald Hebb's first decade as Chair was drawing to a close. In short order his graduate students had made two important advances. First, there had been the finding of a pleasure centre in the brain by James Olds and Peter Milner, and now had come clinical evidence that the hippocampus was essential for memory. There had also been a fine piece of research by another McGill graduate student. Mortimer Mishkin, operating on monkeys in John Fulton's laboratory at Yale, had shown another function for the temporal lobes—they were engaged in visual recognition. It was the first clear evidence that vision involved more than the previously recognized areas at the back of the brain (in the occipital lobes). And then, predating the discoveries in the laboratories and the surgical operating theatre, there had been Hebb's book. *The Organization of Behaviour*, with its tentative ideas as to how neural function might underlie thinking and perception—the book that, in its preparatory stage, had made such an impression on the McGill graduate students, was becoming a classic.

The progress in the university department mirrored changes that were taking place outside, not only in Montreal and Quebec but in the country as a whole. The arrival of the Milners in Montreal in 1944 had been followed by those of tens of thousands of other immigrants to Canada. Most of the initial newcomers had come from Britain and Europe, and were men and women who had tired of rationing and other post-war restrictions, and who considered that there were better opportunities for employment in Canada. In Britain there was disappointment that the building of the new socialist Jerusalem, long a promise of the Labour government, had yet to secure a firm foundation, let alone rise from the ashes of the Second World War. Many of the Canadian immigrants were highly skilled, such as the aviation designers and engineers who would create the world's most advanced fighter plane, the Avro Arrow, at an aircraft factory outside Toronto. Others were involved in the construction of the St Lawrence Seaway, a shipping route connecting all the Great Lakes to the Atlantic Ocean. Yet others were responsible for the Chalk River atomic energy research establishment and ultimately for the construction and world-wide sales of CANDU nuclear reactors. And, inevitably, many of the best brains went to fill vacancies in the already established or newly created Canadian universities. Unlike its European counterparts, Canada was seen as a country with a good future. Optimism was in the air.

But while the Psychology Department at McGill was flourishing, the Montreal Neurological Institute, just a few hundred yards away, had come under attack. It was a literary and scientific attack that had been aimed directly at the Institute's director, Wilder Penfield, and it had come without warning. It had been launched by one of Britain's most distinguished neurologists, Francis Walshe (later, Sir Francis), a consultant at the National Hospital for Nervous Diseases in Queen Square, London (Figure 5.1).

The attack appeared in the form of a lengthy article in the July 1957 number of the world's premier neurological journal, *Brain*.[2] The 29 pages followed a similarly long title: 'The Brain-Stem Conceived as the "Highest Level" of Function in the Nervous System; with Particular Reference to the "Automatic Apparatus" of Carpenter (1850) and to the "Centrencephalic Integrating System" of Penfield.'

What was it about and why had Walshe written it?

The answer to the first question is that Penfield had long been intrigued by the relationship of the brain to the mind; his work and ideas on memory were but one aspect of this interest. A greater issue was the whereabouts of consciousness in the brain—where were the assemblies of neurons, the electrical activity of which was responsible for

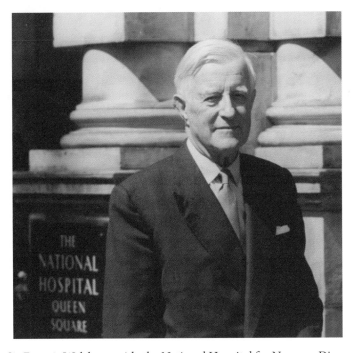

Figure 5.1 Sir Francis Walshe outside the National Hospital for Nervous Diseases, Queen Square, London. Photo kindly supplied by Clare Armstrong, granddaughter.

creating awareness, perceptions, and thoughts? Was the whole brain involved or was there some special region in which the necessary information in the brain was brought together to find expression?

Although it was widely assumed that the great development of the cerebral cortex, and of the frontal lobes in particular, was responsible for human consciousness, Penfield had his doubts—and for good reason. First, there had been his observation that a large part of a frontal lobe could be removed with little apparent consequence. He had observed this when he had operated on his sister's malignant glioma and the story of Phineas Gage would have been well known to him. Moreover, in the patients whose exposed brains he had stimulated in the operating theatre, it was unusual to obtain any response outside the motor and somatosensory strips. While he occasionally evoked 'memories' from the superior and lateral aspects of the temporal lobe, these were the exceptions. In contrast he knew that interference with the brain stem, by injury, disease, or surgical interference, could readily abolish consciousness. And again, the electroencephalography (EEG) studies of Jasper and Pierre Gloor in his own Institute, as well as those of others, pointed to deep structures within the brain as the origin of grand mal epileptic seizures, in which consciousness was lost. Was it not possible, therefore, that the brain stem was where integration of sensory information occurred and where the latter reached consciousness? And where voluntary movements originated?

Penfield had first mooted the idea in an address that he had given in 1936 to the New York Academy of Medicine:

> there is much evidence of a level of integration within the central nervous system that is higher than that to be found in the cerebral cortex, evidence of a regional localization of the neuronal mechanism involved in this integration. I suggest that this region lies not in the new brain but in the old … probably in the diencephalon.[3]

His ideas were undoubtedly reinforced by Hess's animal studies with implanted electrodes showing the importance of midbrain structures in the control of sleeping and waking. And then there had come the 1949 report of the discovery of the ascending reticular activating system in the brain stem by Moruzzi and Magoun; the two neurophysiologists had convincingly shown that electrical stimulation of this structure could awaken a sleeping cat.[4] Indeed, Peter Milner had been stimulating the reticular formation in his rat experiments in the Psychology Department at McGill.

Penfield had continued to advance the concept of the brainstem acting as the 'highest level', including the occasion of the 1953 Laurentian symposium on consciousness.

However, great surgeon and pioneer that he undoubtedly was, Penfield was not a good science writer. The boldness of his centrencephalic idea was diminished by the rather fuzzy language he employed. Nor did he ever specify exactly which structures in the brainstem might be involved.

Penfield's intellectual adversary, Francis Martin Walshe, had been born six years before Penfield. Growing up in London, Walshe had studied medicine at University College and Hospital, where he had gained several prizes. After an unsuccessful attempt at a career in neurophysiology he had become a neurologist instead, betraying his former ambition by insisting that the neurological clinic was a more favourable setting than the laboratory for scientific observation. Walshe's good looks, dignified bearing, and manner of speech made him a patrician figure in the corridors and on the wards of the National Hospital for Nervous Diseases.[5]

With his penetrating logic, attention to detail, use of ridicule, and elegance of language, Walshe was well equipped to act as an iconoclast. In 1942, in another article in *Brain*,[6] he had demolished the novel dual pathway concept of body sensation advanced by Sir Henry Head (Figure 5.2). Head had been a giant in neurology, an original thinker who had been willing to offer his own cutaneous nerves for scientific study, but exclusion from the staff of the National Hospital had helped to make him vulnerable.[7]

In tackling Penfield and his idea of consciousness arising in the 'old brain' rather than in the cortex, Walshe first destroyed any claim that Penfield might have had for originality, pointing out that the same concept had been put forward a century earlier by Carpenter, a professor of physiology at University College London and the author of a widely used textbook. Further, unlike Penfield, Carpenter had specified which neural

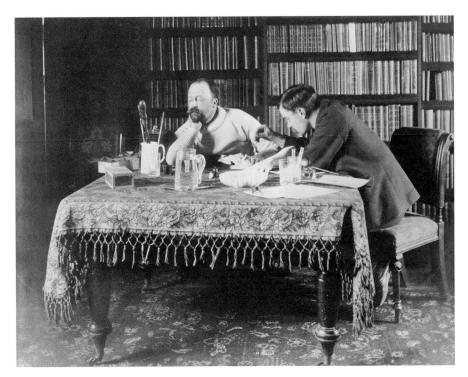

Figure 5.2 Henry Head (*left*) having his touch sensation examined by William Rivers in the latter's rooms at Cambridge University. Despite having been refused a staff appointment at the National Hospital for Nervous Diseases in Queen Square, London, Head remained a brilliant neurologist and general physician, with very original ideas on how the nervous system functioned. Retiring prematurely because of parkinsonism, he was knighted in 1929 and died in 1940. (Wellcome Images.)

structures were involved in generating consciousness—the sensory ganglia in the brainstem and the thalamus. Carpenter considered that although the cerebral cortex was responsible for emotions, ideas, reasoning, and the will to move, none of these activities reached consciousness until the cortex had contacted the sensory ganglia and the thalamus. Walshe argued, however, that while Carpenter's speculations might have been acceptable a century earlier, Penfield's could not be justified in the light of new advances in knowledge involving the sensory and motor cortices.

Yet, devastating as Walshe's paper was, the sharp-edged sentences mostly avoided giving answers to Penfield's observations. In particular, there had been no accounting for the relatively minor consequences of injury or surgery to large areas of frontal cortex or, in the opposite direction, for the ready loss of consciousness produced by seizure activity or damage involving the brain stem. Instead, Walshe's argument was the seeming absurdity of supposing that the relatively large cerebral cortex had little to do with consciousness in contrast to the much smaller brain stem. As regards the inability to evoke anything other than simple responses on stimulating the cerebral cortex, Walshe pointed out that electric shocks were a very abnormal way of engaging cortical activity. Another cause for criticism was Penfield's use of non-physiological terms, such as 'elaboration', 'way-station', and 'stop-over' to describe aspects of cerebral function. Walshe finished his demolition of Penfield's hypothesis:

> [A]s we read it we find ourselves back in the intellectual climate of mid-nineteenth century pre-Jacksonian imaginings. The cerebral cortex, of course, could not be wholly ignored, but it is perhaps not unfair to say that it has been stretched upon the Procrustean bed of a preconceived centrencephalic system, so that we can scarce recognize it.[8]

Inevitably, Penfield was annoyed and dismayed by the nature and tone of Walshe's criticism, and probably surprised as well. In a situation such as this, it should have been a courtesy on the part of the journal editor not only to have given advance notice of the paper but to have provided the recipient of the attack an opportunity for rebuttal. This had not happened. To add to Penfield's surprise, Walshe's onslaught had come twenty years since he, Penfield, had first put forward his idea of a central, conscious-generating integrating system, and this was the first time that he had been challenged over it. Rather than fight back, as he could have done, Penfield claimed that he had been misunderstood and that he had never denied a role for the cortex. At the International Congress of Neurological Sciences, held in Brussels in the same year, 1957, that Walshe's article had appeared, Penfield stated:

> We are not discussing a new or separate block of brain. There is no centrencephalon as distinct to diencephalon … Consciousness exists only in association with the passage of impulses through ever changing circuits of the brainstem and cortex. One cannot say that consciousness is here or there. But certainly without centrencephalic integration it is nonexistent.[9]

But the damage had been done. In three years, at the age of 69, Penfield would retire as Director of the Montreal Neurological Institute and begin writing books. Though he never wrote on the subject again, Penfield remained a believer in his centrencephalic hypothesis until the end of his long life, and, as would appear later, he may have been right to do so.

Meanwhile, Brenda Milner's paper with William Scoville had attracted the interest of a young, newly qualified physician in New York.

Notes

1. W.B. Scoville and B. Milner, 'Loss of Recent Memory after Bilateral Hippocampal Lesions' (1957) 20 *Journal of Neurology, Neurosurgery and Psychiatry* 11–21.
2. F.M.R. Walshe, 'The Brain-Stem Conceived as the "Highest Level" of Function in the Nervous System with Particular Reference to the "Automatic Apparatus" of Carpenter (1850) and to the "Centrencephalic Integrating System" of Penfield' (1957) 80 *Brain* 510–39.
3. W. Penfield, 'The Cerebral Cortex in Man. I. The Cerebral Cortex and Consciousness' (1938) 40 *Archives of Neurology and Psychiatry* 417–42.
4. F. Moruzzi and H.W. Magoun, 'Brain Stem Reticular Formation and Activation of the EEG' (1949) 1 *Electroencephalography and Clinical Neurophysiology* 455–73.
5. Interestingly, Walshe appears not to have been outstanding as a clinician. In his memoir: F.M.R Walshe, *The Spice of Life: from Northumbria to World Neurology* (London: Royal Society of Medicine, 1993), John Walton (later, the Lord Walton of Detchant) recalls an incident at neurology rounds at Queen Square when Walshe had completely misdiagnosed a patient with muscle weakness for want of a simple neurological test (the plantar response—the reflex movement of the big toe when an object is drawn along the lateral sole).
6. F.M.R. Walshe, 'The Anatomy and Physiology of Cutaneous Sensibility: A Critical Review' (1942) 65 *Brain* 48–112.
7. L.S. Jacyna, *Medicine & Modernism. A Biography of Henry Head* (Pittsburgh, PA: University of Pittsburgh, 2016).
8. As described by Jacyna (see note 7), Head had carried out, and published, a detailed study of aphasia affecting officers wounded in the First World War, in which he alluded to the Procrustean bed. Procrustes was a bandit in Greek mythology who would prey on unwary travellers and take them to his stronghold. Were they too small to fit his bed, he would stretch their limbs; if too large, he would amputate the legs accordingly. Walshe would almost certainly have been aware of Head's earlier use of the Procrustean analogy.
9. W. Penfield, 'Consciousness and Centrencephalic Organization' (1957) *Premier Congrès International des Sciences Neurologiques* 7–18.

6

The Path to Psychiatry

(New York, 1957: Eric Kandel)

In 1929 Eric Kandel (Figure 6.1) had been born into a Jewish family in Vienna.[1] His parents had owned and operated a toy and luggage store, and the family had lived in a small apartment not far from the medical school and the residence of Sigmund Freud. The relative order and comfort had come to an abrupt end with the annexation of Austria by Hitler and the Nazis in March 1938. The ready acceptance of the invaders by the Austrian government and by most of the population had been followed by persecution of the Jews, just as had happened in Germany. Eric's family had had their apartment ransacked and their store taken away from them; worse, his father had twice been imprisoned. After a year of hardship and humiliation the family succeeded in escaping to the United States.

Having arrived in New York City by boat, the Kandels adapted quickly to their new home and before long Eric's parents had established a clothing store in Brooklyn. Meanwhile Eric won a scholarship to Harvard College, studying modern European history and literature. The interest in these subjects was accompanied by a fascination with psychoanalysis and with the writings of Sigmund Freud in particular. Eager to enter the field, Eric decided to obtain a medical degree and enrolled at New York University (NYU).

By North American standards, NYU was respectably old. It had been founded in midtown Manhattan by prominent New Yorkers in 1831 and had added a medical faculty a few years later. Though the university had had its ups and downs, it had steadily increased its enrolment and had eventually come to occupy a large site on the bank of the East River. Separated from the latter only by FDR Drive, the campus was within a mile of both the United Nations Headquarters and the Empire State Building.

It was during his second year of medical studies that Eric Kandel had been introduced to the anatomy of the human brain. Wishing to learn more about the way that the nervous system functioned, Kandel received permission to spend a six-month elective with Harry Grundfest at the Neurological Institute of New York. The Institute, situated in Upper Manhattan and on the other side of the island, was associated with Columbia University. It had been created in the 1920s by a group of prominent city neurologists. Had matters turned out differently, Wilder Penfield might still have been a member, having been one of the two original neurosurgeons appointed to the Institute.[2]

Aranzio's Seahorse and the Search for Memory and Consciousness. Alan J. McComas, Oxford University Press.
© Oxford University Press 2023. DOI: 10.1093/oso/9780192868244.003.0008

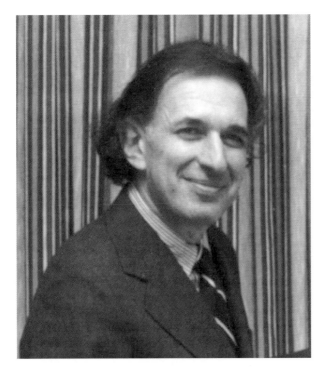

Figure 6.1 Eric Kandel in 1978, at the time he was at Columbia University, New York, and heavily involved in the *Aplysia* work. (Wikimedia Commons file: Eric Kandel 1978.jpg.)

Kandel's choice as his instructor at the Neurological Institute was widely recognized as a gifted experimenter. However, Harry Grundfest[3] had had the misfortune to become a target of Senator Joseph McCarthy's infamous anti-communist witchhunt. Though he had been deprived of national research funding, Grundfest had nevertheless managed to keep his laboratory active at the Neurological Institute and it was there that Kandel would spend his six-month elective. By assisting Dominic Purpura,[4] little older than himself, the young medical student was introduced to experimental neurophysiology for the first time. Purpura and Grundfest had been examining the effects of psychedelic drugs on the brain and their experiments involved recording with very fine glass microelectrodes from single neurons in the cat visual cortex. In addition to the experiments there had been informal and lively discussions of research, not only of the research in the local laboratory but of that elsewhere. Kandel had been fascinated. It was a new world and one very different to that of psychoanalysis.

In keeping with his new interest Kandel, after graduating as a Medical Doctor (MD), was able to obtain a temporary research position at the National Institute of Mental Health in Bethesda, Maryland. The head of the Laboratory of Neurophysiology, Wade Marshall, had made his reputation investigating, in animals, the areas of cerebral cortex responsive to different types of sensory stimulus—tactile, visual, and auditory. Marshall, unusually for a laboratory head, allowed

Kandel to choose his own research topic. And it was a recently published article in *The Journal of Neurology, Neurosurgery and Psychiatry* that influenced his decision. William Scoville and Brenda Milner's paper had, for the first time, clearly linked memory to the hippocampus.

Kandel would study memory and would begin with the cat hippocampus. The hippocampus had already been the object of neurophysiological studies in which recordings had been made from groups of neurons with wire electrodes. Among these investigations had been an especially thorough one by John Green and Arnaldo Arduini in Los Angeles.[5] In several species (cat, rabbit, monkey) they had drawn attention to rhythmic electrical activity in the theta range (5–7 Hz) that appeared when the animal was alert and was usually replaced with desynchronized fast discharges when the animal became sleepy. As the authors pointed out, this was the inverse of what occurred in the cerebral cortex, including that of humans. They also showed that hippocampal neurons responded to a variety of stimuli—olfactory, auditory, visual, and tactile—and that, in return, hippocampal stimulation affected wide areas of cortex. But neither these authors nor those who had preceded them could relate the various observations, striking as they were, to any definite function for the hippocampus.

Kandel's plan was to dispense with recordings from cell groups and, instead, to explore impulse activity in single neurons with glass microelectrodes, the same methodology he had employed while assisting Dominic Purpura in Harry Grundfest's laboratory. Hardly had Kandel embarked on his new quest than he was joined by another young MD, Alden Spencer, who had also come to work in Marshall's unit. Kandel and Spencer's hippocampal project was something of a 'fishing expedition', in that the two had little or no idea as to what they might find. One question they did attempt to answer, however, was whether the hippocampal neurons had the same biophysical properties as motoneurons—the nerve cells in the spinal cord and brain stem that controlled muscles and that had been the subject of a detailed investigation by John Eccles in New Zealand (prior to his move to Canberra).

Kandel's memoir conveys something of the excitement that the two young investigators experienced in the course of their work. The experiments were not easily undertaken, largely because of the difficulty in keeping the tip of the glass microelectrode inside a hippocampal neuron without damaging the cell membrane. But every now and then Kandel and Spencer succeeded and they would not only be able to see the electrical impulses instantly displayed on the oscilloscope screen but also to hear them on the loudspeaker—'*BANG! BANG! BANG!*' Though they were themselves novices, they had experienced neurophysiologists in neighbouring laboratories to advise them on matters of technique and to discuss their results with. As the work progressed Kandel and Spencer found that the hippocampal neurons (Box 6.1) developed and fired impulses in much the same way as the well-studied motoneurons in the spinal cord.

Box 6.1. Hippocampal structure.

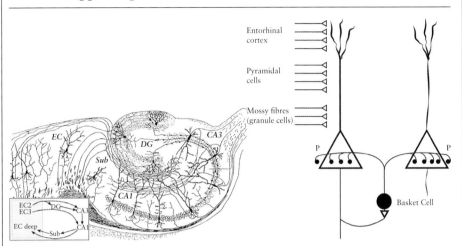

Left. Microscopic appearance of a transverse section of the hippocampus. Some typical neurons have been drawn with their axons and dendrites, others shown simply as ovals. Original by Cajal in his *Histologie du Système nerveus de l'Homme et des Vertébrés* (Paris: A Maloine, 1911) with lettering added subsequently as follows: *CA1*, *CA3*, divisions of hippocampus; *DG*, dentate gyrus; *EC*, entorhinal cortex; *Sub*, subiculum. The pyramidal cell bodies lie in a single curved layer throughout the hippocampus; two are shown below the *CA3* lettering. *Insert* shows the direction of impulse activity in the hippocampus, as determined by Per Andersen and his colleagues. (Wikimedia Commons File: CajalHippocampus (modified).png). *Right*. Synaptic connections on cell body and dendrites of a *CA1* pyramidal cell. Note basket cell with inhibitory synapses on cell body of pyramidal neuron (*P*).

Cells and fibres in the hippocampus

Several types of neuron are found in the hippocampus. The largest and most impressive type is the *pyramidal cell*, so called because of the distinctive shape of its cell body (Figure). Emerging from the top of the pyramid is the *apical dendrite*, a heavily-branched structure with hundreds, if not thousands, of connecting points (*synapses*) with the endings of fibres (*axons*) that have come from other cells inside and outside the hippocampus. In their size, shape, and structure the hippocampal pyramidal cells resemble the pyramidal cells that form the columns of the neocortex (the frontal, parietal, occipital, and temporal lobes). Rather than form columns, however, the hippocampal pyramidal cells exist in a single layer (Figure). Because of their relatively large sizes, these are the cells from which Kandel and Spencer, and later neurophysiologists, would most often obtain their successful recordings.

In the dentate gyrus, the bulge running along the medial border of the hippocampus, the most numerous neurons are granule cells; these also form a layer, one that wraps around the beginning of the hippocampal pyramidal cell layer (Figure).

The granule cell axons (*mossy fibres*) form prominent synapses with the bases of the apical dendrites of the pyramidal cells. The more distant branches of the apical dendrites make synaptic connections with the endings of axons in the *perforant path* from the *entorhinal cortex* and these provide the strongest excitation. In contrast, inhibition of the pyramidal cells is brought about by synapses on the cell bodies that form with the axons of *basket cells*. Complicated though these various arrangements might appear, they are only part of the connections between the hippocampus and cortex, other limbic structures, thalamus, mid-brain, and lower brain stem. An important operating feature of the hippocampus is that the CA4 region, itself influenced by the enveloping dentate gyrus, projects to the *CA3* region, and thence to *CA2* and *CA1* (the *CA* regions differ from each other in their microscopic structure).

There was, however, one important difference. Unlike the motoneurons, the hippocampal cells appeared capable of generating impulses in their dendrites, the branching structures attached to the cell body that received information from other neurons. The dendritic impulses would then generate a flow of electric current through the cell body and its axon attachment, causing the latter to fire a full-sized impulse that could be transmitted to junctions (synapses) with other nerve cells. The results of the experiments, together with detailed analyses, were published in four consecutive papers in the *Journal of Neurophysiology*.[6]

It was an extraordinary achievement by two beginners. Kandel's term at the National Institutes of Mental Health had come to an end, however. While Spencer would turn to the study of spinal reflexes and continue in Bethesda, it was time for Kandel to leave for Boston and the prospect of a career in psychoanalysis.

Notes

1. Kandel's life, including his scientific work, is given in his highly readable autobiography: E.R. Kandel, *In Search of Memory. The Emergence of a New Science of Mind* (New York, NY: WW Norton, 2006). An additional account of his youth and Viennese background is described in the background to his Nobel Prize: http://www.nobelprize.org/prizes/medicine/2000/kandel/biographical accessed 20 April 2022.

2. The merger of the New York neurologists and neurosurgeons to form the Institute had been a move that Penfield had approved of but it had not provided him with the opportunity to pursue and expand either his surgery or his histological research on brain scarring. The inability had proved to be Montreal's gain, Penfield's move to Canada having been followed by the creation of the Montreal Neurological Institute.

3. Harry Grundfest (1904–1983) was a highly original and very productive neuroscientist who spent most of his working career at the Neurology Institute of Columbia University. His work ranged from the properties of cell membranes, cell-to-cell junctions, impulse conduction in nerve fibres (with Herbert Gasser), post-synaptic potentials as generators of EEG waves (with Dominick Purpura), and much else.

4. Dominick Purpura (1927–2019) was an excellent neurophysiologist who became an accomplished administrator. From his early research on interactions between thalamus and cortex, he went on to study brain development and mental retardation. For 22 years he was a highly successful Dean of the Albert Einstein College of Medicine at Yeshiva University (New York).

5. J.D. Green and A.A. Arduini, 'Hippocampal Electrical Activity in Arousal' (1954) 17(6) *Journal of Neurophysiology* 533–7.

6. E.R. Kandel, W.A. Spencer, and F.J. Brinley Jr, 'Electrophysiology of Hippocampal Neurons. I. Sequential Invasion and Synaptic Organization' (1961) 24 *Journal of Neurophysiology* 225–42. E.R. Kandel and W.A. Spencer, 'Electrophysiology of Hippocampal Neurons. II. After-Potentials and Repetitive Firing' (1961) 24 *Journal of Neurophysiology* 243–59. W.A. Spencer and E.R. Kandel, 'Electrophysiology of Hippocampal Neurons. III. Firing Level and Time Constant' (1961) 24 *Journal of Neurophysiology* 260–71. W.A. Spencer and E.R. Kandel, 'Electrophysiology of Hippocampal Neurons. IV. Fast Prepotentials' (1961) 24 *Journal of Neurophysiology* 272–85.

7

A Trip to Australia

(Oslo, Canberra, 1961: Per Andersen, John Eccles)

Kandel and Spencer had not been the first to investigate impulse activity in the mammalian hippocampus. There had been Green and Arduini, already mentioned, while in the Department of Anatomy at University College London, Brian Cragg and Lionel Hamlyn had used fine steel needles to record responses evoked by local stimulation. Indeed, they had succeeded in identifying propagated impulses in the dendrites before the young Americans. Nor had Brenda Milner been the only person at the Montreal Neurological Institute interested in the hippocampus, for Pierre Gloor and his colleagues had been studying its slow-wave electroencephalography (EEG) activity. But there had also been someone else, working mostly on his own in a university outside the mainstream of research.

Per Andersen (Figure 7.1) had been born a year after Eric Kandel, in 1930, and, following the system in the United Kingdom and Europe, had entered medical school straight from high school.[1] At that time Oslo, though the capital of Norway, was still small, with a population of a third of a million. Situated at the mouth of a fjord and with mountains behind it, the attractive city was also a busy seaport. Befitting its status, the city had a university and medical school; there was also the Anatomical Institute that had been founded in the early 1800s. Though he had not been awarded a medical degree, there had been a national hero who had done pioneering histological studies of the brain in the late 1800s. This was the future Arctic explorer Fridtjof Nansen who, having qualified in zoology in Oslo (or Christiana, as it then was), worked for a short time at the university museum in Bergen, Norway's second most populous city. Using silver staining methods, Nansen had shown, independently of Cajal, that neurons were separate from each other rather than being connected by strings of cytoplasm, as was commonly thought. By coincidence, in Vienna, the young Sigmund Freud had been engaged in exactly the same type of work and had reached the same conclusion.

At the time of Per Andersen's entry into Oslo's medical school, the Anatomy Department, with its small staff, was surprisingly strong in neuroanatomy. In Jan Berger Jansen, it had an expert on the structure and connections of the cerebellum. Alf Brodal, at the young age of 38, had published, in English, a very thorough and attractively written *Neurological Anatomy in Relation to Clinical Medicine*.[2] However, it was a third person who would come to influence Per Andersen the most. Birger Kaada had returned to Oslo in 1950 after a two-year period of study in North America. He had divided his time between John Fulton's laboratory at Yale and Herbert Jasper's at the

Aranzio's Seahorse and the Search for Memory and Consciousness. Alan J. McComas, Oxford University Press.
© Oxford University Press 2023. DOI: 10.1093/oso/9780192868244.003.0009

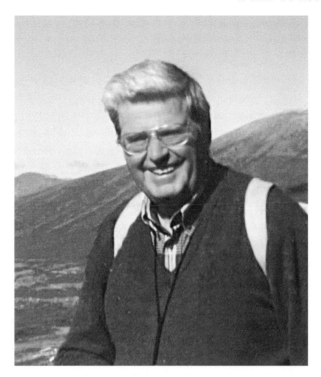

Figure 7.1 Per Andersen hiking in Norway in 1996, long after his period in Canberra. Photograph kindly supplied by Dr Terje Lømo.

Montreal Neurological Institute. The overseas work had mostly been an extension of his doctoral studies and had involved analysing the effects of stimulating different parts of the brain on various body systems. Most of the research had been conducted on animals but in Montreal, Kaada had had the opportunity to work with Jasper on some of Penfield's patients during surgery.[3]

Back in Oslo, Kaada had asked for student help with his neurophysiological studies and Per Andersen had volunteered. Dividing his time between the undergraduate medical programme and laboratory work with Kaada, Andersen had become enthused by the nervous system and especially intrigued by the hippocampus. One of the features of the latter was that, regardless of where the nerve fibres were going, the cell bodies of the pyramidal neurons lay together in a single band.[4] This simple arrangement contrasted with that in the remainder of the cerebral cortex, in which the neuron cell bodies and fibres formed columns that ran perpendicular to the surface of the brain. The difference in anatomy was attributed to the hippocampus having evolved earlier than the rest of the cortex; the two types of cortex were therefore referred to as allocortex and neocortex respectively. As Andersen described it: 'I was captivated by the elegance, the stringency, and the beauty of the hippocampal histology.' It was the elegance of the hippocampus that had attracted Brian Cragg and Lionel Hamlyn at University College London earlier. Only Eric Kandel had chosen it for study because of its importance for memory.

Andersen's enthusiasm was understandable but he was far from being the first medical student to feel the attraction of physiology—the investigation of how the body works. Indeed, many of the leaders in the various branches of physiology, including that of the nervous system, had qualified as physicians or surgeons but not gone on to practise medicine. Andersen became one of them, undertaking an electrophysiological study of the hippocampus for a doctorate. It was not an easy task, for although there were skilled neuroanatomists in Oslo to whom he could turn to for advice, the only neurophysiologist was Kaada—himself a relative newcomer to the discipline and one not well versed in techniques for recording from neurons singly or in groups. Andersen's experiments were physically and mentally exhausting. The electrical activity of the hippocampal neurons was photographed on film that had to be developed before being analysed by eye and ruler, frame by frame, sequence by sequence. And then there was the brain histology that had to be done, laborious but essential if one was to know exactly where the stimulating and recording electrodes had been placed during the experiment.

Though his thesis would be approved by the examiners, Andersen was only too aware of his limitations as an experimental neurophysiologist. He was therefore delighted when it became possible for him to obtain further experience in what was regarded as the most prominent central nervous system laboratory at that time. And so, in 1961, the Andersen family—neurophysiologist husband with wife and three children—duly caught the plane for the first stage of their long journey. To Australia and John Eccles (Figure 7.2).

To someone meeting him for the first time, Eccles could be intimidating. He was tall and well-built, balding, taken to wearing glasses with thick frames, and possessed of a penetrating voice with a strong Australian accent. He had been born in Australia but had gone to the United Kingdom as a newly qualified medical doctor and Rhodes Scholar to study the nervous system under Sir Charles Sherrington at Oxford University.[5] Because of Sherrington's reputation as the leading neurophysiologist of his day, it was a journey that others had taken. Wilder Penfield had been one of them, going as a student before and then immediately following the First World War. John Fulton, the head of the primate laboratory at Yale and the author of the well-received *Physiology of the Nervous System*,[6] had been another Rhodes Scholar.

At Oxford Eccles had worked with Sherrington in the last phase of that great man's experimental career. It was Eccles who had introduced electrical recordings in muscles to complement the measurements of tension. Together, the two had discovered the importance of inhibition in modifying spinal reflexes, had established the presence of an excitatory zone surrounding discharging neurons in the spinal cord, and had estimated the numbers of motor nerve cells (motoneurons) supplying individual muscles. Eccles had then gone on to study how excitation and inhibition was passed across the small gaps (synapses) separating one neuron from another. To Eccles, it seemed most likely that the transmission was electrical, the ionic current of the impulses in the terminals of an axon flowing through the membrane of the receiving neuron and exciting it directly. In this matter, however, he was strongly opposed by Sir Henry Dale and

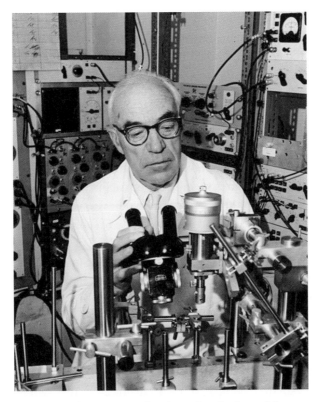

Figure 7.2 Sir John Eccles. This portrait of Eccles in his Canberra laboratory was taken in 1963 at the time of his Nobel Prize. The many electronic instruments in the background (oscilloscopes, amplifiers, timers, stimulators, etc.) are typical of a neurophysiological laboratory prior to the advent of laptop computers. Immediately in front of Eccles is a dissecting microscope, to the immediate right of which is the micrometer drive used to slowly advance a recording microelectrode into the brain or spinal cord. Photograph courtesy of the John Curtin School of Medical Research, Australian National University (Wikimedia Commons file: Eccles.lab.jpg; Creative Commons Attribution 3.0 Unported license).

others who insisted that there must be a chemical mediator involved—that the axon terminal would release molecules that would then act on the membrane of the recipient neuron and change its polarization. It was the 'soup' versus 'sparks' battle[7] that Eccles was thought to have lost, until electrical transmission was shown to be a feature of the especially narrow ('gap') junctions between certain types of cells. That finding was to come much later, however.

Prior to the start of the Second World War Eccles had left his much-loved Oxford for Australia, setting up a neurophysiology research laboratory in one of the Sydney hospitals. Then, in 1944, came an appointment as Professor and Head of The Physiology Department at the University of Otago in New Zealand. Though it was a small and understaffed department that required much teaching on his part, Eccles nevertheless brought off a major scientific coup in making the first systematic study of the membrane properties of a mammalian neuron. To do this, he had employed very fine fluid-filled capillary glass microelectrodes inserted into motoneurons of the cat spinal cord. At Eccles' request, the stimulating and recording system had been designed by a talented university colleague, John Coombs, and was better than any equipment available elsewhere. The new work, conducted on motoneurons, was a logical extension of the voltage-clamp experiments on the giant axon of the squid that had been carried out by Alan Hodgkin, Andrew Huxley, and Bernhard Katz at the Plymouth Marine Biological Laboratory in the United Kingdom immediately after the Second World War. Eccles had been able to extend the work of the Cambridge neurophysiologists, however, by exploring the changes in membrane conductance (ionic permeability) following excitatory and inhibitory messages from other nerve cells.[8]

Following this success Eccles had been invited to become Professor of Physiology at the newly created Australian National University (ANU) in Canberra—then a research university for postgraduates and faculty. Initially working in huts on the campus, Eccles began to attract excellent visiting fellows from overseas, some of them already well established in their own countries and others, like Per Andersen, still in the early stages of their careers.

At the time that Andersen and his family arrived, in 1961, Canberra, like the new national university, was still very much a work in progress. Though the land had been designated as the site of the nation's capital 50 years earlier, the population was less than 60,000, small in comparison with major cities like Sydney or Melbourne. Canberra had good weather, however, and the new city was acquiring charm. With low mountains on either side, a future artificial lake at its centre, and radiating streets lined with fruit trees, the city provided an attractive setting for the new government buildings and the university. Being small, it was a city that could be walked, and in the evenings the visiting academics could meet for dinner and discussion in University House.

Prior to Andersen's arrival, Eccles had brought off a major scientific coup, one that had not been anticipated and was yet another example of neurophysiological serendipity. The crucial observations had been made on the very day that Arthur Buller, a young and relatively untrained physiologist from London, had begun his year of study in Canberra. Eccles, with the invaluable help of his daughter, Rose, had been crossing over the nerves supplying two contrasting leg muscles in the cat. He had anticipated that, after the cut nerve fibres had regenerated, the respective motoneurons in the spinal cord would be altered, having been receiving novel sensory information from 'foreign' muscles. Like all Eccles' experiments this had been a long one and the results had proved disappointing—the electrical properties of the motoneurons were unchanged. By now it was early morning on the following day but, before abandoning the experiment, Eccles had checked to make sure that the divided nerve fibres had managed to grow back. To his surprise, not only had the nerve fibres successfully innervated their new targets but they had transformed the muscles. A muscle that normally had a fast twitch now had a slow one and, conversely, the previously slow-twitch muscle has now become 'fast-twitch'. Not only did the motoneurons excite the muscles and cause them to contract but, through this newly discovered 'trophic' effect, they appeared to control protein synthesis inside the muscle fibres. Within a few hours of his arrival, Arthur Buller had been witness to an important discovery, one that he would successfully pursue for the remainder of his career.[9]

Buller had already left when Andersen had arrived in Canberra, but present on the ANU campus was another visiting neurophysiologist, one with whom Andersen would work closely in some of the experiments. Thomas Sears, already recognized for his research on the peripheral nervous system, had taken leave from the National Hospital for Nervous Diseases in London. First, however, Andersen would work with Eccles and others on a special type of inhibition (presynaptic) that could be exerted on the endings of sensory fibres in the spinal cord following stimulation of the cortex.[10] Then, still exploring sensory pathways, came a study of neurons in the thalamus.[11] Regardless of site, the various investigations followed a formula—first the recording microelectrode would map the flow of synaptic current at different points in the tissue, then an electrode would penetrate the cell body of a neuron and the changes in the electrical polarization of the membrane would be recorded following different types of stimulation. In this way it was possible to show not only whether a neuron was being excited or inhibited by a stimulus but whether the active synapses were situated on the cell body or on the dendrites of a neuron. It was a formula that always worked and would yield results for more than one publication.

The experiments were physically and mentally demanding. The dissections of the nerves or the brain structures began soon after 8:00 a.m. and the recordings often continued into the early hours of the following morning. Eccles himself was often present; he was an expert dissector of the peripheral nerves and of the nerve roots entering the spinal cord. Later, as the experiment progressed, he would sit in front of the oscilloscope, controlling the camera and giving instructions. Whether performing the exhausting experiments by day or discussing the ongoing results with Eccles late at night, Per Andersen found the work exciting. 'From the first to the last day, it was a stay coloured by excitement, intense learning, new discoveries, friendship, and a deep satisfaction with the field as such.'

Knowing Andersen's interest in the hippocampus, Eccles one day suggested that they investigate it. It was probably as a kindness to Andersen that the proposal was made because Eccles was aware of the thorough examination of the hippocampus that had already been made by Eric Kandel and Alden Spencer. Once more the Canberra formula worked, however—Andersen and Eccles were able to show that the pyramidal cells in the hippocampus were inhibited by another type of neuron, the basket cell.[12,13] Further, the inhibitory synapses were clustered around the cell body of the pyramidal cell rather than being on the dendrites. The investigators showed that every time a pyramidal cell fired an impulse, a small branch of its axon would excite a basket cell and the latter would then inhibit the pyramidal cell and its neighbours—an example of negative feedback in the nervous system. With his knowledge of neuroanatomy, Andersen had been able to show Eccles pictures of basket cells embracing the cell bodies of the pyramidal neurons. The pen-and-ink sketches had been made by the great histologist, Santiago Ramon y Cajal, half a century earlier.

Andersen had gone on to investigate the cerebellum with Eccles, exploring the possibility that the cerebellar basket cells were also inhibitory, as they were found to be. The demonstration was another major success; nevertheless, the highlight of Andersen's stay in Canberra had been the discoveries in the hippocampus. Though there had been no mention of the role of the hippocampus in memory in their publications, it was not surprising. The microelectrode investigation, thorough as it was, had not offered any clue as to what made the hippocampus suited for its physiological role. That clue would have to wait for one of Andersen's young colleagues in Oslo to find it.

Notes

1. P. Andersen, *History of Neuroscience in Autobiography*, L.R. Squire (ed.) (Amsterdam: Elsevier, 2004) 4: 2–39.
2. A. Brodal, *Neurological Anatomy in Relation to Clinical Medicine* (Oxford: Clarendon Press, 1948).
3. Having become the first true neurophysiologist in Oslo, Kaada's research would later switch from animals to humans and would include the effect of peripheral nerve stimulation on tissue blood flow and also the mechanism of the sudden infant death syndrome.
4. See Figure in Box 6.1.
5. D.R. Curtis and P. Andersen, 'Sir John Carew Eccles, A.C. 27 January 1903–2 May 1997' (2001) 47 *Biographical Memoirs of Fellows of the Royal Society* 159–87 (doi.org/10.1098/rsbm.2001.0010).
6. J.F. Fulton, *Physiology of the Nervous System* (New York, NY: Oxford University Press, 1938).
7. For a full account of the controversy, see: E. Valenstein, *The War of the Soups and the Sparks: The Discovery of Neurotransmitters and the Dispute over How Nerves Communicate* (New York, NY: Columbia University Press, 2005). Also: J.A. Marcum, '"Soup" vs "Sparks": Alexander Forbes and the Synaptic Transmission Controversy' (2006) 63 *Annals of Science* 139–56.
8. L.G. Brock, J.S. Coombs, and J.C. Eccles, 'The Recording of Potentials from Motoneurones with an Intracellular Electrode' (1952) 117 *Journal of Physiology* 431–60. For a summary of the motoneurone studies, see: J.C. Eccles, *The Physiology of Nerve Cells* (London: Oxford University Press, 1957).
9. In a letter to the author (7 January 1999) Arthur Buller wrote the following about John ('Jack') Eccles remarks during the experiment, following his stimulation of the reinnervated cat muscle: 'Something odd here, that's not a slow twitch.' Then, after searching the laboratory for a strain gauge, and confirming his naked-eye impression: 'There's a good story here, Arthur, we'll concentrate on the muscles of these operated cats.' An account of the work appeared in two papers: A.J. Buller, J.C. Eccles, and R.M. Eccles, 'Differentiation of Fast and Slow Muscles in the Cat Hindlimb' (1960) 150 *Journal of Physiology* 399–416. A.J. Buller, J.C. Eccles, and R.M. Eccles, 'Interactions between Motoneurones and Muscles in Respect of the Characteristic Speeds of Their Responses' (1960) 150 *Journal of Physiology* 417–39.
10. P. Andersen, J.C. Eccles, and R.F. Schmidt, 'Presynaptic Inhibitory Actions: Presynaptic Inhibition in the Cuneate Nucleus' (1962) 194 *Nature* 741–3.

11. P. Andersen, C.M. Brooks, J.C. Eccles, and T.A. Sears, 'The Ventro-Basal Nucleus of the Thalamus: Potential Fields, Synaptic Transmission and Excitability of Both Presynaptic and Postsynaptic Components' (1964) 174(3) *Journal of Physiology* 348–69 (doi:10.1113/jphysiol.1964.sp007492).

12. P. Andersen, J.C. Eccles, and Y. Løyning, 'Hippocampus of the Brain: Recurrent Inhibition in the Hippocampus with Identification of the Inhibitory Cell and its Synapses' (1963) 198 *Nature* 540–2.

13. See Box figure (*right*) for relationship between basket and pyramidal cells.

8

Taking Stock

(Montreal, 1960: Brenda Milner; New Haven, John Fulton)

By 1960 Milners were well settled, both in their professional work and in their Westmount apartment, but major changes were taking place around them. The new decade would witness the election of a progressive provincial government determined to alter the social and political fabric of Quebec. The influence of the Catholic Church, for so long a strength and yet a restrictive force, would be removed. Schools, universities, and hospitals that had been founded and operated by the Church would become the responsibility of government. The 'quiet revolution' was under way and the new secular society had less use for religion. There would be fewer church bells ringing out over the villages and fields along the banks of the St Lawrence, and many church doors, which had previously been open for morning Mass every day of the week, would close forever. Quebec—the 'New France' of its original settlers—had begun to lose its soul.

There were changes elsewhere, including those at the Montreal Neurological Institute. Penfield's chosen successor as director had been one of his fellow neurosurgeons. It would have pleased Penfield that Theodore Rasmussen would continue the brain stimulation studies for which the Institute had become so well known. For Herbert Jasper, however, Penfield's retirement from active research in the operating theatre was a loss. The two men had been together for almost a quarter of a century and, among other achievements, had written a major text on epilepsy.[1] They had enjoyed a friendship that had included dinghy sailing on Lake Memphremagog in the eastern townships where both had cottages within easy reach of Montreal. In a few years Jasper would leave the Neurological Institute to join the francophone Université de Montréal as Professor of Physiology.

There had been changes in the McGill Psychology Department as well. Following his discovery of a pleasure centre in the rat brain, James Olds had spent two years in Los Angeles, working in Horace Magoun's Brain Research Institute. After that, he had gone to the University of Michigan as an assistant professor. Olds' erstwhile partner in the study at McGill, Peter Milner, had continued his interest in the reward system, especially in how it would normally be activated by an animal or human being. Mindful of Hebb's proposal of neural assemblies, he was also applying engineering principles in an attempt to understand how groups of neurons might become established and interact. In *The Organization of Behaviour*, Hebb had not discussed the possible role of inhibition in constraining the sizes of the neural assemblies and this, to Peter, was an

Aranzio's Seahorse and the Search for Memory and Consciousness. Alan J. McComas, Oxford University Press.
© Oxford University Press 2023. DOI: 10.1093/oso/9780192868244.003.0010

important oversight. His theoretical work was one of the first forays into artificial intelligence and would attract the attention of IBM and then the Rand Corporation.

Meanwhile, Hebb, ever loyal to his students, not only continued to lecture but was now writing a textbook for them. The *Textbook of Psychology*[2] was written in simple, direct language that undergraduates could readily absorb. Well illustrated—literally from cover to cover—the book included his tentative diagrams as to how assemblies of neurons might interact. Like *The Organization of Behaviour*, the new book would become a best-seller and run to several editions.

Mortimer Mishkin had been another to leave. Though his PhD was a McGill degree, the experimental work had been carried out on primates in John Fulton's laboratory at Yale. He had then spent five years at the Institute of Living in Hartford, Connecticut, where the enterprising director, Dr Burlingame, had established not only a neurosurgical operating theatre for Dr William Scoville to perform lobotomies but an animal research laboratory as well. It was in the latter that Mishkin had been able to continue his primate work. Later he would move to the National Institute of Mental Health where he would stay for the remainder of his long and distinguished career.

There had been a death, too, though not at the Montreal Neurological Institute. It had been a sad ending for a life that had achieved so much and yet promised more. For many years John Fulton had been the golden 'boy' of neurophysiology (Figure 8.1). As a young man he had, like Penfield and Eccles, been a Rhodes Scholar at Oxford.[3] In studying with Sherrington, Fulton had not only acquired much neuroscientific knowledge and experimental proficiency but had absorbed the older man's love of

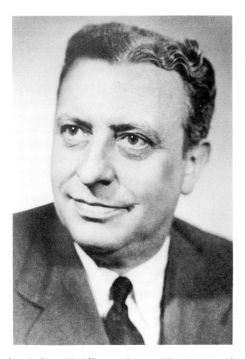

Figure 8.1 John Farquhar Fulton. (Wellcome Image M001079.jpg.)

medical history. On returning to the United States he had trained in neurosurgery under Harvey Cushing, only to leave that discipline for a career in neurophysiology. So great was Fulton's reputation and promise that, at the early age of 30, he had been appointed to a Chair of Physiology at Yale and it was there that he had established the first primate laboratory in the United States. His own work, together with the excellent laboratory facilities, had attracted other neurophysiologists, especially those interested in the functions of the different cortical areas. It was Fulton who had discovered that frontal lobectomy had a calming effect in two aggressive chimpanzees—the observation that would lead to frontal lobotomies being performed on thousands of psychiatric patients across the world.

In addition to his other talents Fulton had been an excellent writer, bringing out the first edition of *The Physiology of the Nervous System* in 1938 and a biography of Harvey Cushing in 1947. He had founded the *Journal of Neurophysiology*, had promoted historical studies in medicine and science, and had been the recipient of no fewer than 35 honorary degrees. All this had been achieved despite an ever-increasing dependence on alcohol, a fact that had become all too obvious to his friends and colleagues. John Fulton had died at the age of 60.

On a happier note, 1963 would see the award of a Nobel Prize to Australia. Per Andersen had still been in Canberra when the news had come of John Eccles' success and it was he who had helped arrange an impromptu celebration in the laboratory. Eccles had shared the Prize with Alan Hodgkin and Andrew Huxley, the Cambridge men now famous for their elegant mathematical descriptions of the membrane conductances responsible for the resting membrane potentials and action potentials (impulses) of nerve fibres.

The new decade would see another major discovery in the understanding of memory mechanisms and once again it would be Brenda Milner who would be responsible. Now firmly established in her office at the Montreal Neurological Institute, she had continued to think about Henry Molaison, the young man whose severe memory loss had been a consequence of the bilateral medial temporal lobectomy performed by Dr William Scoville. That intervention had left him unable to recall events in the years leading up to his surgery, nor could he retain new information for longer than 30 seconds or so—unless he could repeat the key words over and over again in his mind. Once distracted, however, the new information would be gone.

Despite Henry's severe handicap, Brenda had a suspicion that he might, with practice, do better. It was certainly worth making another trip to Hartford, Connecticut, to find out.

As usual Henry was pleasant and cooperative although, of course, he had no recollection of having seen Brenda before. On this occasion Brenda had brought two learning tests with her from Montreal. One of these was a fairly complex maze involving 28 decisions that Henry proved incapable of learning—by the time he had reached the end of the maze with the stylus, he had forgotten how he had started off.

The second test demanded good hand–eye coordination. Henry had been presented with the print of two five-pointed stars, one inside the other. He was then required to trace his way around the figure, keeping his pencil point within the narrow space separating the two stars. The task was made difficult in that he could only observe his hand and the paper in a mirror; the latter had the effect of reversing the apparent direction of his fore and aft movements (Figure 8.2).

Henry was presented with this task 30 times over the course of Brenda's 3-day visit and, to Brenda's astonishment, showed that he was perfectly capable of learning how to accomplish it—yet without having any memory of the previous trials. Though the result has been regarded as the first clear demonstration that there was more than one type of memory, there had been a strong hint of the latter previously. In their classic 1957 paper, Scoville and Milner had stated that, regardless of any effect on memory, the mesial temporal lobectomies performed on their ten patients had '*left technical skills intact*'. Although Henry had lost his memory for facts and events ('declarative' memory), he still knew how to do things and could learn new motor tasks ('procedural' memory). Further, this second type of memory appeared not to involve the hippocampus.

Brenda's discovery was an important one for psychology as well as for neuroscience. And yet, should it have been such a surprise? A patient with a memory loss such as Henry's may still be able to walk, rise from a chair, dress, use a knife and fork, and—if musical—play an instrument. And talk. All of these are skills requiring sensory–motor coordination that have had to be learned and yet can survive a loss of declarative memory. And, of course, the various everyday objects have to have been remembered.

In contrast to the psychologists, the neurophysiologists seemed to have lost interest in the hippocampus, at least for the time being. The work of Eccles and Andersen had revealed the pattern of connections within the structure—the input–output

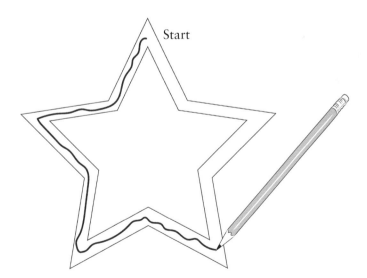

Figure 8.2 Mirror drawing test. The subject is asked to trace a star, keeping the pencil point within the two printed outlines. The task is made difficult since the subject only sees the drawing in a mirror and forward and backward movements of the pencil appear reversed.

relationships—as well as the properties of the hippocampal neurons themselves. That there were few crumbs left for other like-minded investigators was not surprising. Whenever Eccles had moved into a new field, the studies had been conspicuously thorough. This had happened with the reflex connectivity of spinal motoneurons, his original interest, and later with the main sensory pathway from the skin (the dorsal column–medial lemniscal system), presynaptic inhibition, the cerebellum, the thalamus, and, finally, the hippocampus. The Canberra formula had worked every time. But there was another reason for attention being directed away from the hippocampus.

Very exciting discoveries were now being made in the visual cortex and, for many neurophysiologists, this was a more promising part of the brain to study anyway. Not only did the visual cortex have a highly developed structure, one that reflected its later evolution, but it was part of a more discriminating sensory system—one that could detect small changes in size, colour, and movement within the visual field. In contrast, the only sense that might involve the hippocampus was olfaction and, in Brodal's expert opinion,[4] even that was doubtful. Indeed, in John Fulton's *Physiology of Nerve Cells*, the hippocampus had been fleetingly identified as part of the rhinencephalon ('nose-brain') and then dismissed from further comment.

The new work on the visual cortex was a different matter altogether. And, once again, there was a connection to Montreal and its Neurological Institute.

Notes

1. W. Penfield and H. Jasper, *Epilepsy and the Functional Anatomy of the Human Brain* (Boston, MA: Little Brown, 1954).
2. D.O. Hebb, *A Textbook of Psychology* (Philadelphia, PA: Saunders, 1958).
3. G. Shepherd and C. Tsay, 'Triumph and tragedy: the life of John Farquhar Fulton' <http://www.library.medicine.yale.edu/historical/fulton> accessed 20 April 2021.
4. A. Brodal, 'The Hippocampus and the Sense of Smell' (1947) 70 *Brain* 179–222.

9

Visual Focus

(Cambridge, Massachusetts, 1962: Stephen Kuffler, David Hubel, Torsten Wiesel)

David Hubel had been born to American parents in Windsor, Ontario, in 1926. Following the family's move to Montreal, he had attended McGill University, first to study mathematics and physics and then medicine.[1] It was as a medical student that he had encountered Herbert Jasper who, in addition to carrying out an intensive research programme in animals and assisting Penfield in the latter's intra-operative studies, was in charge of the clinical neurophysiology laboratory at the Montreal Neurological Institute. The encounter was to the benefit of both. Hubel became interested in neurophysiology while Jasper, who was studying for a medical degree also—despite his prominence as a neuroscientist—was able to read the lecture notes that Hubel had taken. After qualifying in medicine Hubel had moved to the United States, becoming a resident in neurology at Johns Hopkins Hospital in Baltimore. After military service he had returned to Johns Hopkins, this time to carry out research on vision under Stephen Kuffler.

Though born in Hungary and educated in Austria, Stephen Kuffler (Figure 9.1) had learned to do research in Australia while working as an assistant to John Eccles.[2] This was at the time in the Second World War when Eccles had set up a neurophysiology unit in a Sydney hospital and had taken on Bernard Katz as a junior colleague. Despite a previous dislike of physiology, Kuffler not only absorbed all that Eccles and Katz had been prepared to impart but taught himself to make exquisite dissections of nerve and muscle fibres. Having proven himself imaginative and insightful as a neuroscientist, Kuffler had emigrated to the United States after the war, ending up in Baltimore. It was there, in the basement of the ophthalmology institute at Johns Hopkins, that he had chosen to investigate the visual system. Recording first from cells in the mammalian retina and then in the lateral geniculate body—the next stage in the visual pathway—Kuffler had investigated the kinds of stimuli that would cause the neurons to fire impulses or, alternatively, to stop firing. He had found that some cells responded to white light while others were more demanding, responding to a limited range of wavelengths; that is, to wavelengths evocative of colours. The responses could be excitation or inhibition, depending on exactly where the stimulus—a spot of light—was shining on the retina. Further the cells had concentric receptive fields in the retina, such that a spot falling on the inner field could make a cell fire, whereas on the outer field it stopped any spontaneous discharge (i.e. caused inhibition). In other neurons it could be the reverse

Aranzio's Seahorse and the Search for Memory and Consciousness. Alan J. McComas, Oxford University Press.
© Oxford University Press 2023. DOI: 10.1093/oso/9780192868244.003.0011

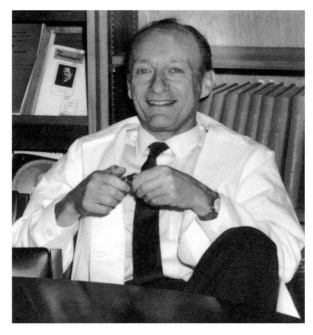

Figure 9.1 Stephen Kuffler, holding forth in the Neurobiology Department at Harvard. Photograph courtesy of Dr UJ MacMahon.

arrangement, such that a central inhibitory zone was surrounded by an excitatory one. And one wavelength could inhibit another (Figure 9.2).

But what might be happening at the next stage in the visual pathway, the cortical receiving area at the back of the brain? In attempting to answer this question Hubel had a partner who had arrived in Baltimore from Sweden three years earlier. Born in Uppsala, Torsten Wiesel had graduated in medicine at the famous Karolinska Institute

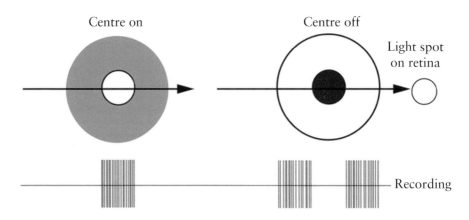

Figure 9.2 Concentric mammalian retinal receptive fields, as determined by Kuffler.

in Stockholm. After a year teaching physiology he had, like Hubel later, decided to join Kuffler and do research.[3]

The two investigators decided to investigate the problem of 'higher' visual processing in the cat, using fine-tipped tungsten wire electrodes of Hubel's design to record from single neurons in the visual cortex. Hardly had they begun, however, than they were obliged to stop and move their equipment to a new location. Kuffler's brilliance had been noted elsewhere and had resulted in an invitation for him to set up a neurobiology division with the Pharmacology Department at Harvard University. Kuffler had taken Hubel and Wiesel with him to Boston.

Hubel and Wiesel resumed their experiments in the new surroundings. The studies entailed the anaesthetized animals facing a curved screen on to which spots of light were projected (Figure 9.3). It was the same type of procedure that had given Kuffler success in his recordings from the retina and the lateral geniculate body. To Hubel and Wiesel's consternation, however, most of the neurons encountered by the recording electrode failed to respond to the spot stimuli. And then, just as it had for James Olds and Peter Milner in the rat, luck intervened. As Hubel and Wiesel inserted a fresh slide into the projector, a cortical neuron fired. Curious, the two investigators puzzled over what had happened and eventually found the reason—the cell had responded to the moving edge of the slide as it had fallen into position. As they carried on with their experiment, it became clear that, rather than respond to spots of light, the cortical cells were only excited by linear stimuli; that is, by edges, illuminated slits or dark bars falling on the retina. Hubel and Wiesel reasoned that each linear 'field' had been pro-duced by a small number of incoming nerve fibres from the lateral geniculate body

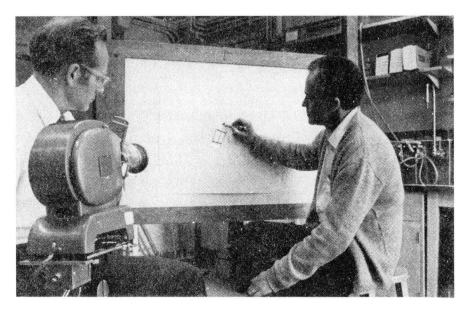

Figure 9.3 David Hubel and Torsten Wiesel mapping out retinal receptive fields in the visual cortex. Photograph courtesy of the late Dr Hubel.

making synaptic connections with a single cortical neuron ('simple' neuron). Several simple neurons could then project to a higher-order neuron ('complex' neuron) that responded to linear stimuli that, rather than being stationary, were moving across the retina (Figure 9.4).

The new findings were the first evidence of sensory information undergoing a major transformation as it was passed from one group of cells to the next. It was a major breakthrough and, through work in a number of other laboratories, would eventually give rise to the concept of parallel processing in the visual cortex. Thus, while one group of neurons could be recognizing linear features in the visual field, as Hubel and Wiesel had demonstrated, another group would be responding to certain wavelengths ('colour-sensitive neurons') and yet another group would be detecting movement. Each type of function would be carried out in a special part of the visual cortex and the results of the different types of analysis would be combined to produce the conscious perception of what had been viewed.

Recognizing that linear features were detected in the visual field was but one of Hubel and Wiesel's accomplishments.[4] They were able to show how information from the two eyes was arranged in the visual cortex of each hemisphere. They also demonstrated the susceptibility of the developing cortex to the visual environment of the animal. Finally, they had evidence that the immediate synaptic connections in the

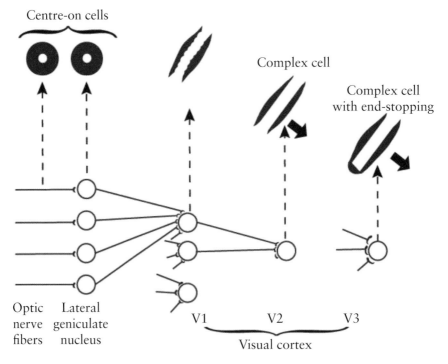

Figure 9.4 Visual cell hierarchy in the lateral geniculate nucleus and visual cortex. The concentric retinal receptive fields are transformed into linear fields (bars, slits, edges) as information flows through the visual cortex.

visual cortex occurred between cells in columns perpendicular to the surface. In fact, the columnar organization had been recognized by Lorente de Nó in his histological study of the cortex and had been described by him in his two invited chapters of John Fulton's *Physiology of the Nervous System* (published in 1938). It had also been found by Vernon Mountcastle at Johns Hopkins Hospital, in his exhaustive study of the somatosensory (body surface) cortex.[5] Apart from the other new findings, the discovery of a columnar organization also helped to make the visual cortex more interesting to neurophysiologists than the hippocampus, in which all the neuron cell bodies were packed into a single layer.

David Hubel would continue to work on the visual system, summarizing his work and that of others in a beautifully written and illustrated monograph.[6] It was largely the work that he and Torsten Wiesel had done that would persuade Francis Crick to choose the visual system for his speculations concerning the neural circuitry responsible for consciousness. Crick's entry into neuroscience was yet to come, however.

Meanwhile, as already noted, research on the hippocampus, at least neurophysiological research, had dwindled. Those who had worked on it previously seemed to have lost interest.

Notes

1. D.H. Hubel, *The History of Neuroscience in Autobiography*, L.R. Squire (ed.) (Washington D.C.: Society for Neuroscience,1998) 1: 294–317.
2. There are several biographies of Kuffler of which the most thorough was written by his friend and collaborator in Australia during the Second World War, Bernard Katz: Sir B. Katz and S.W. Kuffler, '24 August 1913–11 October 1980' (1982) 28 *Biographical Memoirs of Fellows of the Royal Society* 225–9. Kuffler had great scientific curiosity and imagination as well as a gift for exploiting novel biological preparations suited to the question of the moment. A kind and humorous person, Kuffler was liked by everyone who knew him.
3. At the time of writing Torsten Wiesel is still active at the age of 97. After a period as Head of the Neurobiology Department at Harvard, he transferred to the Rockefeller University in New York, serving as its President 1991–1998. He then became President of the International Brain Research Organization (IBRO) until 2004. Wiesel has received numerous awards and other honours, and served on many international committees. In addition to his scientific work he has been active in human rights issues and, on occasion, a public critic of US government.
4. The first publication of Hubel and Wiesel's novel findings was: D.H. Hubel and T.N. Wiesel, 'Receptive Fields of Single Neurones in the Cat's Striate Cortex' (1959) 148 *Journal of Physiology* 574–91. This was followed by a more extensive paper, with many additional findings, three years later: D.H. Hubel and T.N. Wiesel, 'Receptive Fields, Binocular Interaction and Functional Architecture in the Cat's Visual Cortex' (1962) 160 *Journal of Physiology* 106–54. Hubel continued to work on the visual system at Harvard until his death at the age of eighty-seven in 2013. The summation of his work with Wiesel and later collaborators was the very readable and well-illustrated monograph: D.H. Hubel, *Eye, Brain and Vision*, Scientific American Library, No 22 (New York, NY: WH Freeman, 1995). Although the linear detection, parallel processing scheme of vision is now accepted, it is quite possibly incorrect, a clue coming from the flickering zigzags ('fortification spectra') that may enter the visual fields of migraine patients before the arrival of headache (see

Chapter 7 in A.J. McComas, *Sherrington's Loom. An Introduction to the Science of Consciousness* (New York, NY: Oxford University Press, 2019).

5. V.B. Mountcastle, 'Modality and Topographic Properties of Single Neurons of Cat's Somatic Sensory Cortex' (1957) 20(4) *Journal of Neurophysiology* 408–34.

6. Hubel, *Eye, Brain and Vision*, see note 4.

10

Enter the Giant Sea Slug

(Paris, 1962: Eric Kandel, Ladislav Tauc)

Even before Hubel and Wiesel's vision studies, Eric Kandel had been prepared to leave the hippocampus. Though he and Alden Spencer had completed an exhaustive microelectrode investigation of the pyramidal neurons in the hippocampus, the study had not brought him any closer to understanding how the hippocampus stored memories. Rather than apply his newfound expertise with microelectrode recordings to examine other parts of the mammalian brain, as Eccles was doing, Kandel remained committed to the study of memory. He would find the most suitable preparations and learn whatever techniques were necessary; it would prove a long but fascinating path, one that would end many years later in molecular biology and protein chemistry.

In deciding to work on a simpler preparation than the cat brain, Kandel had been influenced by the philosophy of some very successful scientists. Edgar (Lord) Adrian, for instance, had studied vision in eels and smell in hedgehogs, and had used a water beetle to demonstrate the presence of rhythmic electrical activity surprisingly similar to the human electroencephalography (EEG). Also at Cambridge, Alan Hodgkin and Andrew Huxley had chosen the giant axon of the squid for their analysis of the membrane permeabilities and ionic currents responsible for the resting and action potentials of nerve fibres. Nearer home, Kandel had come across Stephen Kuffler's work on the crayfish during the time that he, Kandel, was doing a six-month neurophysiology elective as a medical student in Grundfest's laboratory. In his publications Kuffler had shown that the crayfish had neurons sufficiently large for their dendrites to be visualized under the microscope and studied in detail. Later, while working in Wade Marshall's laboratory at the National Institutes of Health (NIH), Kandel had heard two lectures on the neurophysiology of the giant sea slug, *Aplysia*. Both speakers had been from France; Angelique Arvanitaki-Chalazonitis was the more senior and was based in Marseilles, while Ladislav Tauc, a Czech, was working in Paris at the Institut Marey. Both neurophysiologists had stressed the advantages of using a preparation with a simple nervous system containing relatively large neurons. As Kandel would discover for himself, some of the nerve cell bodies in the ganglia (nerve cell clusters) were 1 millimetre across and could be recognized with the naked eye.

Though it had a simple nervous system, Kandel thought that *Aplysia* might still exhibit basic learning and that this might be explored by microelectrode recordings from the large neurons. After discussion with his wife, Kandel and his family left the United States and took up residence in Paris. He would work with Tauc at the Institut Marey.

Aranzio's Seahorse and the Search for Memory and Consciousness. Alan J. McComas, Oxford University Press.
© Oxford University Press 2023. DOI: 10.1093/oso/9780192868244.003.0012

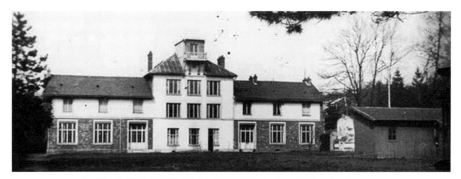

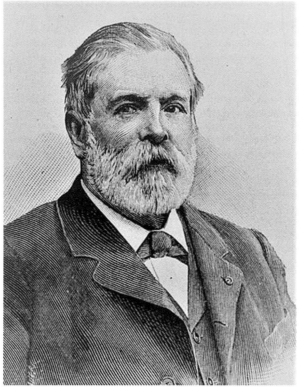

Figure 10.1 *Upper.* The Institut Marey. Photograph kindly supplied by Dr Jean-Gaël Barbara. *Lower.* Étienne-Jules Marey. Gravure photograph by Nadar (Creative Commons CC0 1.0. Universal public domain dedication).

Formerly the Station Physiologique, the Institut Marey had an interesting history. Situated in the Bois de Boulonge next to the Roland Garros tennis stadium, it was a large three-storey villa set in spacious grounds (Figure 10.1, *Upper*). It had been built at the end of the 19th century at the instigation of a commission for standardization of methods and devices used in physiology. Paris was already the home of the standard metre and the standard kilogram, and this may have influenced its choice for an institute dealing with physiological measurement as well. Further, in Etienne-Jules Marey (Figure 10.1, *Lower*), the first director of the Station Physiologique, there was an internationally renowned physiologist who had a number of inventions to his name, including a camera-gun that enabled rapid movements to be photographed.

After completing an extraordinary number of fundamental studies of movement in humans, horses, birds and even insects, Marey had died in 1904. However, the building and its grounds, which now included Marey's grave, continued to be looked after by Marey's last assistant, Lucien Bull. During the difficult days of the Second World War it had become the scientific refuge of a distinguished French physiologist, Alfred Fessard, and his research assistant and future wife, Denise Albe (later Albe-Fessard; Figure 10.2).[1] Chronically underfunded both then and in the post-war years, the two had not only managed to keep the Institut viable but to create a neurophysiological centre of excellence, attracting visiting scientists from around the world as well as young neurophysiologists from their own country. While Denise Albe-Fessard had explored function with microelectrodes in the deep brain nuclei and motor cortex of the cat, her husband was more eclectic, his interests ranging from the EEG and consciousness to muscle fatigue and to such exotic creatures as electric fish and *Aplysia*. This last preparation, a giant sea slug, had been in Alfred Fessard's laboratory when the visiting Czech neuroscientist, Ladislav Tauc, had first encountered it and then used it for his own electrophysiological studies.[2]

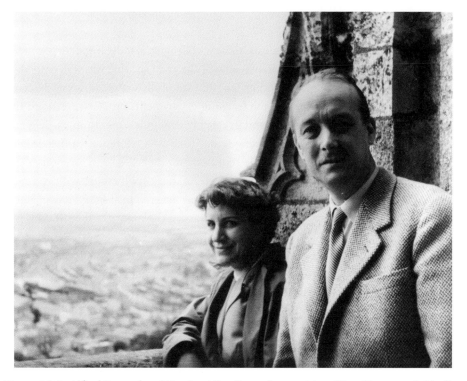

Figure 10.2 Alfred Fessard and Denise Albe-Fessard on a visit to Pisa. Photograph kindly provided by Dr Jean-Gaël Barbara.

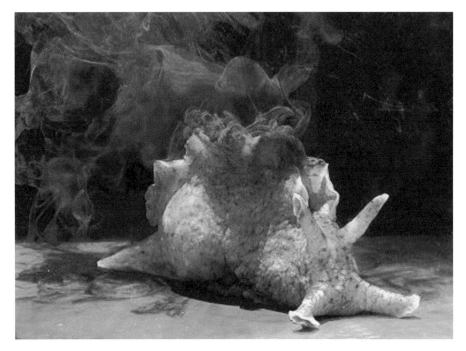

Figure 10.3 *Aplysia californica*, the largest species of sea slug. When threatened, the slug releases a poisonous reddish secretion into the water. Wikimedia Commons (File: Aplysia californica NHGRI-79108.jpg).

Now settled in Paris and with Tauc as his new colleague, Kandel began experiments on *Aplysia*. He would have immediately seen that the giant sea slug was well named, its body weighing up to 7 kilograms and its length, when fully extended, some 30 centimetres (Figure 10.3). Kandel based the learning experiments on electric stimuli that were given in different combinations and in varying strengths. One stimulus, delivered to a nerve branch, was of constant strength and used as a reference. In the simplest experiment the same stimulus would be repeated and the sizes of the responses of a giant neuron in a ganglion would be measured. As the stimuli continued the amplitudes of the responses declined—this behaviour was referred to as *habituation* (Figure 10.4, *left*). It was as if the ganglion neuron had learned the nature of the stimulus and was losing interest in it.

Another experiment of Kandel's mimicked *sensitization* in human beings—how, following a sudden unexpected event (a gunshot, for example) a normally innocuous stimulus (a gentle sound or touch) can be startling. In Kandel's experiment a weak stimulus was given to a nerve and the response of the giant ganglion cell noted. The same stimulus was then delivered immediately after a series of strong shocks to a different nerve and the response was found to be greatly enlarged (Figure 10.4, *right*). In a third type of experiment (not shown) a weak stimulus was quickly followed by a strong one to the same nerve. After this pairing had been repeated a number of times the response to the first (weak) stimulus was seen to have become larger, even when given

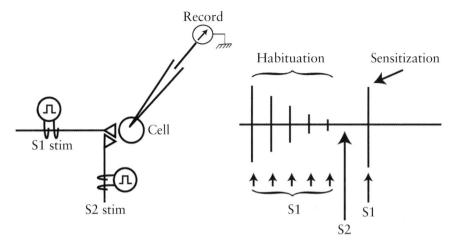

Figure 10.4 Experimental arrangement (*left*) used to elicit habituation and sensitization (*right*). When a nerve is stimulated repeatedly (S1 arrows, *right*), the postsynaptic responses recorded with a microelectrode inside a neuron (*Cell*) become progressively smaller—*habituation*. If a strong shock is then given to a second nerve (S2), the response to a further S1 shock is greatly enlarged—*sensitization*. Kandel later showed in *Aplysia* that there was an interneuron in the sensitization pathway (not shown in figure) and that it released the neurotransmitter serotonin on to the endings of the S1-stimulated nerve fibres.

by itself. Kandel used this experiment as a model for '*aversive conditioning*' in animal experiments—that is, when a normally innocuous event becomes the signal for an unpleasant aftermath. In the early 1900s the great Russian physiologist Ivan Pavlov had performed conditioning studies in dogs, pairing the sound of a bell with a following electric shock.

Though the ideas for the experiments had been Kandel's, Ladislav Tauc had been his partner in the experiments, both at the Institut Marey and, during the autumn, at a marine biological station at Arcachon, near Bordeaux. The work had gone well and a pair of papers by the two investigators appeared in the *Journal of Physiology*.[3] Kandel's gamble had paid off—he and Tauc had shown that electrophysiological changes in a simple nervous system might serve as a model for the development of human behaviours. The fact that the altered amplitudes of the cell responses in *Aplysia* could persist for half an hour or so, strongly suggested that the 'learning' had involved some changes at the synapses on the ganglion cell. The next stage would be to try and find out what those changes were. That, however, would have to await Kandel's return to the United States.

Kandel had been fortunate in choosing to go to Paris when he did. Had he delayed he would certainly have had his plans interrupted by the student unrest of 1968, in which life in the city was brought to a halt by demonstrations, marches, barricades, and occupations. The Institut Marey has not escaped. Students had taken over the building and, in public meetings, had accused staff—even the esteemed Fessards—of errors and improprieties. As Denise Albe-Fessard would write later, it was all nonsense. Nevertheless the damage had been done. Research at the Institut, superb research that was recognized as such by the international community of neurophysiologists, would never fully recover.

In 1978 the Institut Marey would be demolished, its site given over to an expansion of Roland Garros national tennis facility. But the old building and those who had worked in it had left a valuable legacy, a part of which would point another way to learning more about the hippocampus in the years to come. It was the ability to record from single neurons in the human brain.

Notes

1. The difficulties encountered by the Fessards, coupled with a description of the research conducted at the Institute Marey, is described in Denise Albe-Fessard's memoir (the very first in the *History of Neuroscience in Autobiography* series): D. Albe-Fessard, *The History of Neuroscience in Autobiography*, L.R. Squire (ed.) (Washington, DC: Society for Neuroscience, 1996) 1: 2–48..
2. Ladislav Tauc (1926–1999) was a Czech who came to study at the Institut Marey in 1949. His work with Kandel would prove a highlight of his career and was largely responsible for his subsequent appointment as founding director of the Cellular and Molecular Neurobiology Laboratory at the French National Centre for Scientific Research (CNRS).
3. E.R. Kandel and L. Tauc. 'Heterosynaptic Facilitation in Neurons of the Abdominal Ganglion of *Aplysia depilans*' (1965) 181 *Journal of Physiology* 1–27. E.R. Kandel and L. Tauc, 'Mechanism of Heterosynaptic Facilitation in the Giant Cell of the Abdominal Ganglion of *Aplysia depilans*' (1965) 181 *Journal of Physiology* 28–47.

11

Human Neurons—Success and Disappointment

(Paris, Uppsala, 1960s: Denise Albe-Fessard, Karl-Erik Hagbarth)

At the Institut Marey, Denise Albe-Fessard's investigations of the deep brain nuclei in the cat had attracted the attention of Parisian neurosurgeon, Gerard Guiot. Guiot would have been aware of Denise's considerable success, not only in her own research but in directing that of her students and visiting postdoctoral fellows, many of whom had come from abroad. Denise was able to exert her authority without raising her voice; her firmness was reflected in the way she was able to seize a feral cat and anaesthetize it before starting surgery. Respected because of her prowess during the complex experiments, Denise nevertheless maintained a Parisian elegance, complement by an occasional quiet smile.

Guiot asked Denise if it might be possible to make recordings from the thalamus in patients undergoing stereotaxic surgery for parkinsonism. The problem with this type of surgery, as Guiot well knew, was that it was impossible to know exactly where the target nucleus lay even after consulting the best human brain atlas and being able to locate any point in the three-dimensional space that included the patient's head. The imprecision was a consequence of the variation in skull shape—and hence brain shape—between one person and another. Denise (Figure 11.1), ever willing to collaborate in the cause of neuroscience, duly brought one of her recording electrodes to the operating room and supervised its insertion into a micromanipulator mounted on the stereotaxic frame attached to the patient's head.

It was a very different experimental situation to the ones that she had been accustomed to in the Institut Marey. Not only was the subject a human rather than a cat, but, since the stereotaxic procedure had been prepared under local anaesthesia, he or she could respond to the surgeon's instructions. Denise employed the same kind of recording electrode that had brought success in the cat—an insulated copper wire inside a thin steel cannula. As the electrode penetrated the thalamus from the back of the brain, the instructions would begin. 'Do you feel this?', 'Move your fingers', and so on. Eventually a thalamic nucleus would be entered and the oscilloscope and the amplifier would come to life with the discharges of a responding neuron.[1] Sometimes it would be a touch on the patient's skin that was the effective stimulus and sometimes it was the movement of a joint (Figure 11.2). Not uncommonly the neuron would be one firing with the rhythm of the patient's tremor. At this point Denise knew exactly where the tip of the electrode was in the thalamus—and Guiot knew where he had to put his

Aranzio's Seahorse and the Search for Memory and Consciousness. Alan J. McComas, Oxford University Press.
© Oxford University Press 2023. DOI: 10.1093/oso/9780192868244.003.0013

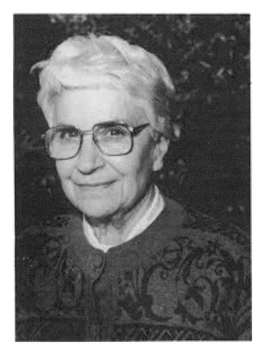

Figure 11.1 Denise Albe-Fessard. Photograph kindly supplied by Dr Jean-Gaël Barbara.

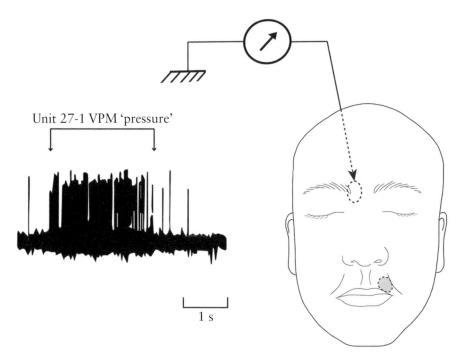

Figure 11.2 Response of somatosensory neuron in human thalamus to touching small area of skin on the opposite side of the face, above the upper lip. Author's recording.

own electrode to destroy the neurons that were part of the tremor circuit. It was skillful and time-consuming work but justified by the results. Soon a number of other neurosurgeons would be calling on neurophysiologists for similar help, including several in Britain. In Canada, at the Montreal Neurological Institute, Gilles Bertrand would have Herbert Jasper as his collaborator.

At the same time the human thalamus was being explored, a novel procedure was being developed for recording from a very different family of human neurons—those whose long axons formed the peripheral nerves of the arms and legs and were responsible for transmitting sensory information from skin, muscles, and joints. To record impulses from a single fibre in a human nerve was a challenge that had been met once before. At the University of Marburg in Germany, Herbert Hensel and Kurt Boman had found medical students prepared to sacrifice part of their radial nerves. Following a surgical incision at the wrist the radial nerve was exposed; one of its branches was then divided and the distal end dissected until only a few fibres lay on the wire recording electrode. The recordings of nerve impulses were of good quality and fibres responding to touch, pressure, and cooling were found.[2] Though it was a unique achievement, the findings had added little to what was already known from animal experiments. Moreover, because of its invasive nature, the technique would not be taken up elsewhere.

In Sweden, however, the problem of recording from single human nerve fibres was being attacked in a different way—one that did not require surgery and that left intact the nerve fibres running to the spinal cord from the skin and muscles in the periphery.

After completing his medical training Karl-Erik Hagbarth (Figure 11.3) had studied neurophysiology under Ragnar Granit at the Karolinska Institute in Stockholm. Granit was a future Nobel Laureate who, like Eccles, had been trained by Charles Sherrington at Oxford. Under Granit's supervision, Hagbarth had studied cutaneous reflexes in humans for a doctoral thesis. Then had followed a year at the Brain Research Institute in Los Angeles, during which time he had investigated the descending control of sensory pathways. On returning to Stockholm he had undertaken more work on human reflexes and motor control. However, Hagbarth's best years were to come following his move to Uppsala, where he had been invited to establish a department of clinical neurophysiology.

Positioned 70 kilometres north of Stockholm and pleasantly situated on the banks of the River Fyris, Uppsala had a much smaller population than the nation's capital. Nevertheless, it had a history that included the founding of Scandinavia's oldest university (in the 15th century) and the building of Sweden's largest cathedral. Among its university faculty had been Carl Linnaeus (famous for the classifications of animals and plants), Anders Celsius (inventor of the temperature scale), and Anders Ångstrom (pioneer in microscopic measurements). Then, as now, student traditions in Uppsala had been observed. It was an ideal setting for the new director of clinical neurophysiology.

Hagbarth's first achievement in his new surroundings was to demonstrate, in certain human muscles, that sustained reflex contraction could be produced by tendon vibration. He had then turned his attention to the possibility of recording from single human nerve fibres and to do this with microelectrodes. Clearly glass electrodes could not be

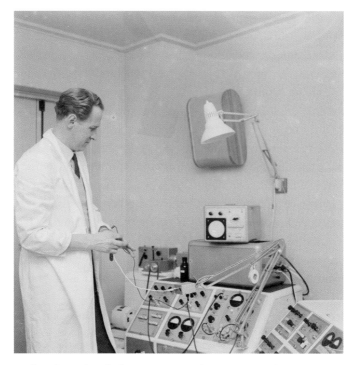

Figure 11.3 Karl-Erik Hagbarth demonstrating electromyography in the university hospital in Uppsala, Sweden, in 1959. Uppsala-Bild/Upplandsmuseet (BY-NC-ND.)

used and steel wires bent, so the eventual solution was to make use of the stiffness of a short length of tungsten wire, just as Hubel and Wiesel had done for their vision experiments. After electrolytic etching of the tip of the wire and coating the shaft with a resin-based lacquer, there was an electrode that was surprisingly easy to slip through the skin and into a nerve trunk. Well aware that the new experiments would not receive ethical approval because of the theoretical risk of nerve damage or infection, Hagbarth decided to experiment on himself. He was not at all confident that the approach would work, largely because the ionic currents flowing around a nerve fibre during an impulse might be too small to be detected. Hagbarth was therefore delighted when, having inserted an electrode into his own ulnar nerve, he was able to hear faint sounds on the loudspeaker whenever he tapped the skin. Having demonstrated the phenomenon to his junior colleague, Åke Vallbo, the two has no hesitation in exploiting the new technique—on themselves.[3]

With increasing success, the two found that they were eventually able to recognize the discharges of single sensory fibres belonging to muscle spindles or to touch and pressure receptors in the skin. Most surprisingly, given their extreme thinness, the slowly conducting sympathetic nerve fibres could also be examined for impulse activity; these were the fibres controlling blood flow and sweat glands[4,5] (Figure 11.4).

The new methodology was soon taken up elsewhere, especially by clinicians with an interest in the autonomic nervous system and its control of blood pressure. For the

The microneurographic technique

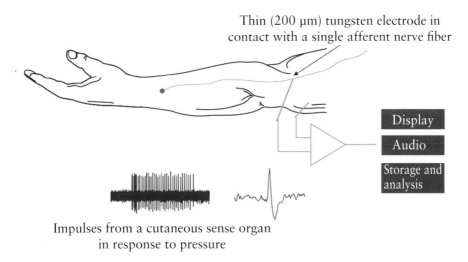

Thin (200 μm) tungsten electrode in
contact with a single afferent nerve fiber

Display
Audio
Storage and
analysis

Impulses from a cutaneous sense organ
in response to pressure

Figure 11.4 Recording from a single human peripheral nerve fibre responsive to touching the skin. Note the similarity of the response to that recorded in the thalamus (Figure 11.2). Creative Commons Attribution-Share Alike 4.0 international. File: Microneurography, experimental setup, schematic.jpg. Author: Whisper viper.

thoughtful neurophysiologist, however, there was something disconcerting about the single neuron recordings from receptors in the skin and joints. It didn't appear to matter whether the recording was being made in the peripheral nerve of healthy subjects or in the thalamus of parkinsonian patients—as far as could be seen, the results were similar. The patterns of impulses, the areas of skin responsive to touch or pressure, the responses to flexing or extending a joint, were indistinguishable when compared at the two recording sites. Moreover, the thalamic responses were unchanged by attracting the patient's attention either towards, or away from, the stimulated part. Surely, it was thought, some sort of analysis would have been carried out once the sensory message reached the brain, an analysis that would be susceptible to the demands of the moment. If not, what could be the function of the prominent nerve fibre pathways descending from the cortex to the sensory neuron populations in the spinal cord and brainstem? The mystery would only deepen when Patrick Wall began to investigate sensory pathways in the spinal cord.

Among those active in the field, the results of depth recordings in the human brain were disappointing. While useful to the neurosurgeon treating movement disorders or pain, the recordings had yielded little of scientific interest and nothing that was not already known from animal experiments. No-one could have foreseen the rich harvest that would come many years later.

Meanwhile, using animals rather than humans, Patrick Wall was well underway with his own investigations of sensory pathways in the spinal cord and brain stem.

Notes

1. D. Albe-Fessard, G. Arfel, G. Guiot, P. Derome, E. Hertzog, G. Vourc'h, H. Brown, P. Aleonard, J. de la Herran, and J.C. Trigo, 'Electrophysiological Studies of Some Deep Cerebral Structures in Man' (1966) 3 *Journal of the Neurological Sciences* 37–51. Later studies in other centres mostly employed fine electrodes of the Hubel tungsten wire type and were able to obtain superior recordings from single neurons.
2. H. Hensel and K. Boman, 'Afferent Impulses in Cutaneous Sensory Nerves in Human Subjects' (1960) 23 *Journal of Neurophysiology* 564–78.
3. Å.B. Vallbo and K.-E. Hagbarth, 'Activity from Skin Mechanoreceptors Recorded Percutaneously in Awake Human Subjects' (1968) 21(3) *Experimental Neurology* 270–89.
4. For a review of the percutaneous recording technique, with its research applications, see: Å.B. Vallbo, 'Microneuronography: How It Started and How It Works' (2018) 120(3) *Journal of Neurophysiology* 1415–27.
5. The most probable answer is that the descending fibres from the brain, by imposing inhibition, serve to focus impulse activity at earlier stages of the sensory pathway. By doing this, they are compensating for the excessive nerve fibre sprouting and synaptic connectivity that remains at the conclusion of embryonic and postnatal development. Wall's own experiments on the effect of spinal cord section in rats provided evidence for such an explanation.

12

Understanding Pain

(Cambridge, Massachusetts, Montreal: Patrick Wall, Donald Melzack, John O'Keefe, Suzanne Corkin)

Patrick Wall (Figure 12.1) had been educated in the United Kingdom and had gone to Oxford University as a medical undergraduate.[1] While studying anatomy he had come to the attention of Paul Glees, whose specialty was the histological staining of degenerating nerve fibres. The latter was the type of work that immediately aroused Wall's interest and led him to improve on existing methods for making small cuts in the brain or spinal cord and then tracing the paths of the degenerating nerve fibres. It was also the type of work that persuaded Wall, like so many others, to reject the practice of medicine for a career in basic science.

After graduating in medicine Wall had crossed the Atlantic to work in John Fulton's department at Yale, where he mingled with the highly talented and well-established neuroscientists that Fulton had gathered together. Wall, in addition to learning some electrophysiology, would have become familiar with the primate lobotomy research and might have met Henry Molaison's surgeon, William Scoville, on one of the latter's visits. Wall next moved to Chicago, attracted by the presence of the energetic but un-orthodox Jerry Lettvin who, while working as a full-time psychiatrist in a mental hospital, was also conducting animal research in a laboratory of his own creation.[2] The next move was to MIT (the Massachusetts Institute of Technology), this time with Lettvin.

For many, MIT is synonymous with Boston and, indeed, the world-famous institute is situated within the Boston metropolitan area. However, MIT lies across the Charles River from Boston and is actually in Cambridge. Though the latter is a small city in comparison with Boston, it has a similarly long history and, if it wished, could make a strong claim to be the intellectual capital of the nation for it was in Cambridge (or 'Newtowne' as it then was) that Harvard College was founded, initially for the education of clergy. If Harvard has the longer history, MIT, founded in 1861, has the better location—a fact appreciated by faculty and students who, on emerging from the institute's Great Dome, can enjoy unobstructed views of lawns and river (Figure 12.2).

It was at MIT that Wall continued his new research on impulse conduction in sensory nerve fibres as they entered the spinal cord. It was not a lone effort, however, for he was joined by Lettvin and others; indeed, it was Walter Pitts, a self-educated genius, who suggested mapping the flow of current in the spinal cord by means of microelectrode recordings at multiple sites and who performed the necessary mathematical analysis afterwards. The result of the study was to show that, following an impulse volley in a

Aranzio's Seahorse and the Search for Memory and Consciousness. Alan J. McComas, Oxford University Press.
© Oxford University Press 2023. DOI: 10.1093/oso/9780192868244.003.0014

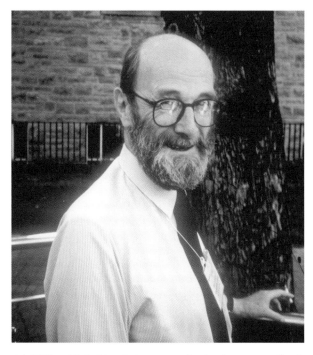

Figure 12.1 Patrick Wall, with habitual cigarette, relaxing between talks during a symposium at Queen's University, Canada, in 1995. Photograph by author.

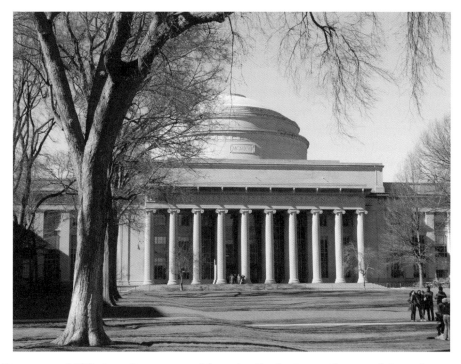

Figure 12.2 MIT's Great Dome, viewed from the Charles River. Photograph by author.

sensory nerve root, the impulses in a second volley were prevented from reaching the terminals of the nerve fibres. It was evidence for a novel type of inhibition—*presynaptic*.[3]

Wall had presented the new work in 1953 at the XIX International Physiology Congress in Montreal and then, intriguingly, had been summoned to Wilder Penfield's office at the Montreal Neurological Institute. To Wall's surprise he had found himself confronted not only by Penfield but by Edgar Adrian, John Eccles, and Herbert Jasper. Wall was even more surprised when the four senior neuroscientists informed him that he was mistaken in thinking there was such a process as presynaptic inhibition and that he should change his thinking accordingly. It would have been small consolation when, five years later, Eccles took over the field himself, publishing a series of papers on pre-synaptic inhibition with Per Andersen in Canberra (!).

Wall's next interaction with Montreal was a happier one, however. In the early 1960s Wall was joined in his MIT laboratory by Ronald Melzack (Figure 12.3), one of Donald Hebb's former graduate students at McGill and a contemporary of Mortimer Mishkin and the two Milners. Melzack's own graduate work had been on the effects of a restricted sensory environment on the behaviour of dogs. Sensory deprivation was a field that Hebb had long been interested in and, while a student of Lashley, had himself studied the effects of rearing rats in darkness. In his own study on dogs, Melzack had noticed that the sensory-deprived animals might repeatedly bang their heads on over-head pipes—it was not that the impacts appeared painless but rather that the animals seemed unable to alter their behaviour. The observation had caused Melzack to con-sider pain as unexpectedly complex; not only did it depend on the immediate injury but also on the circumstances and the previous history of the individual.

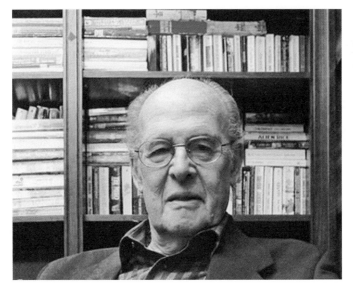

Figure 12.3 Ronald Melzack in his retirement residence in 2010. (Photo by Marty555. Wikimedia Commons file: Melzack Ronald.jpg. Creative Commons Attribution-Share Alike 3.0 Unported license).

Such a conclusion was not surprising. It was a common observation that sporting injuries or wounds sustained in war could be initially painless or even unnoticed. The Battle of Waterloo on 18 June 1815 had provided a memorable example. At one point in the fighting, Lord Uxbridge had had one leg shattered below the knee by a Napoleonic cannonball. Still seated on his horse but looking down at his mutilated leg, Uxbridge was heard to remark: 'By God, I have lost my leg.' (Whereupon the Duke of Wellington is alleged to have replied: 'Have you, by God!' and resumed his survey of the battle through his telescope).[4] And then there was the description of an attack by an African lion, given by the 19th-century medical missionary-explorer, David Livingston in 1857:

> I heard a shout starting, and looking half-round, I saw the lion just in the act of springing upon me. I was upon a little height; he caught my shoulder as he sprang, and we both came to the ground below together. Growling horribly close to my ear, he shook me as a terrier does a rat. The shock produced a stupor similar to that which seems to be felt by a mouse after the shake of the cat. It caused a sort of dreaminess in which there was no sense of pain nor feeling of terror, though quite conscious of all that was happening. It was like what patients partially under the influence of chloroform describe, who see all the operation, but feel not the knife ... The shake annihilated fear, and allowed no sense of horror in looking round at the beast.[5]

Melzack was intrigued by Wall's research. The bearded and bespectacled Englishman, still investigating impulse transmission in sensory nerve fibres entering the spinal cord, had already demonstrated a novel form of inhibition—presynaptic. He had shown that this inhibition could be exerted between incoming large-diameter sensory fibres and that small neurons in the spinal cord acted as intermediaries. It now appeared that the inhibitory neurons could also suppress impulse activity in the cells that informed the brain about potentially painful stimuli. Melzack, responsive to new thinking about pain mechanisms, assisted Wall in proposing a 'gate' theory. Thus, under normal conditions, the continuing flow of impulses in large-diameter nerve fibres (responsive to touch and pressure on the skin) would exert presynaptic inhibition and keep excitability low in the spinal cord. However, in the event of injury, the enhanced flow of impulses in small-diameter nerve fibres would be sufficient to override the presynaptic inhibition. Information from the damaged tissues would then be able to reach the brain and produce pain. A corollary of the gate theory was that pain should be alleviated if the balance of impulse activity between small- and large-diameter nerve fibres could be restored. This thinking, in turn, would lead to repetitive electrical stimulation of the skin as a treatment for pain.

Melzack and Wall published their gate theory in *Science*,[6] one of the two top journals in the world for general science (the other being *Nature*). Though the theory was immediately recognized as exciting and original, it inevitably provoked disbelief in neuroscientists and clinicians beholden to a simple, 'fixed-line' mechanism for pain. But Melzack and Wall had support. In the Netherlands, the neurosurgeon William Noordenbos had independently reached a similar conclusion to Melzack and Wall's, though without the latter's detailed knowledge of the underlying neural mechanisms. Another neurosurgeon, George Rowbotham in Newcastle-upon-Tyne (United Kingdom), had for years recommended the use a commercially available cosmetic vibrator on a painful area, should other measures fail.[7] And was it not a natural tendency to rub the hand over a painful area of the body? Not least, the gate theory was supported by the ameliorative effect of repetitive electrical stimulation, as in the use of the newly developed TENS (Transcutaneous Electrical Nerve Stimulation) devices. The different parts of the new pain story fitted together very nicely.

The publication in *Science*, soon to become a classic citation, represented another success for the McGill Department of Psychology and for Donald Hebb's original graduate students. First there had been Brenda and Peter Milner, then Mortimer Mishkin, and now Ronald Melzack—all had achieved international fame, as had Hebb's postdoctoral fellow, James Olds.

However, the gate theory had made no attempt to deal with another puzzle of pain. How was it that in particularly unfortunate patients, pains persisted even when every stage in the pain pathway had been interrupted—from the peripheral nerves right up to the brain? Related to this question, how was it that patients could continue to have quite complex sensations involving an arm or leg that had been amputated? The latter, the 'phantom limb' phenomenon, was clearly dependent on a form of memory quite different to that responsible for names and events ('declarative' memory) or to that involving physical activities ('procedural' memory). The phantom limb was a topic that Ronald Melzack would continue to explore after his return to Montreal.[8] It was a return made more promising by two developments, of which the first was the award of a generous research grant.

The second development was the arrival of a young doctoral student from New York. John O'Keefe, the son of impoverished Irish immigrants, had been born in Harlem.[9] After graduating from high school he had worked briefly as a clerk and bookkeeper before deciding to study aeronautical engineering at New York University. Though O'Keefe was able to combine evening lessons with daytime work for an aircraft manufacturer, the travelling involved was exhausting. Meanwhile he had become interested in philosophy and, related to that, the possibility of studying the brain. He then became a full-time student at the City College of New York, enthusiastically tackling a wide range of courses and keeping himself solvent by driving a taxi at night. Reluctantly obliged to graduate, he had chosen psychology as his major. The thought of undertaking research on the brain himself, prompted in part by his study of Donald Hebb's *The Organization of Behaviour*, had resulted in an application to graduate school at McGill. With Melzack as his supervisor, O'Keefe had undertaken to investigate neuronal activity in a part of the limbic system related to the hippocampus and, like the latter, situated within the medial temporal lobe—the amygdala. With his engineering background, O'Keefe decided to improve on the recording system that Peter Milner and James Olds had used in their discovery of the pleasure ('reward') centre in the early 1950s. A microdrive mounted on the cat skull now allowed the position of the wire electrodes to be adjusted within the cat brain. A miniature amplifier was also attached to the head, permitting much lighter and more flexible wire connections to the recording and display equipment in the laboratory.

The amygdala recordings were intriguing. Most of the cells were silent, not firing impulses, and only a few were found that would break into activity when the cat was confronted with a highly specific stimulus. For one cell it was the presence of a mouse, for another cell an item of food, and for another the sound of a singing bird.[10] Rather than the recognition of an object or creature being represented by the conjunction of impulse activity in several regions of the brain, individual cells in the amygdala had been given this task. Though the specificity of the neuron responses was a major discovery, the fact that so few cells had been characterized may have denied the study the interest it deserved. In the end it did not matter. O'Keefe's first neuroscientific foray would prove to be the prelude to a line of his work that would attract world-wide attention and the award of a Nobel Prize.

Meanwhile, across the McGill campus in her office at the Montreal Neurological Institute, Brenda Milner had remained active. She had begun to explore other fields in addition to memory. Like Ronald Melzack, she now had her own research grant and was attracting graduate students, one of whom would play a significant role in the study of memory. Suzanne Hammond had come to Montreal in 1961 in order to work for a PhD under Brenda Milner. She, Suzanne, had grown up in West Hartford, Connecticut[11] and, by coincidence, had been a childhood friend of the daughter of Dr William Scoville, the neurosurgeon who had operated on Henry Molaison. Originally intending to study medicine, Suzanne had settled for psychology instead. After graduating from Smith College she had decided to explore, in Penfield's patients and under Brenda Milner's supervision, the effects of brain surgery on the sense of touch.

At a time when her doctoral work was well underway, Suzanne's interest had been piqued by the arrival of Henry Molaison. This had been in 1962 and it had been Henry's only visit to the Montreal Neurological Institute. He had been brought from Hartford by his mother in order to undergo a battery of tests devised by Brenda Milner. The testing would take all week and, in the course of it, Suzanne would repeatedly put Henry through one of the challenges. In the test, Henry was required to manoeuvre a stylus through a maze that was hidden from his view. Suzanne found that, despite repetition, Henry was unable to improve his accuracy, continuing to make as many wrong turns as before. However, though Henry's memory of the previous attempts (episodic memory) was clearly deficient, Suzanne noticed that he had become significantly quicker at getting to the end of the maze—that is, Henry's procedural memory was intact. The same test had shed light on two entirely different forms of memory.

The interaction between the young graduate student and the increasingly famous patient was to have an important consequence. After Suzanne completed her PhD and took a position in the Psychology Department at MIT, she took over Henry Molaison as well.

From now on, it was Suzanne Corkin (her married name), rather than Brenda Milner, who would be responsible for the use of Henry in memory experiments.

Notes

1. P.D. Wall. *The History of Neuroscience in Autobiography*, L.R. Squire (ed.) (San Diego, CA: Academic Press, 2001) 3: 472–501. This must be the most amusing memoir of the many that have been published in the series, and it also captures Wall's scientific originality and defiance of authority. Wall, born in 1925, died in 2001.

2. J. Lettvin. *The History of Neuroscience in Autobiography*, L.R. Squire (ed.) 1008. 2. (San Diego, CA: Academic Press, 2008) 2: 222–43. Like Wall's, this autobiography is humorous, and describes the remarkably free and undisciplined path that Lettvin and others were taking in entering, and then pursuing, neuroscience. The memoir gives a good account of the genius of Walter Pitts. Lettvin, born in 1920, died in 2011.

3. B. Howland, J.Y. Lettvin, W.S. McCulloch, W. Pitts, and P.D. Wall, 'Reflex Inhibition by Dorsal Root Interaction' (1955) 18(1) *Journal of Neurophysiology* 1–17.

4. E. Longford, *Wellington. The Years of the Sword* (New York, NY: Harper & Row, 1969). Later, while the damaged leg was being amputated in a nearby cottage, Uxbridge remained fully conscious, remarking only on the apparent bluntness of the surgical instruments.

5. D. Livingstone, *Missionary Travels and Researches in South Africa* (London: John Murray, 1857). The same account appears in: ER Kandel, JH Schwarz, and TM Jessell, *Principles of Neural Science*, 4th edn (East Norwalk, CT: Appleton & Lange)—which is where the present author first encountered it.

6. R. Melzack and P. Wall, 'Pain Mechanisms: A New Theory' (1965) 150 *Science* 171–9. Though there have been some modifications to the theory subsequently, it is generally regarded as being correct.

7. The author was house-surgeon to Mr Rowbotham for six months in 1960.

8. R. Melzack, 'Phantom Limbs' (2006) 16(3s) *Scientific American Special Editions* 52–9. Ronald Melzack was born in 1929 and died in 2019.

9. <https://www.nobelprize.org/prizes/medicine/2014/okeefe/biographical/> accessed 22 April 2022.

10. J. O'Keefe and H. Bouma, 'Complex Sensory Properties of Certain Amygdala Units in the Freely Moving Cat' (1969) 23(3) *Experimental Neurology* 384–98. Bouma was a visiting Fellow from the Netherlands.

11. Suzanne Corkin's account of her professional interaction with Henry Molaison, including general observations as well as psychological experiments, is given in her beautifully written and highly informative monograph: S. Corkin, *Permanent Present Tense. The Unforgettable Life of the Amnesic Patient, H.M.* (New York, NY: Basic Books, 2013). Suzanne's childhood friendship with William Scoville's daughter is described in: L. Dittrich, *Patient H.M. A Story of Memory, Madness, and Family Secrets* (New York, NY: Random House, 2016). Suzanne died in May 2016.

13

Return of the Slug

(New York, 1965: Eric Kandel)

Following his 14 months of research on *Aplysia* with Ladislav Tauc in France, Eric Kandel had returned to Boston where, as a newly appointed member of the Harvard psychiatry faculty, he had been responsible for training junior residents.[1] One advantage of his new position was that it had given him the opportunity to talk to Stephen Kuffler in the Department of Pharmacology. When Kuffler had been recruited from Johns Hopkins University in Baltimore, David Hubel and Torsten Wiesel had brought their exciting work on vision with them. But there had also been Edwin Furshpan, David Potter, and John Nicholls with their novel experiments on crayfish, goldfish, and leeches. Under Kuffler's guidance, neurophysiology had become but one aspect of neurobiology and the choice of preparation was strictly determined by the type of question being asked. It was a change in direction for neurophysiology which, following the brilliant analysis of their voltage clamp experiments by Hodgkin and Huxley, had for a while become largely mathematical and biophysical. In 1965, Harvard University, recognizing Kuffler's talents, appointed him head of a new department—the world's first department of neurobiology.

Kuffler, knowing of the work that Kandel had carried out in France, had been encouraging and able to see the advantages of using *Aplysia* again for any future experiments on learning. And future experiments were what the young psychiatrist had in mind. After discussion with his wife, Kandel had committed himself to a career in research. Psychoanalysis had been tempting and, indeed, had been the reason for him entering medical school, but it was not enough. Like so many other young clinicians, past and present, Eric Kandel had felt the call of basic science.

It was a good time to pursue basic research, even though there was much disorder in the world outside the laboratory. Indeed, the 1960s would prove the most turbulent decade to follow the Second World War. It was a time when the old order was giving way to the new. Students rioted in Paris and elsewhere in Europe. In the United States the assassination of President John Kennedy was followed by that of Martin Luther King, while the ever-widening war in Vietnam brought protests and demonstrations. There were race riots and burning buildings in major US cities. Yet it was also a period of youthful energy and exuberance, the time of the Beatles and of the half-million attending the Woodstock Festival.

It was very much a boom time for neuroscience. The amplifiers and oscilloscopes of Tektronix and Hewlett-Packard were now supplemented by computers capable of

Aranzio's Seahorse and the Search for Memory and Consciousness. Alan J. McComas, Oxford University Press.
© Oxford University Press 2023. DOI: 10.1093/oso/9780192868244.003.0015

detecting small biological signals and of plotting the numbers and latencies of nerve impulses. Vernon Mountcastle, investigating the somatosensory cortex in his neuro-physiology laboratory at Johns Hopkins Hospital, was among the first to purchase one of the physically imposing LINC computers designed at MIT. A few years later most laboratories would have their own purpose-built CAT (computer of average transients), the portable and less expensive brainchild of the Australian inventor-pianist, Manfred Clynes.

The 1960s were also a golden period when money for computers and other neuro-physiological equipment was plentiful, especially in the United States, where the National Institutes of Health was generous in its awards of grants. It was in the United States, too, where most of the expertise in brain research was to be found. Increasingly, Europeans would travel to America for a year or two of postdoctoral research, often staying for the rest of their careers. In basic science as well in medicine, a BTA (Been To America) was a prestigious if fictitious qualification.

Such was the situation in 1965 when Eric Kandel, with his wife and infant daughter, was back in the nation's largest city, this time as a member of the Physiology Department at New York University. Before long he would be able to recruit Alden Spencer, his former partner in the extensive microelectrode study of the cat hippocampus at the National Institutes of Health (NIH). Another new colleague was James Schwartz, a brilliant biochemist prepared to work on the neurotransmitters employed in the *Aplysia* nervous system. The fourth member of the team was Irving Kupfermann, a young behaviourist with a history of designing and conducting experiments on woodlice.

The new programme of work was intended as a logical extension of the studies in France. There, Kandel and Tauc had shown that *Aplysia* neurons stimulated directly through nerve branches would alter their responses, depending on the nature and pattern of the electrical pulses. But did *Aplysia* have natural behaviours that might be suitable for investigation?

It did. Kandel and his colleagues observed that the giant sea slug was capable of feeding, moving, copulating, laying eggs, secreting mucus, and expelling ink. The most promising behaviour for experimental analysis, however, was a withdrawal reflex involving the creature's siphon and gill (Figure 13.1). It was noted that, whenever touch was applied to the siphon (a duct for removing water and waste), there was a retraction into the body cavity of the gill (an organ for breathing). An advantage of using this reflex for experiments was that it involved neurons in the abdominal ganglion, a part of the *Aplysia* nervous system that Kandel knew well from his earlier investigations with Tauc. In the French studies it had been possible not only to identify the larger neurons in the ganglion under the microscope, or even by naked eye, but to penetrate them with a microelectrode and to obtain stable recordings.

To Kandel's satisfaction, the gill withdrawal reflex was shown capable of both habituation and sensitization. Thus, repeatedly light touches to the siphon lightly produced progressively weaker retractions of the gill (*habituation*) but an exaggerated withdrawal movement resulted if the touch was paired with an electric shock to the body (*sensitization*).

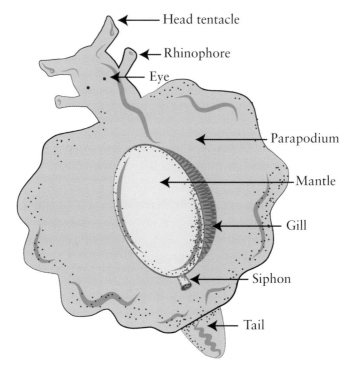

Head tentacle

Rhinophore

Eye

Parapodium

Mantle

Gill

Siphon

Tail

Figure 13.1 *Aplysia*, showing siphon and outermost gill tissue (the latter visible beyond the protective overlying mantle). The function of the siphon is to remove waste; touching it evokes a reflex that causes the gill to withdraw fully under the mantle. Note the prominent rhinophores for detecting molecular signals in the environment and, in contrast, the poorly developed eyes (see Chapter 36).

The next step was to explore the large neurons in the abdominal ganglion to determine whether they might be involved in gill withdrawal reflex. By stimulating the cells individually though a microelectrode, as well as by recording from them, Kandel and his colleagues were able to identify the six neurons (motoneurons) supplying the muscle fibres that retracted the gill. A further six neurons (sensory neurons) would respond to touching a single point on the skin and initiate the reflex. Also present in the ganglion was a small number of interneurons, that is, nerve cells capable of modifying the activities of the sensory and motor neurons.

Kandel and his colleagues now proceeded to show that weakening of the withdrawal reflex with repetition (habituation) was associated with a reduced signal in the motoneurons—that is, the later touches on the skin resulted in progressively smaller changes in the electrical potential across the motoneuron cell membrane. Conversely, the exaggerated withdrawal reflex following a light touch paired with an electric shock (sensitization) was evidently due to an enhanced response of the motoneuron cell membrane. The conclusion from the experiments was inescapable—*Aplysia* had 'learned' by altering the strength of the synaptic connections between the skin neurons and the motoneurons.[2,3]

It was an important result though the findings had been limited to behavioural changes persisting for a few minutes only. Such short effects were due to what had been variously referred to as 'immediate', 'primary', or 'short-term' memory. Many neuroscientists had thought it likely that this type of memory was achieved by continuing impulse activity in neural circuits. Karl Lashley, for one, had written: 'It is highly probable that immediate memory is maintained by some sort of after-discharge of the originally excited neurons.'[4] Kandel's group had shown that this was not true, at least in their preparation. Rather than continuing impulse activity, the synapses themselves had been temporarily altered.

Aplysia had been an obliging preparation and Kandel's choice had been vindicated. Indeed, life must have seemed good for the former psychiatrist, not only as he surveyed his group's achievements but also during the moments of leisure when he might be found at one of New York's many art galleries or, during a special evening, at the Metropolitan Opera House. But could the giant sea slug enable the small group of neurobiologists to go further in their research, perhaps finding out what was happening inside a single neuron at a molecular level? And what sort of changes might be occurring at synapses to account for long-term memory? There was still much to be done.

While *Aplysia* was yielding its secrets in New York, there had been two significant developments elsewhere. One of them was the publication of a book.

Notes

1. Most of the information in this chapter, including the nature and results of the experiments on *Aplysia*, has come from Eric Kandel's memoir: E.R. Kandel, *In Search of Memory. The Emergence of a New Science of Mind* (New York: WW Norton, 2006).
2. I. Kupfermann and E.R. Kandel, 'Neuronal Controls of a Behavioral Response Mediated by the Abdominal Ganglion of Aplysia' (1969) 164 *Science* 847–50.
3. I. Kupfermann, V. Castellucci, H. Pinsker, and E.R. Kandel, 'Neuronal Correlates of Habituation and Dihabituation of the Gill-Withdrawal Reflex in *Aplysia*' (1970) 167 *Science* 1743–5.
4. F.C. Bartlett, 'Karl Spencer Lashley, 1890–1958' (1960) 5 *Biographical Memoirs of Fellows of the Royal Society* 107–18.

14

Polish Insights

(Warsaw, 1967: Jerzy Konorski)

The *Integrative Activity of the Brain*[1] had taken more than three years to prepare, partly because its author had decided to write it in English himself rather than have it translated from his first language, Polish. The invitation to write the book had come from the University of Chicago Press and had followed a successful visit to the United States by the intended author some years earlier.

Jerzy Konorski (Figure 14.1) had been born into a middle-class family in Lodz, Poland in 1903 and, on graduating from high school, had chosen medicine as a career.[2] While studying at Warsaw University the tedium of class work had been alleviated by friendship with a fellow student, Stefan Miller, and by their discovery of the ongoing work of Ivan Pavlov on conditioned reflexes. It was the Russian Pavlov, a Nobel Laureate in 1904 and the head of physiology at the Imperial Institute of Experimental Medicine in St Petersburg, who had demonstrated the formation of conditioned reflexes in the mammalian nervous system.[3] The best-known example had been the automatic salivation of a dog on hearing a bell, the sounding of the bell having previously been associated with the presentation of food. The two young Poles had had ideas of their own, however, and had been able to demonstrate a different form of conditioning. Having no other resources, the impoverished students had used their own limited funds to buy a dog in the Lodz market and toilet paper for their tracings (!).

It had been the start to a remarkable career for Konorski, one that had taken him to St Petersburg to work under Pavlov and then, following his return to Warsaw, to the Nencki Institute. The outbreak of the Second World War and the subsequent Nazi invasion had brought his work to a halt: nevertheless, through the intervention of friends, he had managed to flee the country and to start some research in Russia. Journeying back to Poland at the end of the war he had been confronted by the total destruction of Warsaw, including the Nencki Institute. Most of the former staff had been killed, and Stefan Miller was among the dead. Despite the many obstacles, however, a new Nencki Institute would be built and Konorski would be appointed Head of the Neurophysiology Department. Starting with a skeleton staff, most without a formal university education, Konorski had quickly established teaching and research programmes. The new work and the publication of an earlier book, *Conditioned Reflexes and Neuron Organization*,[4] had brought him to the attention of Western neuroscientists and had resulted in invitations to speak, not only in the United States but elsewhere as well. Curiously, Konorski appears never to have visited Donald Hebb in Montreal, though the work of the McGill

Aranzio's Seahorse and the Search for Memory and Consciousness. Alan J. McComas, Oxford University Press.
© Oxford University Press 2023. DOI: 10.1093/oso/9780192868244.003.0016

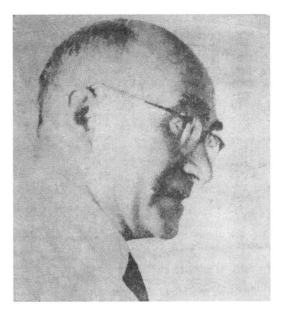

Figure 14.1 Jerzy Konorski (1903–1973) photographed in 1970, three years after the publication of his book and his return to the Nencki Institute in Warsaw (Author unknown. Wikimedia Commons).

psychologists, with their emphasis on finding the neural basis for behaviour, would have attracted him.

Konorski's new book, the 1967 *The Integrative Activity of the Brain*, combined observations in the laboratory with those in the neurology clinic and bulged with original ideas, one of which had to do with memory. It was the concept of gnostic units.

Konorski's proposal was that a sensory system operated as an 'analytic analyser' and consisted of several stages. In the first, information about the environment involved various forms of energy (mechanical, electromagnetic, chemical) being transduced into nerve impulses by sensory receptors (touch domes; Meissner's corpuscles and free nerve endings in the skin, rods, and cones in the retina; taste buds in the tongue; and olfactory receptors in the nose). When the impulse message reached the appropriate receiving area in the brain, some selectivity would occur. In the visual system, for example, there would be a group of neurons only responsive to circular or ovoid objects. These cells, in turn, would pass their information to other populations, one of which would respond only if the oval was a face. This last population would then send impulses to a yet 'higher' set of neurons, of which only one cell (or a small number) would respond, depending on whose face was being viewed. Other sets of neurons would recognize rounded objects as, for example, balloons, car tyres, or dinner plates. The neurons in the final stage of a sensory pathway would be the 'gnostic' (knowing) units and would function as memories (for persons, objects, places, certain sounds, etc.).

The successive categorization of sensory information, with gnostic units at the top of the system, was a bold idea—bold not only because of the way it had been stated but

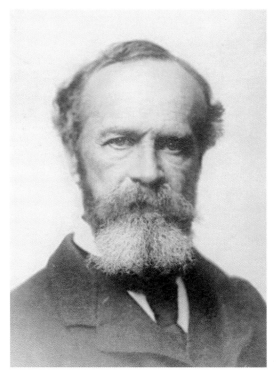

Figure 14.2 William James (1842–1910), a Harvard graduate and later professor, regarded as the founder of American psychology. (Wikimedia Commons.)

also because it ran counter to a popular hypothesis. The latter supposed that information about different aspects of an object or person (colour, shape, movement, etc.) were analysed by different populations of neurons ('parallel processing'). The results of the various analyses were then combined, possibly by the different groups of cells firing impulses rhythmically and synchronously, so as to give the complete perception.

The two contrasting ideas had a long history. In 1890 William James (Figure 14.2), the founder of academic psychology in the United States, had postulated the existence of 'pontifical' cells 'to which our consciousness is attached'.[5] Fifty years later, Charles Sherrington (Figure 14.3), having retired from his position as head of physiology at Oxford to write *Man on his Nature*, would promote the opposite view, that information about any given subject was distributed within the brain.[6]

The matter had been taken up again, this time by a neuroscientist investigating vision. Jerry Lettvin[7] had been a colleague of Patrick Wall at MIT, when they and others had been mapping current flows in the spinal cord. Lettvin had then turned his attention to the visual system of the frog, noting that the ganglion cells in the retina responded most vigorously when shapes suggestive of flies were presented to the eye. The observation suggested that the different types of neuron in the retina interacted in such a way that individual cells became able to recognize meaningful stimuli.

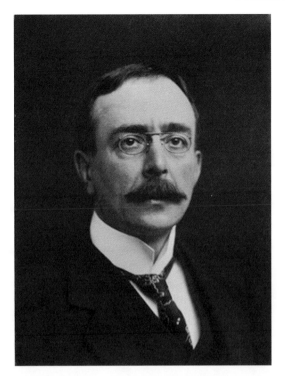

Figure 14.3 Charles Sherrington (1857–1952) photographed in mid-career, probably before his move to Oxford. (Wellcome Images.)

It was he, Lettvin (Figure 14.4), who had impressed upon his students the likelihood of the brain containing pontifical cells, doing so by means of a clever fable of his own invention. The hero of Lettvin's fable was a Russian neurosurgeon capable of ablating each and every neuron containing information about a particular individual—in this case, the patient's mother.[8] Rather than 'mother' cells, however, Lettvin's fictitious neurons became known within the neuroscience community as 'grandmother' cells. At the University of Cambridge Horace Barlow, another vision scientist and one known to Lettvin, had also posited the existence of pontifical cells.[9] He had pointed out, however, that the serial processing of categories would involve ever greater numbers of neurons at each stage. Counter to the hierarchy in the Catholic Church, where a single pope exerted ultimate (pontifical) authority, in a sensory system there would be more 'bishops' than 'parish priests', more 'cardinals' than bishops, and more 'popes' than cardinals.

Though the rival parallel processing scheme had powerful support in the neuroscience community (including that of Francis Crick), there were already a few observations that favoured its alternative. First, neurologists would occasionally encounter patients with an inability to recognize individual faces (*prosopagnosia*). Indeed, the case of one such patient had attracted wide interest, having been described at length by Oliver Sacks ('*The Man Who Mistook His Wife For a Hat*')[10]—the author later

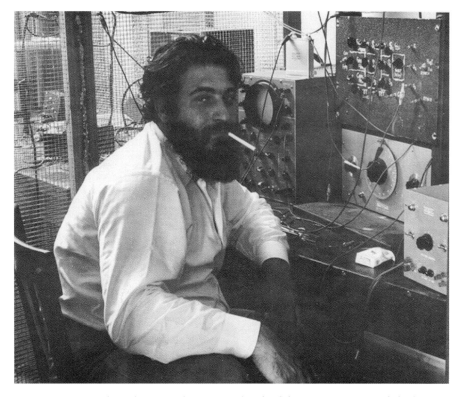

Figure 14.4 Jerome (Jerry) Lettvin (1920–2011) in his laboratory at MIT. While the electrophysiological equipment is similar to that in Eccles' laboratory (see Figure 7.2), Eccles' appearance gives the impression of serious intent whereas Lettvin's, with its relaxed posture and cigarette, suggests a more laid-back approach. The wire mesh is part of a Faraday cage, built to exclude electromagnetic interference. (Creative Commons File: Lettvin Faraday cage.jpg. Attribution-ShareAlike 3.0 License.)

confessing, in his autobiography, that he had been born with the same embarrassing problem. Support for the existence of pontifical cells, though sparse, was also starting to come from the laboratory. Thus Charles Gross, the head of psychology at Harvard, had encountered a neuron in the inferior temporal lobe of a monkey that responded specifically to the shape of a hand.[11] And then there had been the handful of highly selective cells in the cat amygdala that John O'Keefe had found responsive to such diverse stimuli as birdsong, an item of food, or the presence of a mouse.

But back to Konorski's book. Following its publication, the *Integrative Activity of the Brain* had been favourably reviewed (by Charles Gross) and then … nothing. Despite its originality and the high professional standing of its author, the book did not sell well, at least in the West. Commenting afterwards, Konorski concluded that he had packed too much information into a single volume and admitted that it would not have been easy reading. For the few that had struggled through it, however, the concept of 'gnostic units' was powerful and the term would eventually find its place in contemporary neuroscience alongside its cousins, the pontifical cells of William James and the grand-mother cells of Jerry Lettvin.

It would take a further 40 years before the question of gnostic units was finally re-solved, however.

Notes

1. J. Konorski, *Integrative Activity of the Brain: An Interdisciplinary Approach* (Chicago, IL: University of Chicago Press, 1967).

2. J. Konorski, *A History of Psychology in Autobiography*, G Lindzey (ed.) (Engelwood Cliffs, NJ: Prentice-Hall, 1974) 6: 185–217..

3. Ivan Pavlov (1849–1936) was influenced by his eminent countryman Ivan Sechenov (1829–1905) to pursue physiology as a career. Pavlov's greatest success was the experimental production of conditioned reflexes in dogs, and this led him to an explanation of human behaviour. Despite his public criticisms of the Soviet government, Pavlov managed to escape Stalin's purges of the country's intelligentsia. No doubt the applicability of Pavlov's ideas to government control and his award of a Nobel Prize in 1904 assisted in his survival.

4. J. Konorski, *Conditioned Reflexes and Neuron Organization* (Cambridge: Cambridge University Press, 1948).

5. W. James, *The Principles of Psychology* (New York, NY: Dover, 1890).

6. C.S. Sherrington, *Man on His Nature* (Cambridge: Cambridge University Press, 1940).

7. J. Lettvin, *The History of Neuroscience in Autobiography*, L.R. Squire (ed.) (San Diego: Academic Press, 1998) 2: 222–43.

8. The fable has been reproduced in: A.J. McComas, *Sherrington's Loom. An Introduction to the Science of Consciousness* (New York, NY: Oxford University Press, 2019).

9. H.B. Barlow, 'Single Units and Sensation: A Neuron Doctrine for Perceptual Psychology' (1972) 1 *Perception* 371–94. (Other than being remarkable for his research on vision and on sensory mech-anisms generally, Horace Barlow, a great-grandson of Charles Darwin, has continued to teach at Cambridge into his late nineties).

10. O. Sacks, *The Man Who Mistook His Wife for a Hat and Other Clinical Tales* (New York, NY: Simon & Schuster, 1985).

11. C.G. Gross, D.B. Bender, and C.E. Rocha-Miranda, 'Visual Receptive Fields of Neurons in Inferotemporal Cortex of the Monkey' (1969) 166 *Science* 1303–6.

15

Continuing Excitation in Norway

(Oslo, 1968: Terje Lømo, Timothy Bliss)

Per Andersen had returned to Oslo after working with Eccles in Australia. He could have stayed longer in Canberra had he wished because Eccles had appreciated the advantages of having a knowledgeable neuroanatomist in his department. Though more a neurophysiologist, Andersen's familiarity with brain structure had ultimately been responsible for Eccles turning his attention to the hippocampus and cerebellum.

Back in his home city, Andersen was now in a position to exploit the knowledge and the experimental techniques acquired in Canberra and, in turn, to pass these on to younger scientists. One possible recruit had been encountered while walking in the city. Terje Lømo, a medical graduate of Oslo University, had been on leave from the Norwegian Navy and was looking for a job. Aware that Lømo had done a year's research in Pisa following his medical graduation, work that had entailed recording from single neurons in the visual cortex of awake rabbits, Andersen suggested that Lømo study for a PhD under his, Andersen's, supervision.

The doctoral research would be on the hippocampus, specifically on the responses of cells in the dentate nucleus to stimulation of afferent nerve fibres in the perforant pathway. Andersen had already looked at this system and had found that, if the electrical stimuli had been delivered in a high-frequency burst, the responses of the dentate neurons remained enlarged for several seconds, even half a minute. It had been an interesting finding but not unlike the kind of result obtained in experiments elsewhere—in the spinal cord, for example. The phenomenon had been termed post-tetanic potentiation (PTP) and David Lloyd, while working at the Rockefeller Institute, had shown that, even in the case of a simple monosynaptic reflex (the circuit responsible for the knee-jerk), the potentiation could last for three to four minutes.[1] By the simple expedient of testing with a nerve that had not been stimulated repetitively as well as with one that had, Lloyd had further demonstrated that a change in the tetanized nerve endings was the most likely cause of the potentiation. John Eccles, in a study with Krešimir Krnjević in Canberra, had confirmed Lloyd's finding and extended it by inserting recording microelectrodes inside the sensory nerve fibres.[2] The two had observed transient increases in the membrane potentials of the fibres and speculated that these might result in additional chemical transmitter being released at the synapses with the motoneurons—thereby accounting for the potentiation. The importance of the spinal cord reflex experiments had not attracted much attention at the time the results had been published, however, possibly because there were so many other parts of

Aranzio's Seahorse and the Search for Memory and Consciousness. Alan J. McComas, Oxford University Press.
© Oxford University Press 2023. DOI: 10.1093/oso/9780192868244.003.0017

the nervous system waiting to be explored with the new technique of microelectrode recording.

By the time he embarked on work for his thesis, Lømo (Figure 15.1) had already gained useful laboratory experience, having participated in experiments on the thalamus with Per Andersen. For his new studies, he decided to experiment on anaesthetized rabbits and to stimulate the nerve fibres entering the hippocampus repetitively, but using repeated bouts rather than the customary single one.[3] It was immediately clear from the first results that something important was happening to the synapses in the hippocampus—the evoked responses became larger, added new components, and shortened their latencies. However, these change were not only observed during the course of a single bout of stimulation but were still detectable after a seven-minute period of rest. And, as the bouts of stimulation continued, the changes remained well-developed for at least an hour, much longer than the few minutes of potentiation that Lloyd and Eccles had observed in their respective spinal cord reflex studies. Lømo had discovered a new phenomenon—*long-term potentiation* (LTP)—and shown it to be a property of the mammalian hippocampus.

The new findings were presented as a communication, given by Lømo to the Scandinavian Physiological Society at a meeting in Finland in 1966. With the claim to the discovery of LTP established, albeit in a short abstract,[4] it would have been natural for an investigator, especially a young one like Lømo, to drop all his/her other interests

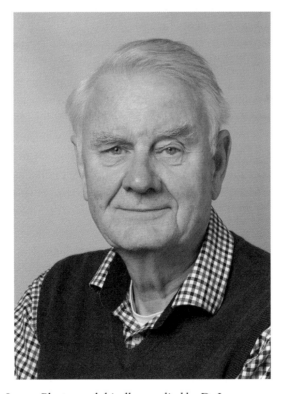

Figure 15.1 Terje Lømo. Photograph kindly supplied by Dr Lømo.

and to work night and day building on the early results and exploiting the new finding to the full. Though Lømo appreciated that LTP could be important for learning and memory, he did not change direction, partly because he was not yet confident in his understanding of the neural mechanisms involved. There was also the doctoral thesis that had to be written and for which Lømo was obtaining good experimental data, data suggestive of the pattern of excitation within the hippocampus following electric stimulation of the perforant pathway. Besides, as Lømo was to remark afterwards, there was no sense of urgency over the newly found LTP phenomenon, even though he had recognized its possible significance for memory. In the end a full paper on LTP did not appear until 1971.[5]

It was while he was still experimenting for his PhD that Lømo was introduced to a visitor from Canada. Timothy Bliss had been born and raised in the United Kingdom but had gone to Montreal for doctoral studies under Ben Delisle Burns. The latter, a member of the physiology department at McGill, was well known for his research on the electrical activity generated in isolated slabs of cerebral cortex. It was a preparation that Burns had perfected, one that remained in good condition despite having had all the nerve fibres entering and leaving the slab severed. Bliss' interest had been in learning and memory, however, and for these the slab preparation had no particular advantages. After graduation, Bliss had approached Per Andersen with the intention of working in Oslo. He had known of Andersen's experience with the hippocampus, including the work with Eccles in Australia, and Bliss suspected that its simpler structure, in comparison with cortex elsewhere, would be an experimental advantage. Andersen, in turn, had brought Bliss to see Lømo.

Though Lømo was still writing his thesis, he was able to spare time to experiment on the rabbit hippocampus with Bliss. Once again, when repeated bursts of high-frequency stimuli were delivered to incoming fibres, the hippocampal neurons gave larger and more complex responses that were maintained for long periods. Lømo's earlier findings that were indicative of LTP were confirmed and extended. By 1969, however, the experiments were over. His thesis submitted and successfully defended, Terje Lømo was off to University College London to broaden his research experience. Timothy Bliss was in London, too, having returned to his laboratory at Mill Hill. While there, he would see Lømo from time to time but also a third person who had become interested in LTP and was investigating it—Tony Gardner-Medwin in the Department of Physiology at University College London (UCL). With Bliss as his partner, Gardner-Medwin had been looking for potentiated responses in rabbits that differed from Lømo's in not being anaesthetized. In order to do this, stimulating and recording wire electrodes had been implanted in the hippocampus and cemented in place during a preliminary procedure. As in Lømo's rabbits, potentiation of responses following earlier stimulation was evident and could even be detected after three days, but it was much more variable and in some experiments appeared to be absent altogether. Had it not been for Gardner-Medwin's energy and drive, Lømo and Bliss might have delayed writing up their own hippocampal work still further. As it was, two papers, one by Bliss and Lømo and the other by Bliss and Gardner-Medwin appeared in the *Journal of Physiology* in 1973.[6,7]

At UCL Lømo's new scientific home was the Biophysics Department. This department, founded by the Nobel Laureate AV Hill, was now headed by Bernard Katz. Like Eric Kandel, Katz had been a Jewish refugee from Europe prior to the outbreak of the Second World War.[8] Almost penniless, he had been taken on by AV Hill[9] and, following a PhD, had gone to Australia to help John Eccles set up his neurophysiology research unit in a Sydney hospital. At the end of the war Katz had returned to UCL and was now a departmental head. Very active in research, especially on the neuromuscular junction, Katz was attracting outstanding research fellows and even senior scientists to work with him.

One of Katz's achievements had been to show that neurotransmitter molecules were stored in small vesicles within nerve endings. When an impulse invaded the nerve terminals, it allowed calcium ions to enter and to release neurotransmitter from the vesicles into the narrow cleft which, in the case of the neuromuscular junction, separated the nerve ending from the muscle fibre membrane. Though so much of the pioneering work was being done on the neuromuscular junction, it had enabled the general rules of chemically mediated synaptic transmission elsewhere in the nervous system to be determined. Katz had been awarded a Nobel Prize in 1969, the year that Lømo had come to work in his department.

Sharing a laboratory with his collaborator, Jean Rosenthal, Terje Lømo was soon immersed in his new research. It had nothing to do with the hippocampus but everything to do with the relationship between muscle fibres and their nerve supply. Was the prevailing belief really true, that the nerve fibres not only excited the muscle fibres but, through the release of special 'trophic' molecules, governed many of the features of the muscle fibres? The new field of enquiry had originated as an unexpected result of the muscle cross-innervation experiments that John Eccles, Rose Eccles, and Arthur Buller had conducted in Canberra in 1958.[10] The topic was much to Lømo's liking and he became ever more skilled at devising methods to explore neurotrophism.

When not experimenting he had the opportunity to meet and observe a number of eminent neuroscientists in the department. There was his own supervisor, Ricardo Miledi, widely respected for his original ideas and fine dissections. Among others there was the future Nobel Laureate, Bert Sakmann, from Germany[11]—and, of course, the Head of the department, Bernard Katz. Then, if he worked his way through a warren of stairs and corridors, the young Norwegian would have found himself in the UCL Department of Physiology among yet more neuroscientists. It was a department that valued tradition, having been the first of its kind in Britain, and the names of two of its most illustrious members (William Bayliss and Ernest Starling)[12] were still visible in gilt lettering on the doors of their former laboratories. Like Biophysics, the department was headed by a Nobel Laureate—Andrew Huxley, a winner in 1963 with Alan Hodgkin and John Eccles. Were he to push further on inside the building, Terje Lømo would have entered the Anatomy Department and in one of its rooms might have met John O'Keefe. That young man, an American, was, like Lømo, at an early stage of his research career but had come to UCL to work under Patrick Wall in the Cerebral Functions Unit.

Back in his own laboratory, engaged in his muscle studies and never far from a famous neuroscientist, it is unlikely that Lømo would have been giving much thought to the fate of his publication with Bliss in the *Journal of Physiology*. Perhaps it would not have surprised or disconcerted him to learn that hardly anyone had bothered to read it—and to appreciate its great significance for memory research. Had they, Bliss and Lømo, not shown that granule cells in the hippocampus could hold the memory of an earlier stimulation for hours?

If Terje Lømo had continued hippocampal research, or had talked and written about what he and Bliss had observed, attention might have been directed much sooner to long-term potentiation and its likely role in the creation of memory (this would have been the strategy of the 'Bellman Principle').[13] On the other hand, Lømo could not be faulted for switching fields. Muscle and its control by the nervous system had become a very exciting area of research. As already noted, there were possible trophic factors involved, the contrasting effects on muscle of exercise and disuse, and perhaps application of the new findings to diseases such as muscular dystrophy and spinal muscular atrophy. Indeed, both at UCL and after his return to Oslo, Lømo would continue to make important contributions to neuromuscular research.

There is also this—the hippocampus would probably not have yielded much more information with the classical electrophysiological techniques of electrical stimulation and recording that Lømo, Bliss, and Gardner-Medwin had used. As Kandel had concluded years before, if one wished to obtain detailed information, including changes at a cellular or molecular level, it would be better to study memory in a simple organism such as *Aplysia*.

When the next big advance in hippocampal research came, it was not through any result of electrical stimulation, but rather through the observation of a rat wandering round its cage. It did involve the recording of impulses, however, and it did involve someone working in the same building as Terje Lømo at UCL. Someone that Lømo had already met.

John O'Keefe.

Notes

1. D.P.C. Lloyd, 'Post-Tetanic Potentiation of Response in Monosynaptic Reflex Pathways of the Spinal Cord' (1949) 33 *Journal of General Physiology* 147–70.
2. J.C. Eccles and K. Krnjević, 'Presynaptic Changes Associated with Post-Tetanic Potentiation in the Spinal Cord' (1959) 149(2) *Journal of Physiology* 274–87.
3. Lømo's life and research is given in: T. Lømo, *The History of Neuroscience in Autobiography*, L.R. Squire (ed.) (San Diego, CA: Academic Press, 2011) 7: 382–436.
4. T. Lømo, 'Frequency Potentiation of Excitatory Synaptic Activity in the Dentate Area of the Hippocampal Formation' (1966) 68(Suppl 277) *Acta Physiologica Scandinavica* 128.
5. T. Lømo, 'Potentiation of Monosynaptic EPSPS in the Perforant Path-Dentate Granule Cell Synapse' (1971) 12 *Experimental Brain Research* 46–63.
6. T.V.P. Bliss and T. Lømo, 'Long-Lasting Potentiation of Synaptic Transmission in the Dentate Area of the Anaesthetized Rabbit Following Stimulation of the Perforant Path' (1973) 232 *Journal of Physiology* 331–56.

7. T.V.P. Bliss and A.R. Gardner-Medwin, 'Long-lasting Potentiation of Synaptic Transmission in the Dentate Area of the Unanaesthetized Rabbit Following Stimulation of the Perforant Path' (1973) 232 *Journal of Physiology* 1973; 357–74.

8. Sir Bernard Katz (1911–2003) tells of his early years in Germany, move to the United Kingdom, Second World War experience in Australia (after working there with Eccles and Kuffler), and return to the United Kingdom and to neuromuscular research in: B. Katz, *The History of Neuroscience in Autobiography*, L.R. Squire (ed.) (Washington, DC: Society for Neuroscience, 1996) 1: 348–81.xyz

9. Archibald Vivian Hill (1886–1977) was an early British biophysicist who studied heat production in muscle and peripheral nerve, as well as muscle contraction. He was awarded a Nobel Prize for his work in 1922. Hill was also involved in politics and was an outspoken critic of Hitler and Nazism prior to the Second World War. In the First World War he had carried out important gunnery research.

10. See Chapter 7.

11. Bert Sakmann (1942–) is a German neuroscientist who shared the 1991 Nobel Prize in Physiology or Medicine with Erwin Neher. Together they introduced 'patch clamping' for investigating single ion channels in membranes; the technique was to enclose the channel within the tip of a microelectrode sealed to the membrane and then to measure the ionic current flowing through the channel.

12. In 1902 William Bayliss and Ernest Starling discovered a chemical messenger in the bloodstream, one that was released from the duodenal mucosa to produce a flow of digestive secretions from the pancreas. The UCL physiologists gave the name 'secretin' to this particular chemical messenger and 'hormone' to the class of substances with similarly remote actions.

13. The Bellman is the character in Lewis Carroll's nonsense poem, 'The Hunting of the Snark' who declares 'What I tell you three times is true'. It was Sir Andrew Huxley who introduced the term 'Bellman Principle' in a historical essay on research into muscle contraction.

16

Revelation on Gower Street

(London, 1971: Patrick Wall, John O'Keefe)

When John O'Keefe had met Terje Lømo for the first time at University College London (UCL), it was because the Norwegian had sought advice on implanting electrodes in freely moving animals. That O'Keefe should have been in the Anatomy Department was Patrick Wall's doing.

Patrick Wall had returned to the United Kingdom in 1967. His time in the United States had been scientifically profitable. Among other achievements he had discovered presynaptic inhibition in the mammalian spinal cord and, with Ronald Melzack, had gone on to develop the gate theory of pain. He had enjoyed the intellectual freedom of the US university system and the generous research funding. And there had been the delightful eccentricity of some of his colleagues—Jerry Lettvin, for example.

The invitation to return had come from one of Britain's intellectual giants. John Zachary Young ('JZ' to his colleagues; Figure 16.1) was a descendant of Thomas Young, the 19th-century amateur scientist. Independently of Helmholtz in Germany, the illustrious ancestor had been responsible for proposing a trichromatic theory of human colour vision; he had also, with enviable versatility, helped to decipher the Rosetta Stone.[1] And were that not enough, there had been the investigation of elasticity and discovery of (Young's) modulus. JZ Young, the descendant, had been a contemporary of John Eccles, though not in Sherrington's laboratory, when the two had studied at Oxford for their D.Phil degrees in the 1920s. With a strong interest in the nervous system, JZ Young had worked on peripheral nerve injuries and nerve regeneration during the Second World War. He had then turned his attention to the nervous system of the octopus, recognizing the intelligent behaviours of which the creature was capable. In the course of the latter work he had discovered (independently of Harvard's Leonard Williams earlier) the giant axon of the squid, drawing attention to its potential for electrical studies of nerve membranes. It was this preparation that Alan Hodgkin and Andrew Huxley has exploited so brilliantly in their voltage clamp experiments, work that had gained them Nobel Prizes (with John Eccles) in 1963.[2]

At the time of his approach to Patrick Wall, Young had been Head of the Anatomy Department at University College London for 20 years. His appointment had been controversial because of his non-medical background and lack of any training in gross anatomy. Nevertheless, it had been an inspired move on the part of the university. JZ Young was an academic star, one well known to the public through his Reith

Aranzio's Seahorse and the Search for Memory and Consciousness. Alan J. McComas, Oxford University Press.
© Oxford University Press 2023. DOI: 10.1093/oso/9780192868244.003.0018

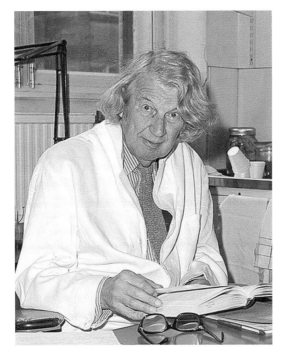

Figure 16.1 John Zachary ('JZ') Young in his room at the Wellcome Institute following his retirement from University College London. (Creative Commons Attribution 4.0 international license.)

Lectures for the BBC. Even before Wall's recruitment, the Anatomy Department had several prominent members. Lionel Hamlyn and Brian Cragg had made their neuro-physiological study of the mammalian hippocampus (preceding Eric Kandel and Alden Spencer's), David Sholl had computed the excitatory contributions of dendritic branches, while George Gray had shown it possible to distinguish between excitatory and inhibitory synapses with the electron microscope and to identify synapses respon-sible for the newly discovered presynaptic inhibition.[3]

Physically, JZ Young and Patrick Wall made an interesting contrast. The former was a large, untidy man, given to wearing a white coat in the department. With a full head of grey hair, irregular teeth, and usually sporting a red tie, Young had an aura of great energy. Patrick Wall was rather smaller, wore spectacles, and had a bushy beard to compensate for his baldness. Rather than vigour, one was struck by Wall's deep thought and his carefully considered way of expressing ideas and opinions. A chain smoker, he would invariably have a cigarette in one hand while gesturing with the other. Both men were excellent speakers; indeed, Wall's students were known to some-times applaud him at the end of a lecture, having recognized the originality of his ideas and his way of inviting the audience to think as he did. It was more than an enthusiasm for neuroscience that the two men shared, however, for both were far to the left in their politics. Wall had been a member of the Communist Party while Young's socialism was reflected in his red ties.

It was to this environment that John O'Keefe (Figure 16.2) had come in 1967, having been recommended by his PhD supervisor, Ronald Melzack, co-founder of the gate theory of pain. London was far from Montreal and New York, but his new environment suited O'Keefe. For one thing, University College, more than any of the other London University colleges, was a hot bed of scientific research. By 1967 there had already been 16 Nobel Laureates in science, all of them men who, like AV Hill and Andrew Huxley, had either been educated at UCL or who had worked there for varying periods of time.

Despite all its academic activity, the College, in the northern fringe of Bloomsbury, looked much as it had in 1836, the year of its founding. On the opposite side of Gower Street was the imposing red-brick Gothic oddity of University College Hospital where, among others of distinction, William Gowers had taught neurology, Victor Horsley had operated, and Francis Walshe had acquired his clinical skills. Further down the street were the elegant grey Georgian terraces, a number of them distinguished by blue historical plaques.[4]

Running parallel with Gower Street, just beyond the hospital and nurses' home, was Tottenham Court Road, a busy street that had three Underground stations and, almost as important, several stores selling second-hand electronic equipment. It was in these Aladdin's caves that an earlier generation of researchers had been able to buy ex-War Department oscilloscopes, amplifiers, motors, meters, solenoids, and gauges. Building one's laboratory equipment had been a rite of passage for an aspiring electrophysi-ologist but, by the time of O'Keefe's arrival, the beautifully engineered amplifiers and

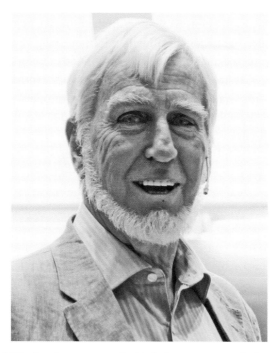

Figure 16.2 John O'Keefe, after winning the Nobel Prize. Original photo in colour. (Author, Per Henning/NTNU; Wikimedia Commons CC BY 2.0.)

oscilloscopes of Tetronix and Hewlett-Packard, and the stimulators and strain gauges of Grass, had made this task unnecessary.

Entering the large UCL quadrangle though the wrought iron gates, O'Keefe would have been confronted by the handsome colonnaded portico and domed roof of the main building (Figure 16.3). Inside, he might have been astonished to find a glass-fronted wooden cabinet housing the clothed body of Jeremy Bentham, the 18th-century social reformer and agitator for higher education.

London, then. Still preoccupied with the function of the descending nerve fibre pathways from the cortex to sensory nuclei, Patrick Wall had suggested to O'Keefe that he make recordings from single sensory neurons in the brainstem of freely moving rats. The unanswered question in Wall's mind concerned the possibility that the descending fibres controlled the flow of information to 'higher' processing sites in the brain. Having settled into his office, John O'Keefe, the newest member of UCL's Cerebral Functions Unit, attempted to find the answer.

O'Keefe had developed expertise in Montreal for recording from single cells in the amygdala of unrestrained cats and Patrick Wall had already had some success with similar technology in the rat spinal cord. Soon O'Keefe had a rat moving around in its cage. A plastic block cemented to its head gave the rat an unusual, top-hatted, appearance. A hole in the skull enabled passage of one or more stiff tungsten wire electrodes, their joint movement controlled by a microdrive attached to the block; independent electrode adjustments could then be made by screws. The potentials from the rat brain

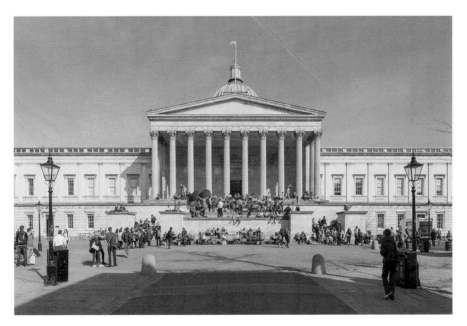

Figure 16.3 University College London. The view is of the Wilkins Building; the anatomy, physiology, and biophysics departments are off to the right and front directly on to the Gower Street sidewalk. (Photograph by David Iliff; Wikimedia Commons file: Wilkins Building 1, UCL, London-Diliff.jpg. License CC BY-SA 3.0.)

were fed into a miniature amplifier on the microdrive and then through a light and flexible cable to larger equipment in the laboratory. It was a very elegant system.

And so the search for responsive neurons began.[5,6]

Disappointingly, the experiments, first in the dorsal column nuclei and then in the thalamus, yielded little of interest. And then, just as had happened with James Olds and Peter Milner in Montreal, with David Hubel and Torsten Wiesel in Boston, and with Arthur Buller, John and Rose Eccles in Canberra, there was a chance observation that would prove a turning point. As with Olds and Milner, it was a misplaced recording electrode. Rather than entering the thalamus, as intended, the tip of the electrode had penetrated the hippocampus. O'Keefe was immediately struck by the behaviour of one of the hippocampal neurons, noting that it fired impulses whenever the animal moved and that the impulses coincided with the appearance of 7–10 Hz electric oscillations in cells surrounding the electrode tip.

His interest piqued, O'Keefe abandoned the thalamus for the hippocampus. It was at this time that he was joined by Jonathan Dostrovsky, a Master's student from Canada. The two would spend hours observing their top-hatted rats as the animals went about their daily business—searching for food, grooming, drinking, pressing a lever, and exploring. It eventually became clear that there were at least two types of (pyramidal) neuron in the hippocampus. One type, the 'theta' neuron, was frequently active, firing whenever the rat moved. It was the vigour rather than the nature of the movement that seemed to matter, and, as with the first such cell encountered, the impulses were associated with electrical oscillations in neighbouring units.[7]

The second type of neuron presented a puzzle. Unlike a theta cell, it would only discharge occasionally and then less strongly. After many days of rat-watching, O'Keefe finally realized what it was that made such a cell fire—it was the position within its surroundings that the rat happened to be in. Whenever the animal returned to the same position, the same cell would fire. When it moved to another position, a different neuron would discharge, and do so consistently. The behaviour of the cells was a totally unexpected solution to the mystery. 'Place' cells had been discovered in the mammalian hippocampus. Further, O'Keefe realized that information from a number of place cells would enable the rat to construct a spatial map in its hippocampus, the extent and orientation of the map depending largely on what the animal could see.

The finding of place cells and of their employment in creating a map of the space surrounding an animal would be recognized as a major advance in brain science, one that would eventually lead to a Nobel Prize for John O'Keefe. And yet, as sometimes happens, the importance of the discovery was not obvious at the time. A paper by O'Keefe and Dostrovsky, published in *Brain Research*,[8] barely attracted attention in the neuroscience community.

But it was not completely ignored. In New York Jim Ranck was doing similar experiments but interpreting the results rather differently. He would subsequently discover in the entorhinal cortex, adjacent to the hippocampus, neurons responsive to the direction of the rat's head. Meanwhile O'Keefe realized additional information for a spatial map could come from some of the 'theta' cells firing impulses when the rat moved to a new position; the speed of the movement would be proportional to the distance travelled between the two points. O'Keefe termed these the 'displace' cells. Another category was 'misplace' cells—those neurons that fired when the rat visited an earlier location, apparently in the expectation of finding a familiar object there. Yet another category to be identified was the 'boundary' cell, a neuron that fired as the rat approached a limiting wall. At a behavioural level, O'Keefe was able to show that rats with hippocampal lesions were no longer able to navigate a water maze successfully—further evidence supporting the idea of the intact hippocampus creating spatial maps.

It was exciting work and the excitement was felt by anyone fortunate enough to see John O'Keefe's video of a rat exploring its environment. As one watched, and as the place cells fired in response to the various locations of the animal, there it was, taking shape before the observer's eyes—a spatial map in the hippocampus. But, as would become evident in the years to come, the hippocampus, and the structures around it, had other secrets awaiting discovery.

Notes

1. Discovered in 1799 during Napoleon's invasion of Egypt, the Rosetta stone was inscribed in 196 BC with a Ptolemaic royal decree written in two Ancient Egyptian and one Ancient Greek languages. The decipherment enabled the Ancient Egyptian hieroglyphic system to be understood for the first time.

2. A recent account of the Hodgkin–Huxley studies on the giant axon, and of preceding and later research on the nature of the nerve impulse is given in: A.J. McComas, *Galvani's Spark. The Story of the Nerve Impulse* (New York, NY: Oxford University Press, 2011).

3. George Gray had been appointed as research assistant to JZ Young but his brilliance in developing electron microscopic techniques for examining the central nervous system and his important discoveries relating to synaptic structure led to his eventual appointment as Professor of Anatomy at UCL and to Fellowship of the Royal Society. See: R.W. Guillery, 'Edward George Gray. 11 January 1924–14 August 1999' (2002) 48 *Biographical Memoirs of Fellows of the Royal Society of London* 151–65.

4. Charles Dickens had lived on Gower Street as a boy and for three years Charles Darwin had rented a cottage, long since demolished.

5. The best account of the O'Keefe's initial and subsequent research at UCL is given in his Nobel lecture: J O'Keefe, 'Nobel Lecture. Spatial Cells in the Hippocampal Formation' <https://www.nobelprize.org/prizes/medicine/2014/okeefe/lecture> accessed 22 April 2022.

6. O'Keefe's autobiography until the award of the Nobel Prize is: O'Keefe J. Biographical. Nobel Prize in Physiology or Medicine, 2014 <https://www.nobelprize.org/prizes/medicine/2014/okeefe/biographical> accessed 22 April 2022.

7. In his Nobel Lecture and in other publications, O'Keefe refers the 6–10 Hz oscillations as 'theta' oscillations, and this designation has been used by others in the field. In fact, the oscillations are as much 'alpha' (7.5–13 Hz) as 'theta' (3.5–7.5 Hz), using the standard electroencephalogram definitions of brain rhythms.

8. J. O'Keefe and J. Dostrovsky, 'The Hippocampus as a Spatial Map. Preliminary Evidence from Unit Activity in the Freely-Moving rat' (1971) 34 *Brain Research* 171–5.

17

Mathematics and the Hippocampus

(Cambridge, United Kingdom, 1971: David Marr)

While John O'Keefe and Jonathan Dostrovsky were discovering place cells in the hippocampus, a young man working not far away had seen his paper on the hippocampus appear in print. Unlike previous publications on that structure, it had not involved any laboratory work. Nevertheless, the paper was immediately recognized for its originality and for its importance for understanding how the hippocampus might operate. Almost a half-century later it would still be cited frequently and it might have occurred to more than one reader that, were it possible for scientific genius to be revealed in biology (as opposed to mathematics and physics), the paper by David Marr would be a prime example.

Marr (Figure 17.1) was 26 when his paper on the hippocampus had appeared in the July 1971 issue of the *Philosophical Transactions of the Royal Society of London*.[1] It followed publications on the cerebral cortex (1969)[2] and cerebellum (1970)[3] that were similarly original. All three were the outcome of work that he had carried out as a graduate student at Cambridge.

As a schoolboy Marr had become keenly interested in the brain and influenced by books such as Grey Walter's *The Living Brain*.[4] With his flair for mathematics, Marr was already wondering if it might be possible to produce a mathematical description of the way the brain operated.[5] Having been awarded an open scholarship, he went to Cambridge in the fall of 1963 as a member of Trinity College (Figure 17.2). The College was the best possible choice for a young person with scientific ambition. Founded by Henry VIII in 1546, it had become the largest, wealthiest, and most scientifically accomplished of all the Cambridge (and Oxford) colleges. It was where Isaac Newton had had his rooms and where, centuries later, its Fellows had included JJ Thompson (discoverer of the electron), Ernest Rutherford (structure of the atom), and the Braggs, father and son (X-ray crystallography). By the time of Marr's admission, Trinity College had already been credited with 21 Nobel Prizes, the last two having been awarded to Alan Hodgkin and Andrew Huxley for their discovery of the ion fluxes through nerve membranes that enabled nerve impulses to be created and transmitted. Andrew Huxley had been a strong mathematician himself and it is likely that David Marr would have appreciated the derivation and implications of the Hodgkin–Huxley equations.

At the time of Marr's entry, Cambridge, despite the presence of the university, was still a small town in the Fens, yet to expand with high-tech companies around its periphery. As they had done for centuries, the market area and the university formed its

Aranzio's Seahorse and the Search for Memory and Consciousness. Alan J. McComas, Oxford University Press.
© Oxford University Press 2023. DOI: 10.1093/oso/9780192868244.003.0019

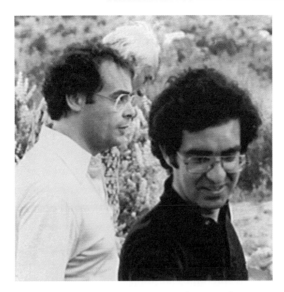

Figure 17.1 David Marr (left) and Tomasio Poggio, after Marr's move to the United States; part of Francis Crick's head is also shown. Courtesy of Dr Vaina Lucia.

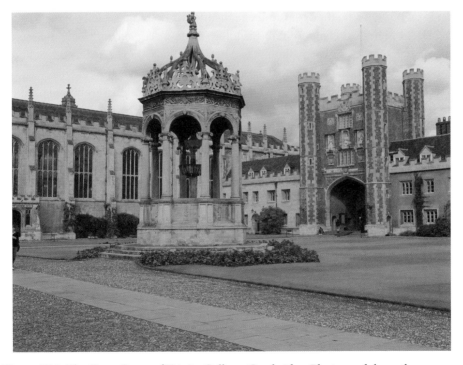

Figure 17.2 The Great Court of Trinity College, Cambridge. Photograph by author.

core. All the old colleges are beautiful, the weathered stonework of the buildings complementing the strong but tasteful colours of the perennials in the gardens and the deep green of the manicured lawns within the courts. Like its college neighbours, Trinity backs on to the river and the meadows while at the front the Great Court separates it from the narrow Trinity Lane.

After obtaining a Bachelor of Arts (BA) in mathematics David Marr, still with a keen interest in the brain, studied physiology and anatomy before electing to work for a PhD in physiology under the guidance of Giles Brindley. For David Marr it would have been a short walk from the college through the market and Corn Exchange to the Physiological Laboratory in Downing Street where Brindley had an office and laboratory. The choice of Brindley as supervisor was a good one. A lean, energetic, and highly intelligent man, one able to combine theory with practical skill in the workshop, Brindley had shown himself capable of tackling many types of problem.[6] As an undergraduate he had had a piece about the scintillations of stars published in *Nature* and as a musician he had designed and built a computer-operated bassoon. As a physiologist he had made original observations on colour vision, and would later stimulate the visual cortex of a blind person with an implanted electrode array, and design and build neural prostheses for bladder emptying in patients with spinal cord injuries. Famously, there had been an occasion when, in front of an audience of surgeons, Brindley had demonstrated on himself a method for producing penile erection in disabled patients. At the time David Marr had come to him, Brindley was preoccupied with neural circuitry and especially that of the cerebellum. It had been his suggestion that Marr might like to apply his mathematical prowess to the cerebellum.

The cerebellum ('small brain') had, like the frontal lobes, long been an enigma to physiologists. Situated at the back of the brain under the cerebral hemispheres, it covered the posterior surface of the brain stem. The grey matter forming its heavily wrinkled surface contained far more neurons than the cerebral cortex and, under the microscope, the arrangement of cells and fibres was uniform throughout. Damage to the cerebellum by injury or disease, or maldevelopment during infancy, caused voluntary movements to become clumsy and tremulous but left consciousness unaffected. It was a structure that had attracted the interest of the Master of Trinity College, Edgar Adrian, during the difficult Second World War years when he had been in charge of the depleted Cambridge Physiological Laboratory. By recording from cats and monkeys Adrian had shown that there was a map of the body surface in the cerebellum, just as there was in the cerebral cortex.[7] The cerebellar studies had come towards the end of Adrian's long and successful career, a career that had brought him a Nobel Prize in 1932 and a baronetcy in 1955.[8]

Marr might have seen Adrian (Figure 17.3) during his occasional appearances in the Physiological Laboratory and, like other Trinity undergraduates, would certainly have witnessed him presiding at the college dinners, sitting at the centre of the High Table with the full-length portrait of Henry VIII, the College's founder, on the wall behind him. Looking at the frail elderly man, with the gaunt cheeks and gold-framed spectacles, few could have imagined the young lion of Adrian's youth. He had been

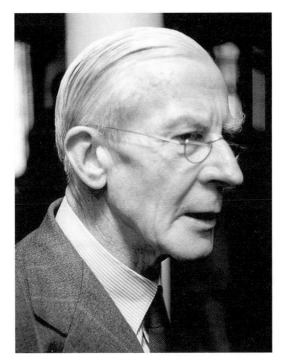

Figure 17.3 Edgar, Lord Adrian, at the time he was Master of Trinity College and following his retirement from the Cambridge Physiological Laboratory. (Wellcome Images. Creative Commons Attribution 4.0 International license.)

one of the daring few who had climbed the Cambridge college walls at night, he had fenced for the university and he had been an accomplished mountaineer. As a neuro-physiologist his skill had been in asking a question of the nervous system and then carrying out an experiment that was sufficient to answer it. The experiments were never elegant—bits and pieces of equipment were strung together and the recordings were often poor—but they were good enough to answer Adrian's question. Indeed, 'simple but good enough' was very much the Cambridge scientific credo at the time. Adrian's other skill was in his writing; there was an elegance of expression and a profundity of thought that none of his contemporaries could match.

David Marr's approach was very different to Adrian's. Whereas Adrian had delighted in laboratory work, Marr would not do any experiments but would draw on the results of others. Instead of electrodes, Marr would probe the nervous system with mathematical equations.

Initially with Brindley's guidance, Marr had tackled the cerebellum and would then move on to the neocortex and, finally, the hippocampus. In each instance his approach had been the same. First, he described in mathematical terms the problem(s) that had to be solved by the brain structure. After the *computational level* came the *algorithmic level*; here he considered how the information in the nervous system was represented and the operations required for processing it. Finally, there was the *implemental level*, when Marr made use of the known neuroanatomy and neurophysiology to suggest how the algorithms might be executed.

In the case of the cerebellum Marr had drawn heavily on the experimental work of Eccles and his group in Canberra.[9] For the neocortex he had been influenced by its columnar structure (the arrangement of the neuron cell bodies and fibres in columns perpendicular to the surface of the cortex) and by the recent, exciting results from the visual cortex by David Hubel and Torsten Wiesel. From the microelectrode recordings by the two Harvard neurophysiologists, it appeared that the first task undertaken by the cortical receiving area was the detection of linearities in the visual field (slits, bars, edges).[10]

As others had done, Marr regarded the hippocampus as 'archicortex' on account of its simpler structure and earlier evolutionary development in comparison with the neocortex. He had studied the writings and the drawings of the hippocampal cells and fibres by Ramon y Cajal and the later ones by Cajal's former student, Rafael Lorente de Nó. He was also aware, largely from the study of Henry Molaison by Brenda Milner, that the hippocampus was concerned with memory. The outcome of Marr's three-level approach was the proposal that the hippocampus served as a 'simple' memory, events being represented first by patterns of synaptic activity in 'input' neurons and thence in 'output' neurons; the output neurons were connected back to the input neurons. The resulting memory of a stored event could be retrieved whenever its input neurons were excited by neural activity associated with a related event. Marr calculated that it would require one second for the hippocampus to memorize a single event and that 100,000 events would be the theoretical maximum stored in the course of a day. He then proposed that the information would be transferred from the hippocampus to the neocortex at night, a time when there would be no interference from incoming sensory information. The hippocampus, then, was envisaged as an essential albeit temporary holding station for memories of events pending their transfer to the neocortex for long-term storage.

Marr's approach had been a unique and powerful contribution to computational neuroscience. By the time his hippocampal paper was published Marr had left the Physiological Laboratory to join Sydney Brenner at another Cambridge institution, the Medical Research Council's Laboratory for Molecular Biology. Founded by Lawrence Bragg, the Laboratory had specialized in the study of proteins by X-ray crystallography and had been where Francis Crick and James Watson had had their phenomenal success in deducing the two-stranded helical structure of DNA in 1953. Brenner, who would become a Nobel Laureate himself, was then devoting himself to unravelling the mysteries of a nervous system by studying the 302 neurons of the worm, *C elegans*. Recognizing the special talents of David Marr, Brenner suggested he visit MIT and talk to Marvin Minsky and Seymour Papert. It was good advice. Though there had been mathematical wizards interested in the brain elsewhere, notably the late Alan Turing (Manchester, United Kingdom) and John von Neumann (Princeton, New Jersey), MIT had Claude Shannon, the founder of information theory. In addition, under the direction of the former mathematical prodigy, Norbert Wiener, MIT had become the world's leading centre for the new discipline of artificial intelligence. It was at MIT that Marr would work closely with Tomasio (Tommy) Poggio, concentrating on computational theory rather than its implementation by the brain. By 1980 he had become a tenured full professor in the Department of Psychology.

It was to be his last year. At the age of only 35, and with the promise of so much more science to come, the extraordinarily gifted David Courtney Marr would die from leukaemia.

Notes

1. D. Marr, 'A Theory of Cerebellar Cortex' (1969) 202 *Journal of Physiology* 437–70.
2. D. Marr, 'A Theory for Cerebral Neocortex' (1970) 176 *Proceedings of the Royal Society of London*, B 161–234.
3. D. Marr, 'Simple Memory: A Theory for Archicortex' (1971) 262 *Philosophical Transactions of the Royal Society of London* 23–81.
4. W.G. Walter, *The Living Brain* (New York, NY: WW Norton, 1963).
5. For a biography of David Marr, see: S. Edelman and L.M. Vaina, 'David Marr' <http://www.kyb ele.psych.cornell.edu/~edelman/marr/marr.html> accessed 22 April 2022.
6. J. Kan, T.Z. Azziz, A.L. Green, and E.A.C. Pereira, 'Biographical Sketch. Giles Brindley, FRS' (2014) 28(6) *British Journal of Neurosurgery* 704–6.
7. E.D. Adrian, 'Afferent Areas in the Cerebellum Connected to the Limbs' (1943) 66 *Brain* 289–315.
8. A. Hodgkin, 'Edgar Douglas Adrian, Baron Adrian of Cambridge, 30 November 1889–4 August 1977' (1979) 25 *Biographical Memoirs of Fellows of the Royal Society* 1–73.
9. The work carried out in Canberra is summarized in: J.C. Eccles, M. Ito, and J. Szentágothai. *The Cerebellum as a Neuronal Machine* (Berlin: Springer Verlag, 1973). However, Marr would have seen the earlier papers before publication of the book.
10. Although the Hubel and Wiesel scheme of linear detection continues to be widely regarded as the first step undertaken by the cortex in the recognition of objects, this may be mistaken; see A.J. McComas, *Sherrington's Loom. An Introduction to the Science of Consciousness* (New York, NY: Oxford University Press, 2019).

18

1980: Departures

(Montreal, 1980; Penfield's death; Hebb's retirement)

The last decade had brought changes.

In a bed in the Royal Victoria Hospital in Montreal, Wilder Graves Penfield had died at the age of 85. In his last years he had been writing his autobiography, finishing it a bare three weeks before his death. Entitled *No Man Alone*, it recounted the story of Penfield's life up to the opening of the Neurological Institute 42 years earlier, drawing upon the author's frequent letters to his mother for the recall of events and dates.[1] It was a fine work, recapturing a full and successful life, one rich in personal and professional adventure. Though there was mention of an early disagreement with Francis Walshe, the British neurologist who would become his nemesis, Penfield showed no rancour in the telling. Walshe, the recipient of a knighthood and revered by his fellow neurologists, had died three years earlier.

Well before his death Penfield had been succeeded as Director of the Neurological Institute by Theodore Rasmussen and he, in turn, would be followed by a third neurosurgeon, William Feindel. Nevertheless, the loss of Penfield and the departure of Jasper to the Université de Montréal had left the Institute without its two most prominent members. On the other hand, the Institute was becoming known for more than its neurosurgery and clinical neurophysiology. Among its recruits had been Eva and Frederick Andermann (neurological disorders of childhood), George Karpati and Stirling Carpenter (neuromuscular diseases), and Pierre Gloor (epilepsy and electroencephalography (EEG)). And the example of the Montreal Neurological Institute had been copied elsewhere. Even in Britain, where all consultant positions in the National Health Service were controlled by government, there was now a Regional Neurological Centre in Newcastle-upon-Tyne and an Institute of Neurological Sciences in Glasgow.

Away from the Montreal Neurological Institute, across the McGill campus, there had been changes in the Department of Psychology. Donald Hebb had retired as Head in 1972 but was still giving seminars to graduate students. Relaxed and popular, the new emeritus professor might have been found at lunchtime playing billiards in the Faculty Club. During the quarter-century that he had been at McGill, all but one year of which he had been Chair, the Department of Psychology had become one of the best in the world, in many eyes *the* best. Apart from the influence of Hebb's books, especially *The Organization of Behaviour*, there had been the successes of former graduate students—including Brenda and Peter Milner, Mortimer Mishkin, Ronald Melzack, Suzanne Corkin, and John O'Keefe. And, of course, the postdoctoral fellow, James Olds,

Aranzio's Seahorse and the Search for Memory and Consciousness. Alan J. McComas, Oxford University Press.
© Oxford University Press 2023. DOI: 10.1093/oso/9780192868244.003.0020

co-discoverer of the brain's pleasure centre. It is fair to note, however, that although Hebb's presence had brought the students to Montreal, and though he had taught them and been available to give advice, Hebb had not involved himself directly in the various research projects. In this there is a comparison with Eccles who, as Per Andersen recounted, would not only carry out much of the dissection needed for an experiment but later perch himself in front of the oscilloscope, enthusiastically giving instructions and operating the camera.

Hebb's last academic years, those spent at Dalhousie University, would not be entirely peaceful, however, for he found himself implicated by the media as having performed Central Intelligence Agency (CIA) -funded experiments on brainwashing (a potential torture method) in the early 1950s.[2] The accusations were false for, while some of his graduate students had certainly studied the behavioural effects of sensory deprivation, it had been for sound scientific reasons and the research had never received US government support. Moreover, the McGill studies had been fully described in the scientific literature and, far from being the objects of torture, the student volunteers had been free to end their confinement whenever they wished.[3] It appeared that the journalists and others had confused Hebb's work with that of another Montreal investigator, the psychiatrist Donald Ewen Cameron–, who had indeed been performing CIA-funded 'brainwashing' on patients at the Allan Memorial Hospital. The false accusation had angered Hebb when it had first appeared in the 1950s and it would have bothered him when it had surfaced again in his retirement.

Meanwhile one of Hebb's former graduate students was adding to her fine body of work at the Montreal Neurological Institute. Brenda Milner had expanded her study of memory by investigating patients who had undergone temporary amobarbital suppression of function in one or other cerebral hemisphere. The drug had been given by injection into the common carotid arteries of patients who were to undergo temporal lobe resection for epilepsy. Initially, the test had been applied to left-handed patients in order to determine which hemisphere was dominant for speech (in right-handed subjects the left hemisphere is dominant, but in left-handed subjects dominance may reside in either hemisphere). Subsequently the injection technique was combined with a memory test, the purpose being to detect any pre-existing temporal lobe damage on the side opposite to that being considered for surgery. For some time Brenda had also been studying function in the frontal lobes. Unlike the situation for patients with surgery or damage to their temporal lobes, the patients who had undergone frontal lobectomy had not shown any inability to remember—though there was confusion in the ordering of memories.[4]

As for Brenda's former subject, Henry Molaison, the patient who had suffered severe amnesia following bilateral medial temporal lobectomy, it was now Suzanne Corkin who was continuing the investigation of his memory mechanisms. His father having died, Henry was now totally dependent on his mother for his care; from time to time, however, he would be taken by car from his home in Hartford for several days of study as an in-patient at MIT's new Clinical Research Center. It had been hoped that a computed tomography (CT) scan might clarify which structures had been resected in the original surgery but this had not been possible, the scans merely showing loss of deep tissue in both temporal lobes.

Elsewhere there had been other deaths. Stephen Kuffler had died unexpectedly at the age of 67, having suffered a massive heart attack on returning from a swim in the ocean at Wood's Hole. Had he lived another year it is likely that he would have shared the 1981 Nobel Prize in Physiology or Medicine with David Hubel and Torsten Wiesel. The new work on visual processing in the brain, for which the award was given, had been a continuation of the research that Kuffler had started long before in Baltimore. Eric Kandel had suffered a loss, too. Alden Spencer, Kandel's great friend and his partner in the microelectrode study of the cat hippocampus, had succumbed to amyotrophic lateral sclerosis (Lou Gehrig's disease, ALS). Yet another premature death had been that of James Olds, the discoverer of a pleasure centre in the brain. Olds, aged 54 and at the pinnacle of his career, had been the victim of a swimming accident (Figure 18.1).

There had also been a notable retirement. John Eccles would have been obliged to give up his laboratory in Canberra on account of age but chose to continue his research in Chicago instead. The move had not been successful and so, after two years, he had transferred to Buffalo in 1968. After seven productive years of research in an appreciative environment, research that had centred on the cerebellum, he had finally retired to Switzerland. There, living quietly in a villa with his wife, Helena, the former Nobel Laureate had been free to think and write again about the brain, consciousness, and the place of humanity in the universe. The thoughts were a continuation of those that had

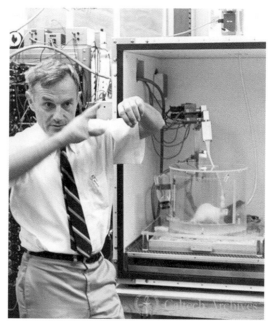

Figure 18.1 James Olds. Olds was a faculty member at the California Institute of Technology in 1971, the time of the photograph (reproduced courtesy of Caltech Archives).

prompted him, as a newly qualified physician, to set off to Oxford and to learn from Sherrington a half-century earlier. What a journey it had been!

Notes

1. W. Penfield, *No Man Alone. A Neurosurgeon's Life* (Boston, MA: Little Brown, 1977).
2. R.E. Brown, 'Alfred McCoy, Hebb, the CIA, and Torture' (2007) 43(2) *Journal of the History of the Behavioral Sciences* 205–13.
3. A prominent account of the sensory deprivation experiments at McGill was given by Woodburn Heron, one of the investigators: W. Heron, 'The Pathology of Boredom' (1957) 196 *Scientific American* 52–6. One of the interesting findings was that, in the absence of information from the external world, subjects would hallucinate.
4. This later research of Brenda Milner is summarized in her autobiography: B. Milner, *The History of Neuroscience in Autobiography*, L.R. Squire (ed.) (San Diego, CA: Academic Press, 1988) 2: 276–305.

19

Hidden Faces

(Oxford, New York, 1980: Edmund Rolls, Eric Kandel)

In Oxford University neuroscience had moved on from Sherrington's time. When the great man had finally retired, in 1936, his team of young collaborators had dispersed. One of those who had studied spinal cord reflexes with him, the New Zealander Derek Denny-Brown, had chosen to make his career in neurology and had moved to Boston. John Eccles, as already noted, had spent the Second World War in Australia (with Bernard Katz and Stephen Kuffler). The precocious John Fulton had become Professor of Physiology at Yale University at the unprecedented age of 30, and had there embarked on his study of function in the different lobes of the cerebral cortex. The departures had left Edward Liddell as the sole survivor of the experimental group and the natural successor to Sherrington as head of the department. With the end of the Second World War neuroscience had been resurrected, with important contributions coming from the departments of anatomy and experimental psychology, as well as from physiology. One of the many who had contributed to the renaissance was Charles Phillips, who had made some of the earliest intracellular recordings in the mammalian cortex. And it was through his exposure to the nerve degeneration studies of Paul Glees in the Oxford Anatomy Department that Patrick Wall, then a young medical student, had started his research career.

When he began his microelectrode examination of the monkey cortex, Edmund Rolls (Figure 19.1) had been a member of the Department of Experimental Psychology at Oxford. Like all studies that combined behaviour with delicate recordings from single neurons, the experiments were complex. The small surgery giving access to the brain having been performed on a previous occasion, it was possible to examine the operation of the brain without the contamination of an anaesthetic. During the experiment the monkey looked through a shutter that opened for one second. The view could be that of a three-dimensional object of some kind, a drawing, a geometric shape, a real human or monkey face, or the projected image of a face. Rolls and his colleagues found that, of the large number of neurons encountered with the recording electrode, roughly one in ten fired trains of impulses whenever the monkey was shown faces or even parts of faces. The responding neurons were on the outer surface of the temporal lobe, in and around the uppermost cleft (the superior sulcus).[1]

The Oxford neuroscientists had obtained the first convincing evidence of visual processing at a much higher level than the discrimination of lines and edges discovered by Hubel and Wiesel in the primary and secondary visual receiving areas in the occipital

Aranzio's Seahorse and the Search for Memory and Consciousness. Alan J. McComas, Oxford University Press.
© Oxford University Press 2023. DOI: 10.1093/oso/9780192868244.003.0021

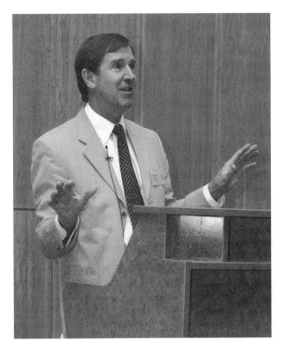

Figure 19.1 Edmund Rolls. Photograph courtesy of Dr Rolls.

lobe. The research had provided a function for the nerve fibre bundles connecting the occipital and temporal lobes, the projection demonstrated by Mortimer Mishkin. In addition, it could now be said that the superior temporal lobe had a memory for faces, though in these experiments, not for any specific faces. Much later research, notably by Doris T'sao at Harvard, would show that it was in another part of the temporal lobe, one situated more inferiorly, that such face-selective neurons were to be found. In these cells the seeming recognition of a real or fictitious face persisted even when the viewed head was tilted in different directions.[2] The findings had an additional significance in that they had identified the probable locus for the curious neurological condition, *prosopagnosia*, in which—usually as a result of stroke or tumour—a patient becomes incapable of identifying faces.

In New York, memory was also being addressed in the laboratory, though in nerve circuits far less elaborate than those of the primate brain. To the enquiring mind of Eric Kandel, *Aplysia* was continuing to reveal its secrets. Kandel had felt the loss of Alden Spencer keenly but there were others who were willing to collaborate in the investigation of the giant sea slug. One of these was James Schwartz, a well-established biochemist who was prepared to help identify the chemical neurotransmitters involved in the neural circuits responsible for habituation and sensitization. Using the gill withdrawal reflex as his model, as before, Kandel discovered that glutamate was the transmitter released by the endings of the siphon sensory nerve fibres at their synapses with the motoneurons.[3] However, there was another transmitter, serotonin, that could control the amount of glutamate released. The serotonin was produced by the interneurons in the reflex circuit, the cells that modified the strength of the response. Thus, when the reflex was enhanced ('sensitized') by an electric shock to the tail of *Aplysia*, it was because the interneurons had released serotonin and this transmitter, in turn, had increased the amount of glutamate released by the sensory neuron at the synapses with the motoneurons.[4] In the other direction, habituation—the lessening of response with repetition—was caused by diminished transmitter release from the sensory nerve terminals following events within the terminals themselves.

The discovery of the modulatory action of serotonin explained much of short-term memory, at least in *Aplysia*, but there was now the question as to how serotonin achieved its effect. What happened after serotonin had combined with receptors on the surface of the sensory neuron? Kandel and Schwartz speculated that this next step might involve cAMP (cyclic adenosine monophosphate), a molecule already known to act as a 'second messenger' within cells, and so it proved. The most direct evidence was that the direct injection of cAMP into the sensory neuron increased the release of glutamate from its endings on to the motoneuron.[5] As Kandel's group showed later, cAMP achieved its effect by activating a phosphorylating enzyme (protein kinase A) inside the sensory neuron.

Following the success with short-term memory, it was now time to tackle the problem of the cellular mechanisms responsible for long-term memory. It was also the time for Kandel to make a career move, though one which enabled him to remain in New York. In 1974 he accepted an appointment at the Columbia University College of Physicians and Surgeons, following the retirement of Harry Grundfest—his former supervisor when he, Kandel, had been a student wishing to learn something about the nervous system. In his new position, that of founding director of the Center for Neurobiology and Behavior (later, the Howard Hughes Medical Institute), Kandel was able to collaborate with scientists familiar with genetic engineering, notably Richard Axel and Richard Scheller, and to attract new recruits.

It was also time to simplify his experimental preparation. Kandel's young colleague, Craig Bailey, had already shown that long-term memory in *Aplysia* involved the growth of nerve endings by the sensory neuron and the formation of additional synapses with the motoneuron. The new tissue would have involved the synthesis of proteins and that synthesis, in turn, would probably have been brought about by switching on genes in the nucleus of the sensory neuron. However, the concept of protein synthesis being necessary for long-term memory had been explored previously by others and the experimental results had not been convincing one way or the other. For example, in one of the earliest studies, Louis Flexner and his colleagues in Philadelphia had given the antibiotic, puromycin, to mice both subcutaneously and by injection into the cerebral ventricles. Using radioactive valine (an amino acid) as a marker, they showed that protein synthesis was largely suppressed in various areas of the brain, including the hippocampus. Yet despite this inhibition the mice, when tested in a cage or in a T-maze, were still capable of learning to avoid electric shocks. When higher doses of puromycin were employed, the mice did show impairment of memory but the results were attributed to drowsiness following the injections.[6]

Later experiments from the same laboratory were interpreted differently, however, and were suggestive of interference with learning. As the field expanded through the work of others, it was pointed out that the protein-inhibiting drugs, including the antibiotic actinomycin, had unintended metabolic side-effects and that the latter would complicate interpretation of the laboratory findings.

In thinking about his own approach to protein synthesis and memory, Kandel recognized the need for a different experimental preparation. While the intact *Aplysia* had been ideal for linking activity in individual neurons to changes in the behaviour of the animal, the exploration of gene expression would require a preparation enabling higher visual resolution and simplified neural circuitry: tissue culture.

Another student, Samuel Sacher, became responsible for growing sensory and motor neurons in culture, together with the modulatory interneurons responsible for releasing serotonin. It was now possible, under the microscope, to see the three types of cell forming synapses with each other. Further, by means of an optogenetic technique,[7] the phosporylating enzyme, protein kinase A, was observed to move into the nucleus of the sensory neuron under the influence of serotonin. Once in the nucleus, protein kinase A was shown to combine with a gene-regulatory protein (CREB), thereby switching on the gene(s) controlling protein synthesis in the now-forming synapses.[8] And, in an intact animal, once the new synapses were established and functioning, so was the corresponding long-term memory.

It had taken a long time, four decades of research since the original microelectrode studies on the cat hippocampus with Alden Spencer, but Eric Kandel had succeeded in identifying the cellular mechanisms enabling a nervous system to form short- and long-term memories. It was research that had begun with little outside help, had necessitated the development of novel techniques, and, in its later part, had included many collaborators. Unlike the chance finding of place cells in the hippocampus or of a pleasure centre in the nucleus accumbens, there had been little luck involved; each stage in the scientific journey had been carefully thought out in advance. Long before his research had reached its conclusion, Kandel had started to receive honours, among them the prestigious Lasker Prize in 1983. Through Kandel's work *Aplysia* had also achieved scientific fame though there was a certain irony. At the very time that Kandel had begun to use the exotic sea slug at the Institut Marey in Paris, Gerald Kerkut and Roger Thomas in Southampton (United Kingdom) were making intracellular recordings from large neurons in the abdominal ganglion of a common garden snail.[9] Had an alternative preparation ever become necessary for the New York researchers, Central Park could have provided a ready source.

There had been another triumph quite apart from the research on memory, however, and it was one that would have a considerable impact in attracting undergraduate and graduate students into neuroscience. In the late 1970s Eric Kandel had enlisted James Schwartz's help in writing a textbook. The first edition of *Principles of Neural Science*[10] had appeared in 1981 and had been an instant success. After 40 years, additional contributors, and five editions, 'Kandel and Schwartz' would continue to hold its place as *the* neuroscience reference book.

While Eric Kandel had been in the midst of his research on long-term memory, there had been a patient on the other side of the Atlantic with a quite extraordinary illness, one that would prove to have profound implications for understanding the neural mechanisms not only of memory but of consciousness itself.

It was a story that deserved to be told in full.

Notes

1. D.I. Perrett, E.T. Rolls, and W. Caan, 'Visual Neurons Responsive to Faces in the Monkey Temporal Cortex' (1982) 47 *Experimental Brain Research* 329–42.
2. E.M. Meyers, M. Borzello, W.A. Freiwald, and D. Tsao, 'Intelligent Information Loss: The Coding of Facial Identity, Head Pose, and Non-Face Information in the Macaque Face Patch System' (2015) 35 *Journal of Neuroscience* 7069–81.
3. N. Dale, and E.R. Kandel, 'L-glutamate May Be the Fast Excitatory Transmitter of Aplysia Sensory Neurons' (1993) 90 *Proceedings of the National Academy of Sciences, USA* 7163–7.
4. M. Brunelli, V.F. Castellucci, and E.R. Kandel, 'Synaptic Facilitation and Behavioral Sensitization in Aplysia: Possible Role of Serotonin and Cyclic AMP' (1976) 194 *Science* 1178–81.
5. V.F. Castellucci, E.R. Kandel, J.H. Schwartz, F.D. Wilson, A.C. Nairn, and P. Greengard, 'Intracellular Injection of the Catalytic Subunit of Cyclic AMP-Dependent Protein Kinase Simulates Facilitation of Transmitter Release Underlying Behavioral Sensitization in Aplysia' (1980) 77 *Proceedings of the National Academy of Sciences, USA* 7492–6.
6. J.B. Flexner, E. Flexner, E. Stellar, G. De la Haba, and R.B. Roberts, 'Inhibition of Protein Synthesis in Brain and Learning and Memory Following Puromycin' (1962) 9 *Journal of Neurochemistry* 595–605.
7. Optogenetics is described in Chapter 26. Briefly, a gene for a light-sensitive protein is inserted into a genome, enabling the target tissue to fluoresce on receiving a light pulse.
8. P. Goelet and E.R. Kandel, 'Tracking the Flow of Learned Information from Membrane Receptors to Genome' (1986) 9 *Trends in Neurosciences* 472–99. For a later review on this topic, see: P.J. Hernandez and T. Abel, 'The Role of Protein Synthesis in Memory Consolidation: Progress Amid Decades of Debate' (2008) 89(3) *Neurobiology of Learning and Memory* 293–311.
9. G.A. Kerkut and R.C. Thomas, 'Acetylcholine and the Spontaneous Inhibitory Post Synaptic Potentials in the Snail Neurone' (1963) 8 *Comparative Biochemistry and Physiology* 39–45.
10. E.R. Kandel and J.H. Schwartz, *Principles of Neural Science* (Amsterdam: Elsevier, 1981).

20

More than a Headache

(London, 1985: Clive and Deborah Wearing)

The handsome, black-haired man was happily married and had a job that he enjoyed (Figure 20.1). For almost as long as he could remember, music had been Clive Wearing's life. Classical music, that is, and especially medieval church music—he was probably the world authority on the life and compositions of the 16th-century Flemish composer, Orlande de Lassus. Among his many accomplishments Clive had formed, directed, and conducted his own choir, the Europa Singers, and he was chorus master for the London Sinfonietta. He had recently been appointed Early Music Producer for the BBC's Radio 3 Channel, a position that he relished and in which he worked tirelessly.

And then, in March 1985, disaster struck.

In her 2005 book *Forever Today*,[1] Deborah Wearing describes the sequence of events that befell her husband, taking away almost everything that had made him so special, not only to her but to the world of music.

It had started with a fever and headache following grocery shopping at the local supermarket. The symptoms had persisted through the weekend and into the beginning of the following week. Then, feeling rather better, Clive had been able to return to work, attending a conference and rehearsing his choir for a concert. The reprieve was short. By the following weekend the fever was back, as was the headache. The pain, which felt like a tight band round the head, was now so severe as to prevent sleep. There was also vomiting and, for the first time, clear evidence of confusion. He had been unable to remember Deborah's telephone number and the name of a close musical colleague. A little later it was worse—Clive had even forgotten Deborah' name.

The name of his wife.

There followed two visits to the apartment by doctors. Clive was thought to be suffering from influenza, and surely it was this that accounted for all his symptoms; sleeping pills were prescribed. Not entirely reassured, Deborah had left for work only to find, on returning, that her husband was missing from the apartment. Missing and wandering the streets.

Having been picked up by a kindly taxi driver and taken to a police station, where his identity was obtained from inspection of his wallet, Clive was taken home by Deborah and put to bed again. On the way back he had failed to recognize the house in which they had an apartment. Over the next two days there were more visits by doctors but the diagnosis remained the same—the intermittently feverish but continually confused

Aranzio's Seahorse and the Search for Memory and Consciousness. Alan J. McComas, Oxford University Press.
© Oxford University Press 2023. DOI: 10.1093/oso/9780192868244.003.0022

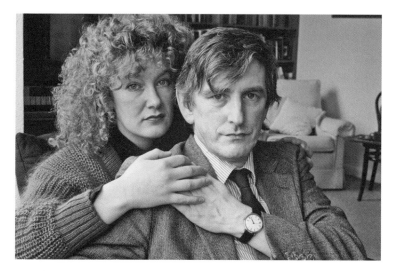

Figure 20.1 Clive and Deborah Wearing. Photograph taken after Clive's illness by Ros Drinkwater (Alamy Stock Photo).

Clive had contracted a severe attack of 'flu and would probably require to be off work for several weeks.

On the following day, there was a rapid deterioration in Clive's condition. Lying in bed, he was now barely conscious, unable to speak, his body limp and floppy. This time the visiting general practitioner took one look and called for an ambulance. Almost three weeks since the first symptoms had appeared, Clive was admitted to St Mary's Hospital, one of the major London teaching hospitals. Over the next eleven hours Deborah would provide a history of Clive's illness while Clive himself would be examined, have blood taken, undergo a lumbar puncture, and have his brain imaged with a computed tomography (CT) scanner. At the end of the eleven hours, there was a new diagnosis—Clive was thought to be suffering from herpes simplex encephalitis.

The herpes simplex virus (HSV-1) is an infectious agent that most of the population carries around. Residing in neurons (like the varicella-zoster virus), its continued dormancy ensures no trouble for most people, but in some the virus is the cause of cold sores. In a very few, perhaps no more than one in 20,000, it produces a rapidly developing inflammation of the brain—as in Clive Wearing. Untreated, most patients with herpes encephalitis die and those who survive are left with severe neurological deficits. Even with treatment, roughly a third will still succumb and full recovery is rare. Why the virus should suddenly become active is unclear, nor is it known why the inflammation should first appear, and be most severe, in the medial temporal lobe—and in the hippocampus in particular.

The diagnosis made, Clive was started on Acyclovir. It was a new drug, the first true antiviral medication, and it had only recently become available. Even with the drug, however, survival was touch and go during the ensuing week. Clive was confined to bed with drips and drainage tubes, completely unable to respond or react to those around him. In the following week, however, he was able to feed himself, though with little or no recognition of what he was eating. Then he was able to walk again, only to get lost in the hospital and incapable of finding his bed on being returned to his ward. Utterly confused, he was now able to speak though the words and sentences, spoken clearly and with authority, made no sense. A sense of mischief appeared, such that he would imitate the posture and portentous walk of a doctor, much to the amusement of the nurses. The only beacon, the only stable reference in his new life, was Deborah and it was she who, with considerable courage, would take Clive away from the hospital for visits to their apartment. On such occasions there was a need for constant vigilance for, now that he had recovered his strength, there was the constant likelihood that Clive would suddenly bolt.

The underlying problem, the reason for Clive's extraordinary, almost primal, behaviour was frighteningly simple. *He no longer had a memory.* In destroying the hippocampus and neighbouring structures, the viral encephalitis had left him with no recollection of the events, people, or places in his previous life. Equally devastating, Clive was unable to form new memories. Though awake, his life now consisted of a series of brief moments of consciousness, each lasting no more than a few seconds and containing no memory of its predecessor. For the remainder of his life he was doomed to be a prisoner of the moment, captive to the present.

It was understandable that Clive's extraordinary condition should attract scientific curiosity and the attention of the media. At a time when his speech had improved sufficiently for his memory deficit to be even more noticeable, he became the subject of a TV documentary by Jonathan Miller.[2] Filmed at King's College, Cambridge, it included the result of an experiment that Miller had devised, an experiment that would determine whether or not Clive had retained any musical memory. Led into the college chapel, Clive was confronted with his former singers, the London Lassus Choir. With a previously familiar Lassus score in place on the lectern, Clive was asked if he would conduct the piece. And he did, his arms moving and directing the choir, phrase by phrase, as fluently and as easily as before. His declarative memory might have gone but his procedural memory was still present.

Since the discovery of Henry Molaison, Brenda Milner's patient, there had been other patients with memory loss following hippocampal brain damage, but none with a deficit as severe as Clive Wearing's. And whereas Henry Molaison still possessed short-term memory, with an ability to remember people and events for half a minute or so, Clive Wearing had no memory beyond a few seconds. Further, Henry could recall some of the events of his childhood and could sometimes camouflage his amnesia for others by prefacing his answer with a phrase such as: 'I 'm having an argument with myself' or 'I keep debating with myself'.

Why should there have been this difference between the two men? Why did one have short-term memory and not the other? It was a question that brain imaging would eventually answer and the answer would have important implications.[3]

Notes

1. D. Wearing, *Forever Today. A Memoir of Love and Amnesia* (New York, NY: Doubleday, 2005).
2. Sir Jonathan Miller (1934–2019) was, like his school friend Oliver Sacks, a physician. However Miller made his brilliant career from comedy ('Beyond the Fringe'), and then, more ambitiously, as an innovative director of opera and theatre, a TV producer, and commentator on the sciences and arts.
3. The matter is discussed again in Part II.

21

Unexpectedly, a Grid

(London, Oslo, 1996: Edvard and May-Britt Moser)

Twenty-five years had passed since John O'Keefe and Jonathan Dostrovsky's discovery of place cells in the rat hippocampus. Inevitably, there had been changes at University College London, including one that had affected the Cerebral Functions Unit of which O'Keefe was a member—Patrick Wall, the Unit's director, had retired in 1992. Wall was not done with research though; he had been offered laboratory space at St Thomas' Hospital Medical School, the same school in which Charles Sherrington had been a pupil more than a century earlier. When not experimenting, Patrick Wall could have looked across the Thames at the Houses of Parliament—but then Wall had had little time for politicians. There were experiments to be carried out and, for those students wise enough to attend them, lectures to be given.

There had been other changes at University College London. Of its three Nobel Laureates in the life sciences, two had left and one had died. The Head of the Physiology Department, Andrew Huxley, had departed to Cambridge, having been elected Master of Trinity College in succession to his friend and former colleague, Alan Hodgkin. The two had exploited the size of the squid giant axon in determining the ionic basis of the nerve impulse. Having shared the 1963 Prize in Physiology or Medicine with John Eccles, all three had been knighted subsequently.

Within the same building on London's Gower Street Sir Bernard Katz was sometimes to be found in the Biophysics Department. The 1970 Nobel Laureate was now an emeritus professor but would still come into the department, though it was more for coffee or tea and the chance to chat rather than for the opportunity to talk neuroscience.

The third Laureate, Archibald ('AV') Hill, had died in 1977. His had been an especially full life. He had been awarded the Nobel Prize in 1922 for research on the contraction and heat production of muscle. Previously, in the First World War, he had invented a rangefinder for anti-aircraft gunnery. Prior to the Second World War he had written a letter to *The Times* deploring Hitler and the National Socialist Party. He had been instrumental in finding employment for Jewish scientists fleeing Germany, one of whom had been the young Bernard Katz. Hill had been a Member of Parliament during the Second World War and had acted for the UK government in the sharing of military research with the United States. The grand old man of British biophysics had kept active in his laboratory almost to the end, dying at the age of 90.

Meanwhile, there was O'Keefe in the Cerebral Functions Unit. Following his discovery of the place cells he had intensified his research, inviting collaboration, and

Aranzio's Seahorse and the Search for Memory and Consciousness. Alan J. McComas, Oxford University Press.
© Oxford University Press 2023. DOI: 10.1093/oso/9780192868244.003.0023

continuing to train young neuroscientists. In the summer of 1996 he had welcomed two young Norwegians to his laboratory. It was a visit that would have consequences.

Edvard and the future May-Britt Moser (Figure 21.1) had been born on different islands off the North Sea coast but had attended the same high school.[1] After graduation they had gone independently to the University of Oslo. On renewing acquaintance they had fallen in love and decided to study psychology together. The study of behaviour was not enough in itself, however, and both students felt the urge to explore the underlying neural mechanisms. With hopes of being accepted for postgraduate studies the two had approached Per Andersen, aware of his international reputation. In order to be taken on, however, the couple were given the task of constructing a water maze. The maze was necessary for a new type of study that Andersen had in mind. If rats could learn to solve the puzzle of the maze despite most of the hippocampus having been removed, then the neurons in the remaining part should exhibit marked long-term potentiation—the phenomenon discovered by Terje Lømo and exploited with Timothy Bliss.

Having sensibly decided to buy an aquarium rather than construct a tank themselves, Edvard and May-Britt set up the maze. In this test, originally devised by Richard Morris in Edinburgh, a rat was required to swim to a submerged platform rendered invisible by the opacity of the water (to which milk had been added). Making lesions that spared a small part of the hippocampus proved more difficult, however, though the Mosers were able to show that it was the dorsal part of the hippocampus, rather than the ventral part, that was necessary for a rat to learn how to navigate.

Edvard and May-Britt were able to present a poster of their work at a meeting of the European Neuroscience Association in Sweden where it attracted the attention of the inventor of the water maze—Richard Morris. Having been submitted and accepted as a joint Master's thesis, the research was published in *The Journal of Neuroscience*.[2] The next step would be gaining doctorates, again in Per Andersen's laboratory. For her research topic May-Britt chose to compare the hippocampi of rats that had been living in standard cages with those of animals that had access to a larger space, one that had multiple floors and home-made toys to explore. The experiments involved injecting individual neurons with a yellow dye and then, with a special microscope, counting the numbers of spines (synaptic projections) on the dendrites. There was a clear difference—the rats exposed to the enriched environment had more dendritic spines. The results were evidence that hippocampal neurons had formed more synapses as the rats learned about their surroundings. It was an important finding, one that extended an earlier study by Greenough and Volkmar that had shown increased dendritic branching in rats reared in a complex environment.[3] And, of course, the result was in keeping with Kandel's discovery of new dendritic spines in the experiments with *Aplysia*. Edvard Moser, meanwhile, was researching what had become Per Andersen's favourite topic, the likely importance of long-term potentiation for learning.

Newly married, it was now time for the Mosers to broaden their research experience by working and studying elsewhere. Their choice was Edinburgh. Richard Morris (of the water maze) was already known to them and his laboratory had expertise in making lesions in the rat hippocampus that were more precise than those of the Mosers. It was

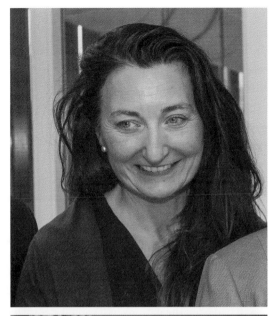

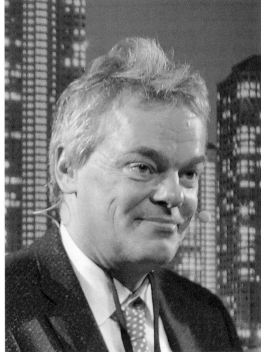

Figure 21.1 *Upper.* May-Britt Moser, 2014. (Wikimedia Commons File: May-Britt Moser 2014.jpg. Creative Commons Attribution-Share Alike 2.0 Generic license.) *Lower.* Edvard Moser, 2015. (Wikimedia Commons file: Edvard Moser 2015.jpg. Author: Bengt Oberger. Creative Commons Attribution-Share Alike 4.0 International license).

now possible to make better comparisons of the functioning of the dorsal and ventral parts of the hippocampus.

Important though the work in Edinburgh was, it was a side-visit to London that would have the greatest consequence. Over a period of three months John O'Keefe spent long hours with the Mosers, teaching them everything he knew about recording from single cells in the hippocampus. It was a generous action and of a kind not always exhibited in scientific communities; with fame so dependent on precedence in discovery, laboratory expertise can be jealously guarded.

As their time in Britain was coming to an end, the Mosers had their attention drawn to a vacancy in the Psychology Department at the Norwegian University of Science and Technology. The university was not in Oslo, where the Mosers had carried out their graduate studies with Per Andersen, but in Trondheim.

Situated midway between Oslo and the Arctic Circle, Trondheim would have been known to the Mosers. Despite its high northern latitude, it was the country's third largest city, with a population of some 150,000 at that time—many of them young people attending the university. It was an old city, at least for Norway, and could claim the Vikings as its founders. It had been the nation's first capital, centuries before Bergen and Christiana (Oslo), and so had the largest cathedral in Norway. Situated on the banks of a large fjord and at the mouth of a river, Trondheim was largely protected from the North Sea storms by the mountains guarding the entrance to the fjord. The fjord had long provided a refuge for shipping and a base for warships, from the Viking long boats to the German battleships and U-boats of the Second World War. Throughout its history Trondheim had been a city of long summer nights and dark winter days, but also of rain, fog, and snow. Yet despite the weather it had become an attractive city, partly on the account of the energy of its youthful population and partly because of the old timbered buildings along the quayside. And then, on all sides as far as the eye could see, there was the magnificent Norwegian scenery.

Trondheim, then. Though both Edvard and May-Britt had still to defend their doctoral theses, they applied and were sufficiently impressive at interview for each to be offered a faculty position. With money provided for equipment and with a former underground bomb shelter as their laboratory, the husband-and-wife team were now free to concentrate on their own projects. Additionally, they would be able to take graduate students and so move the research along faster.

The problem they chose was the nature of the synaptic connections that enabled the hippocampus to contain neurons that were sensitive to the position of an animal in its environment—the place cells that had been discovered by John O'Keefe and Jonathan Dostrovsky in 1970. By making small lesions, they showed that place cells were still present in a part of the hippocampus that had been disconnected from the remainder of the structure. This unexpected finding prompted the Mosers to examine a neighbouring region, the entorhinal cortex. To their surprise, they found individual neurons that were responsive not to a single position of the animal in its environment, but to many. Even more surprising, the positions for each cell formed a hexagonal array (Figure 21.2). The size of each hexagon was proportional to the extent of the rat's

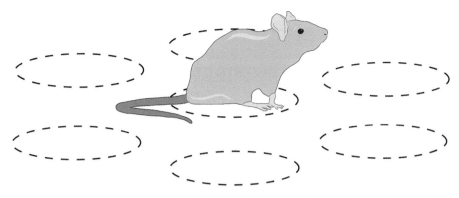

Figure 21.2 Rat standing on one of the loci in the hexagonal arrays of a single entorhinal grid cell.

immediate surroundings, and the complete array for one neuron would overlap with those for other cells. Because each array resembled a grid, this was the name given to the neurons involved—'grid' cells. Somehow the output of the entorhinal grid cells enabled the hippocampus to form its 'place' cells, the neurons that coded for precise locations in the surroundings of a rat.

The hippocampus and its neural neighbourhood had become even more fascinating to the investigators, and there would be rich prizes awaiting those who had made the fundamental discoveries.

Notes

1. The Moser's life histories and research accomplishments are given in their respective Nobel autobiographies and lectures: <https://www.nobelprize.org/prizes/medicine/2014/edvard-moser/biographical/>; <https://www.nobelprize.org/prizes/medicine/2014/may-britt-moser/biographical/>; <https://www.nobelprize.org.uploads.2018/06/edvard-moser-lecture.pdf>; and <https://www.nobelprize.org.uploads.2018/06/may-britt-moser-lecture.pdf> all accessed 22 April 2022.
2. M.-B. Moser and E.I. Moser, 'Distributed Encoding and Retrieval of Spatial Memory in the Hippocampus' (1998) 18(18) *Journal of Neuroscience* 7535–42.
3. W.T. Greenough and F.R. Volkmar, 'Pattern of Dendritic Branching in Occipital Cortex of Rats Reared in Complex Environments' (1973) 40(2) *Experimental Neurology* 491–504.

22

A Telephone Call

(Stockholm, New York, Cambridge, Massachusetts, 2000: Eric Kandel)

The new Millennium had started well for Eric Kandel. On 9 October 2000 there had been an early morning telephone call, the call that every scientist might wish for but that only a handful ever receive. The call was from Stockholm. Eric Kandel, the person who, in his youth, had intended to become a psychoanalyst, had been awarded the 2000 Nobel Prize for Physiology or Medicine. The Prize was to be shared with Arvid Carlsson and Paul Greengard and had been given 'for their discoveries concerning signal transduction in the nervous system'.

It was dopamine that had made the 2000 award possible for all three men. Arvid Carlsson had shown that dopamine was a transmitter in the mammalian brain some 40 years previously, using a novel formaldehyde fluorescence method developed with Nils-Åke Hillarp. Shortly after, others had shown it was a deficiency of dopamine in the human brain that was responsible for the neurodegenerative disorder, parkinsonism; this discovery, in turn, had led to treatment of affected patients with L-DOPA, a chemical precursor of dopamine.

Paul Greengard had trained as a physicist but had become interested in neural research after hearing a lecture on the ionic basis of the membrane potential by Alan Hodgkin. Working at the molecular level he had shown that cAMP (cyclic adenosine monophosphate) acted as a second messenger in nerve cells. Following the combination of dopamine with its receptor on the surface membrane, cAMP was mobilized and able to activate the enzyme, protein kinase A. By attaching a phosphate group, the kinase could activate a protein molecule—an enzyme, for example. It had been Greengard's help that had been so valuable to Kandel when the protein synthesis needed for long-term memory in *Aplysia* had been shown to be initiated by the dopamine: dopamine receptor: cAMP: protein kinase A sequence. Kandel and Greengard had been more than colleagues, they had become good friends.

As it happened, the Nobel announcement was made on 9 October; it was Yom Kippur, the Day of Atonement and the most solemn day of the year for a practising Jew, as Eric Kandel was. There had been a certain irony in the timing, an irony deepened by receipt of a congratulatory telegram from the Austrian government. As Kandel would point out, had it not been for the embrace of Hitler and the Nazis by the Austrian government prior to the Second World War, his family would not have fled to the United States and he would not have had the opportunity for a successful career in neuroscience.

Aranzio's Seahorse and the Search for Memory and Consciousness. Alan J. McComas, Oxford University Press.
© Oxford University Press 2023. DOI: 10.1093/oso/9780192868244.003.0024

Though he would later accept an honour from the Austrian government, his gratitude to America was unwavering.

In 2000, higher up the Atlantic coast, in Cambridge, Massachusetts, Henry Molaison was still participating in tests of his memory. It had been just over 20 years that Suzanne Corkin (Figure 22.1) had taken over the investigation of Henry from Brenda Milner, her former doctoral supervisor in Montreal.[1] The continuing experiments were carried out in the Clinical Research Center, a separate building that was part of MIT. The Center had become Suzanne's academic home soon after its founding in 1964 and, following the death of the Center's first director, Hans-Lukas Teuber, in 1977, Suzanne had become the founding head of the Behavioral Neuroscience Laboratory. In addition to her own experiments, she had been responsible for training graduate students in research; for these, as for herself, Henry Molaison was a prized resource.

When it was time for a new experiment Henry would be collected by Suzanne or one of her graduate students and driven to Cambridge, where he would be admitted to the Clinical Research Center for a few days of study. At the time Henry was a resident in a long-term care facility in Windsor Locks, Connecticut. His mother had been admitted to a nursing home in 1977, being no longer able to care for herself or her son, and would die at 96. Though Suzanne Corkin was not Henry's legal conservator (guardian), she nevertheless felt a responsibility for his health and well-being. More than anyone else, she was acquainted with Henry's past and present life and the cognitive handicap that was his daily burden.

In Suzanne's expert hands, Henry continued to provide valuable new information about brain function—and not just about memory. Suzanne had wondered whether, following removal of large parts of his limbic system, Henry was still capable of

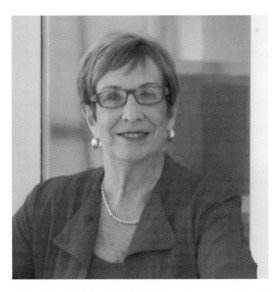

Figure 22.1 Suzanne Corkin. (Wikipedia file: Photo of Suzanne Corkin.jpg.) The photograph is reproduced as an instance of fair use, based on the fact that it is essential to the present narrative and that the copyright holder is unknown.

experiencing such basic sensations as pain and hunger. Regarding the latter, Suzanne concluded that feelings of hunger and its opposite, fullness, were seriously impaired. If, at the end of a meal, a fresh tray of food was placed in front of Henry, he would eat his way through the new offering as steadily as he had consumed the first. Again, when asked to rate his feeling of hunger on a scale of 0 to 100, he would invariably give '50' as his answer, regardless of whether he had just eaten or had been without food for hours.

In relation to pain, Suzanne tested Henry by heating a spot of skin on his forearm, using a contraption resembling a hairdryer. Henry proved incapable of assessing the intensity of the applied heat, or of differentiating between weak and strong heating, nor did he withdraw the heating device from his arm, even with the most intense stimuli.

The further testing of Henry's memory had also paid dividends. When he had been investigated earlier by Brenda Milner his results had shown that there were two types of memory. One type, 'declarative memory', was an ability to recall events form one's past as well as information about people, places, and objects in the external world. The other type of memory, 'procedural memory', enabled coordinated mental and physical activity—riding a bicycle, putting on clothes, eating with a knife and fork, for example. Using his procedural memory, Henry Molaison had learnt to trace a continuous line in the space separating inner and outer star figures. More dramatically, Clive Wearing's procedural memory had enabled him to conduct choral music in King's College, Cambridge.

Suzanne's new experiments had shown that declarative memory contained at least two subtypes. She had discovered that while Henry was unable to recall events from his own past, he was surprisingly successful in identifying previous happenings in the world. He was, for example, knowledgeable about the stock market crash of 1929 (he had been three years old at the time) and familiar with the Second World War. He could also recognize photographs of well-known scenes and famous people (Neil Armstrong taking the first steps on the Moon, for example). Perhaps more surprisingly still, Suzanne found that Henry was able to name persons in old photographs of his family. On the other hand, he was still virtually incapable of remembering any personal happenings from his youth.

The conclusion from this dichotomy was that there were two parts to 'declarative' memory, as had been recently suggested by the cognitive scientist, Endel Tulving. One part was the ability to recall facts about the world—the names and pictures of buildings, cities, and people, as well as a memory for important events—wars, stock market crashes, elections, environmental disasters. This type of memory was 'semantic'; the knowledge had been registered at the time and then reinforced by multiple exposures (discussion, reading, films, TV, radio) over ensuing years. The other type of memory was 'episodic' and referred to particular incidents in the life of the individual—a serious accident, a first visit to the seaside, the loss of a wallet, the death of a parent. It was episodic memory that Henry had lost.

Suzanne thought that the nature of Henry's condition was also helpful in deciding between two theories of memory, the 'Standard Model of Consolidation' and the 'Multiple Trace Theory'. Both theories attempted to account for the way in which an amnesic subject may often retain some memory of the distant past while being unable to recall anything more recent. The explanation provided by the Standard Model was that the hippocampus was necessary for the initial storage and retrieval of an item of information but that, over months and years, areas of cerebral cortex took over this function—the memory had been moved to another part of the brain. If the hippocampus was then damaged by disease or injury, any recent information would be lost but that already stored in the cerebral cortex (frontal, temporal, parietal, and occipital lobes) might still be retrieved.

The Multiple Trace Theory, in contrast, supposed that it was the reiteration of specific information over the years that enabled it to survive; the hippocampus directed the information to sites in the cortex and whenever the same information was repeated, the linkage between hippocampus and cortex was reinforced. When the hippocampus was damaged only the strongest links would survive.

As Suzanne Corkin recognized, if the Standard Model was correct, Henry's amnesia should be equally severe for semantic information (world events, famous people and places, etc.) as for particular happenings in his own life (episodic memory). But this was not the case. The only two events remembered in his entire boyhood were lighting his first cigarette at the age of 10 and having a local ride in a small aeroplane at 13. In contrast, Henry had a good recollection of world events that had occurred in his youth (and after).

Importantly, the cerebral cortex had become accepted as the repository of long-term memory, as David Marr and others had proposed, and this was a feature of both the Standard Model and the Multiple Trace Model; the cortex was also thought to be site of short-term memory and working memory. However, these conclusions were based, to a considerable extent, on the premise that most of Henry Molaison's two hippocampi had been removed during William Scoville's surgery in 1953.

But had the surgery been as radical as Scoville had claimed? Had there been some hippocampus left, enough to have still had some function? It was a hugely important question that Suzanne Corkin had considered and had attempted to resolve with brain imaging. Meanwhile, there was another matter for her attention. As the new Millennium started she, Suzanne, had come to a firm conclusion concerning her prize subject.

Sadly, though inevitably, Henry Molaison's usefulness for an understanding of memory mechanisms was nearing its end.

Note

1. For Henry Molaison's care and further studies see: S. Corkin, *Permanent Present Tense. The Unforgettable Life of the Amnesic Patient, H.M.* (New York, NY: Basic Books, 2013).

23

Death and Disorder

(Bickford, Connecticut, San Diego, 2008: Henry Molaison, Suzanne Corkin, Jacopo Annese)

On 8 December 2008, Henry Gustave Molaison died at the age of 82.

It was late in the evening and he had been failing for some time. Indeed, when Suzanne Corkin had visited him in the long-term care facility some two months earlier, Henry had only been able to look back at her and give a faint smile.

The physical decline had started much earlier, however. In 1985 he had fallen, fracturing his right ankle and left hip and requiring the hip to be replaced the following year. He had begun to be troubled by severe tinnitus and there were still occasional grand mal seizures. He had frequently complained of stomach pains, sometimes refusing meals. Sleep apnoea had become a problem, as had hypertension. There had been another fall and another broken ankle. Having been using a walker, by 2001 he had become dependent on a wheelchair for getting around. It had become difficult for him to travel to MIT, so Suzanne and her graduate students would drive to the nursing home if further cognitive testing were to be done.

By 2000 there had been definite changes in Henry's personality as well. Normally sociable and pleasant, there had been a period when he had become reluctant to take part in social activities and would easily become irritable and angry. His speech, previously fluent, had begun to slur. Suzanne's suspicion that Henry was now exhibiting features of dementia were consistent with the results of new magnetic resonance imaging (MRI) scans, the latter providing evidence of multiple small strokes.

Henry had undergone brain imaging before. As long ago as 1977 he had had a CT scan but it had not been possible, from the scan, to determine how much of the hippocampus and its neighbouring structures had been removed on the two sides. In 1992, however, Henry had had an MRI scan and, with its higher resolution, it showed that some hippocampus remained on both sides. At the time of Henry's operation, his surgeon, William Scoville, had estimated that the anterior two-thirds of both hippocampi had been removed; the MRI revealed that, although some five centimetres (cm) of medial temporal lobe had been taken out, there were 2 cm or so of hippocampus remaining on both sides. It had been an important finding at the time since it could have offered an explanation for the residual declarative memory that Henry still possessed;[1] it was Suzanne's belief, however, that the residual hippocampal tissue was non-functioning. The MRI scan, like the CT scan before it, exhibited some atrophy of the

Aranzio's Seahorse and the Search for Memory and Consciousness. Alan J. McComas, Oxford University Press.
© Oxford University Press 2023. DOI: 10.1093/oso/9780192868244.003.0025

cerebellum; most likely it had been caused by the Dilantin medication that Henry had continued to take for his seizures.

Long before Henry's death Suzanne had appreciated that, useful though the MRI scans had been, there was the need for a careful post-mortem study of his brain by an expert neuroanatomist. From Henry's official guardian she had obtained approval for his, Henry's, brain to be removed after death for research purposes. She had also thought about whom to entrust with the delicate anatomical examination, and had asked Jacopo Annese (Figure 23.1), a young researcher at the University of California, San Diego. Before Annese would begin, however, there were numerous other steps to be taken with Henry's brain. Suzanne had thought them all out, had taken advice when necessary, and had given instructions to everyone who would be involved. When the time had come for her own actions, she had not forgotten to telephone Brenda Milner with the news of Henry's death.

Following Suzanne's meticulous plan, which included the packing of ice around the head, Henry's body had been taken from the nursing home to Boston; there a team had been assembled to take ultra-high resolution MRI scans of the brain. After transfer to a hospital morgue, the brain had been carefully freed and placed in a bucket of formalin, a preservative that would harden the brain and make it easier for sections to be cut later. After a month in the preservative, Henry's brain was temporarily removed for a further ultra-high resolution MRI scan before being taken to San Diego by Jacopo Annese. There Henry's brain (after Einstein's, the most famous brain in the world) was prepared for sectioning. It was soaked in formaldehyde and sugar solution (to prevent ice crystals from forming), embedded in gelatin (to give it support), and then frozen. Starting at the front of the brain and working backwards, more than 2,000 sections were cut, each no more than 70 microns thick—the width of a human hair. It was an astonishing technical feat. Importantly, before each stroke of the microtome knife, the surface of

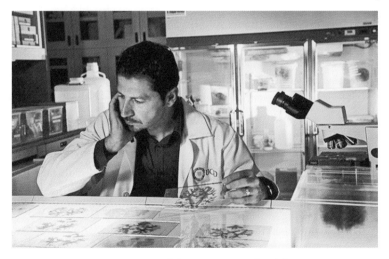

Figure 23.1 Jacopo Annese. Courtesy of the University of California, San Diego. Since this photo was taken, Dr Annese has left the university and founded The Brain Observatory.

Henry's brain was photographed, a step needed for a subsequent reconstructed image of the brain. The sectioning, which took 53 hours, was watched by many, some of them leading neuroscientists and psychologists, some of them members of the media, and some of them people simply interested in what had become a major scientific event. The brain cutting could even be seen on the Internet.

One of those who watched on the Internet was a middle-aged journalist in Whitehorse, a small city in Canada's Yukon Territory, in the country's far north. Luke Dittrich was a grandson of William Scoville[2] and had known of the existence of Henry Molaison and of the latter's participation in memory research, but the sight of Henry's brain now being meticulously sliced had come as a surprise. His interest in Henry having been rekindled, Dittrich resolved to find out more about the life of the famous patient. An accomplished writer, Dittrich would produce a best-selling book, one that would provoke controversy because of its criticism of Suzanne Corkin.[3]

That was for the future, however. The sections of Henry's brain having been cut, it was time to start staining them; that is, to apply various dyes that would colour the tissues, making them more readily visible and distinguishing the various parts from each other. Jacopo Annese also began constructing three-dimensional images of Henry's brain, using the serial photographs that had been taken during the cutting procedure. Meanwhile Suzanne Corkin was preparing a book that would describe Henry Molaison's life and the way in which scientific investigation of his damaged brain had led to major discoveries concerning the nature and underlying neural mechanisms of memory.

Everything was going well until, suddenly, it wasn't.

The trouble began when Suzanne Corkin had unexpectedly asked Jacopo Annese for all the photographs taken of the cut surface of Henry's brain, this at a time when Annese was using them for his three-dimensional reconstructions. It is not known why Suzanne should suddenly have made this demand though, in the light of what was to follow, it is possible that she may have heard rumours of some unexpected findings by Annese. Be that as it may, the increasing tension between the two was compounded when Annese wrote an account of some of the work already accomplished with Henry's brain. He had made three novel observations. One was that the residual hippocampal tissue left from the surgery did not show the damage that Suzanne had anticipated; on the contrary, it looked healthy enough to have been functional during Henry's lifetime. The second observation was of some damage to the undersurface of the left frontal lobe; the damage would most likely have occurred some 50 years earlier when William Scoville had raised the front of the brain in order to gain access to the hippocampus on that side. The third abnormality was the presence of diffuse pathological changes in the white matter (nerve fibres) of the brain, changes associated with aging and most likely responsible for Henry's declining mental abilities in his last years. A fourth observation, one that had also been apparent in MRI scans, was of cerebellar atrophy, most likely a consequence of the anticonvulsant medication Henry had taken for most of his life.

In the manuscript reporting his findings Annese had named as co-authors all those in his laboratory who had been working on Henry's brain. Suzanne Corkin had not been included, nor had she been told of the manuscript, but the editor of *Nature Communications* had invited her to act as one of the reviewers. Corkin, clearly annoyed, had advised rejection of the paper.

Matters had only worsened afterwards, with legal advisors and heads of the respective institutions becoming involved; there had even been a judicial committee formed to settle the dispute. In the end, Annese had been ordered to give up all Henry's brain material, including every one of the thousands of sections and photographs. It was a wretched outcome for the countless hours of patient work and for the considerable research grant money that had been expended. As regards the manuscript, Suzanne Corkin's name had been added to the list of authors; of the 12 names, hers was the last.[4]

The removal of the brain material from the San Diego laboratory and her inclusion as a co-author would prove a pyrrhic victory for Suzanne Corkin. Within three years of the publication of the *Nature Communications* article and the appearance of her own book, *Permanent Present Tense. The Unforgettable Life of the Amnesic patient, H.M.*,[5] Suzanne would die of cancer. It was a sad end to a fine career, one made possible by a young man who had undergone unique and radical surgery for treatment of his epilepsy. The importance of Suzanne's study of Henry Molaison was brought out in the extensive obituary that was given her in the *New York Times*. Her death would only heighten the controversy that had arisen from the publication of Luke Dittrich's book as others came forward to defend her reputation.[6]

There had been another book about memory, one that had appeared two years before Henry Molaison's death and that had attracted much critical praise. Entitled *In Search of Memory. The Emergence of a New Science of Mind*, the author was Eric Kandel.[7] The book had come out six years after the award of the Nobel Prize and it had had two interwoven themes. One was the story of Kandel's life, from his disrupted boyhood in Vienna to his professional success as a neuroscientist in the United States. The other theme was the nature of the electrophysiological and molecular events underlying memory that Kandel had studied so thoroughly in the giant sea slug. Microelectrode recordings had been a large part of that work, and it was microelectrode recordings that would lead to the next great advance in understanding memory.

The recordings would be made in the human brain. Unlike the thousands of thalamic recordings that had been made during stereotactic surgery and had yielded little information of interest, the results of the new studies would be spectacular.

Notes

1. Interestingly, by itself, the hippocampal resection could not explain Henry's retention of semantic, but not episodic, memory.
2. Luke Dittrich's life, the curious and rather alarming Scoville family history, William Scoville's career, and the alleged interactions between Suzanne Corkin and Jacopo Annese, and later between Dittrich and Corkin, are all taken from Dittrich's best-selling book: L. Dittrich, *Patient H.M. A Story of Memory, Madness and Family Secrets* (New York, NY: Random House: 2016).

3. In both his book and in an article in the *New York Times Magazine* (7 August 2016), Dittrich made several serious criticisms of Suzanne Corkin. One was that she had taken Henry Molaison over from Brenda Milner, Suzanne's former PhD supervisor and the psychologist who had explored Henry's amnesia so effectively. However, the transfer made good sense, since Hartford, Connecticut, where Henry resided, was a full day's journey from Montreal but a mere 90 minute drive from MIT, where Suzanne worked. Further, it was still possible for Brenda Milner, by travelling to MIT, to carry out further investigations of Henry, as she did. A second criticism was that, other than by Brenda Milner and doctoral students in Suzanne's own laboratory, access to Henry for scientific purposes was usually denied. This may have been true but was understandable—Henry, like a piece of very expensive equipment, was a valuable resource and had to be handled carefully. Another concern was the dispute with Jacopo Annese over ownership of Henry's brain following the latter's death, a dispute heightened by Annese's submission of a manuscript for publication. The manuscript described unsuspected pathology in Henry's brain, lesions that called into question some of Suzanne's interpretations of Henry's amnesia. Given that Suzanne had dedicated the greater part of her career to the investigation of Henry and had entrusted the histological study of his brain to Annese, the failure to notify her of the impending publication, let alone invite her co-authorship, seems difficult to justify. The brain ownership issue, however, seems to have involved faults on both sides, though Suzanne's increasing ill-health could have been a mitigating factor. Finally, there had been an allegation that Suzanne had shredded scientific notes and records pertaining to Henry. When challenged, Dittrich had been able to release a recording of an interview with Suzanne that bore out his claim. A defence of Suzanne Corkin's reputation appeared six weeks after an article by Dittrich in the *New York Times Magazine*, and was written by two former colleagues: H. Eichenbaum and E. Kensinger, 'In Defense of Suzanne Corkin' *Association for Psychological Science* (30 September 2016) <psychologicalscience.org/observer/in-defense-of-suzanne-corkin/> accessed 22 April 2022. An overview of the dispute had appeared the previous month, however, prompted by letters written to the *New York Times* by 200 supporters of Corkin: S. Begley 'MIT Challenges the New York Times over Book on Famous Brain Patient' *Scientific American Stat Neuroscience* (10 August 2016). <scientificamerican.com/article/mit-challenges-the-new-york-times-over-book-on-famous-brain-patient/> accessed 22 April 2022.

4. J. Annese, N.M. Schenker-Ahmed, H. Bartsch, P. Maechler, C. Sheh, N. Thomas, J. Kayano, A. Ghatan, N. Bresler, M.P. Frosch, R. Klaming, and S. Corkin, 'Postmortem Examination of Patient H.M.'s Brain Based on Histological Sectioning and Digital 3D Reconstruction' (2014) 5 *Nature Communications* 3122 <https://doi.org/10.1038/ncomms4122> accessed 22 April 2022.

5. S. Corkin, *Permanent Present Tense. The Unforgettable Life of the Amnesic Patient, H.M.* (New York, NY: Basic Books, 2013). Suzanne's book had been dedicated 'To the memory of Henry Gustave Molaison. February 26, 1926–December 2, 2008'.

6. See note 3, earlier.

7. E. Kandel, *In Search of Memory. The Emergence of a New Science of Mind* (New York, NY: WW Norton, 2006).

24

Jennifer Aniston Discovered

(Los Angeles, 2005: Itzhak Fried, Christof Koch, Rodrigo Quian Quiroga)

In his delightful part-autobiography *Consciousness. Confessions of a Romantic Reductionist*,[1] Christof Koch recounts that his first encounter with Francis Crick took place in a German orchard, where the co-discoverer of the DNA double helix was to be found lying under an apple tree. The famous Nobel laureate had come to the small university town of Tübingen to discuss biophysical research being undertaken by Koch and his PhD supervisor, Tomaso Poggio. The two had been working on a theoretical model to explain how excitatory and inhibitory inputs might interact in a single neuron, a model that took into account the branching structure of the dendrites. It was 1980 and four years since Crick had declared his intention to devote the remainder of his scientific career to exploring the neural basis of consciousness.

At the time of their meeting, Koch had been 23 (Figure 24.1). He had been born in the United States, in Kansas City. As the son of a German diplomat, Koch's next years would be spent successively in Amsterdam, Bonn, Ottawa, and, finally, Rabat (Morocco). Throughout this peripatetic childhood he had been interested in science, had excelled in physics and mathematics, and had ultimately become fascinated by quantum mechanics and cosmology. Like Peter Milner many years before him, Koch had, as a boy, experimented and built electric devices in the family home.

After gaining his PhD at Tübingen in non-linear information processing, Koch had left Germany for the United States; there, at MIT in Cambridge, his skill in writing computer algorithms was put to use in the Artificial Intelligence Laboratory. Then had come a move to Caltech (the California Institute of Technology), a relatively small but high-powered university in Pasadena that was, or had been, the academic home of no fewer than 39 Nobel Laureates (!) It was at this time that Koch's research with Shimon Ullman on theoretical aspects of vision had attracted the attention of Francis Crick at the Salk Institute. Invited to La Jolla, Koch had been questioned intensively about his work by the older man. The two had quickly established a rapport and from then until Crick's death in 2004, had collaborated closely in a search for what they termed the NCC (Neural Correlates of Consciousness). Never a modest person, Crick had largely dismissed all previous work in the field, claiming that he and Koch were the instigators of a new type of study, the science of consciousness. With their entry into the field, they held that consciousness had finally become a legitimate field of enquiry.[2]

Aranzio's Seahorse and the Search for Memory and Consciousness. Alan J. McComas, Oxford University Press.
© Oxford University Press 2023. DOI: 10.1093/oso/9780192868244.003.0026

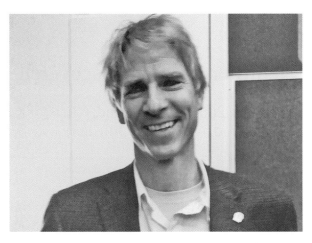

Figure 24.1 Kristof Koch. Having collaborated extensively with the late Francis Crick, Koch remains a major authority on conscious mechanisms and is currently President and Chief Scientist of the Allen Institute for Brain Science, based in Seattle. (2008 photo by Romanpoet, from Wikimedia Commons.)

It would have been difficult not to disagree with this statement, especially after studying *Brain Mechanisms and Consciousness*,[3] the proceedings of the 1953 Laurentian symposium that Herbert Jasper had organized. How could one disregard the work of Adrian, Penfield, Jasper himself, Magoun, Bremer, and Grey Walter, to name but a few of the previous workers.

With a number of wrong turns, the course of the new science of NCC proved difficult to follow. Despite the ability of frontal lobotomized patients to see perfectly well, the front of the brain was identified as the site where information in the visual pathway finally achieved consciousness.[4] Attention was brought about by a thalamic 'searchlight'.[5] The deep pyramidal neurons in the neocortex were the cells generating consciousness.[6] Different aspects of a sensory stimulus (a visual scene, for example) were linked together by repetitive synchronous firing of neurons in different regions of the brain (despite solid evidence of sensory cortex operating in brief 'chunks' of time).[7] Finally, in their last paper together, one that Crick was still working on during his last hours of life, he and Koch proposed that the seat of consciousness might be the claustrum, a thin sheet of cells underlying the main cortex.[8] Many of Crick's ideas were contained in *The Astonishing Hypothesis. The Scientific Search for the Soul*,[9] a book presumably intended for the public rather than for a neuroscientist with a copy of Eric Kandel and James Schwartz's *Principles of Neuroscience* on his or her bookshelf.

The approach of Crick and Koch to explaining the mind was very much 'top-down', one that considered the way the brain *ought* to work, had it been designed by an engineer. Nevertheless, Crick and Koch did succeed in generating discussion and experiment, and valid questions were raised that have yet to be answered. For example, what *was* the function of the hitherto neglected claustrum?

In 2005, however, speculation was replaced by fact. Christof Koch co-authored one of the most important papers ever written about consciousness. It had to do with what he and his co-authors termed 'concept' cells, but which the lay public have come to refer to as 'Jennifer Aniston' neurons. To some neuroscientists, especially those of an older generation, the same neurons would be 'gnostic units' or 'grandmother cells'. Had he still lived, the great pioneering US psychologist William James would have recognized them as his 'pontifical' neurons.[10] It was a type of cell that Koch and his colleagues had discovered in the human hippocampus and, less frequently, in neighbouring structures (parahippocampal gyrus, entorhinal cortex, amygdala).

The subjects for these experiments had been epileptic patients under consideration for temporal lobe surgery, in the tradition of Penfield, Foerster, and others. It was hoped that recording from electrodes implanted in the temporal lobe would assist in lo-cating the origin of the seizure activity. With stereotactic guidance, a leash of nine fine platinum-iridium wires was inserted into the target structure in the medial temporal lobe, the uninsulated ends of wires acting as the recording surfaces. One of the authors of the paper, Itzhak Fried, was a leading Los Angeles neurosurgeon under whose care the patients were being investigated and treated. Alone of the authors, Fried had had experience in this type of recording, having employed them for other cognitive tests.

A problem that Fried had encountered, one common to all experiments with re-cording with electrodes positioned outside the cells, was that more than one neuron could be active at any given time, giving rise to a confusing pattern of impulses. In the Los Angeles studies this was true for each of the wire electrodes inserted in the patient's brain. It was the same type of problem that had been encountered by electromyographers during needle examinations of contracting muscles—as the voluntary effort increased, so did the recording become ever more complex until it was impossible to recognize the contributions of the various muscle fibres (or fibre groups). The solution had been to write computer software that could make the distinctions using differences in the amplitudes, steepness, and shapes of the electric potentials. This is what Rodrigo Quian Quiroga now attempted for the brain recordings, though the small sizes and profusion of the potentials made the task a difficult one.

It was the kind of challenge that Quiroga (Figure 24.2) was well equipped to meet. He had been born in Argentina and had attended the University of Buenos Aires. As a young man, his admiration for the literary work of Jorge Luis Borges,[11] especially in relation to memory, was combined with a strong scientific interest in chaos theory. As a student exercise he had applied chaos theory to the interpretation of the EKG (elec-trocardiogram) before realizing that the electrical activity of the brain (EEG) offered more interesting opportunities. He had then gone to Lübeck in Germany for advanced study, obtaining a PhD in Applied Mathematics. During that time he had developed a highly effective mathematical treatment for distinguishing EEG potentials, based on 'wavelet' analysis; it was not an elegant method, he would say, but it was very efficient nonetheless. Next had come a move to the United States, to the California Institute of Technology, where he had joined Christof Koch in the study with Itzhak Fried. Sorting

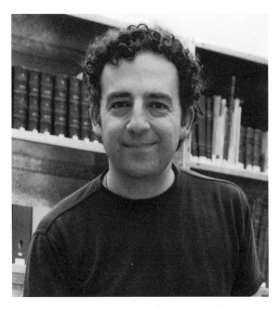

Figure 24.2 Rodrigo Quian Quiroga. Photograph courtesy of Dr Quiroga.

out the discharges of individual neurons was far more difficult than the earlier EEG analysis had been but, as the published illustrations would show, Quiroga's eventual method would work perfectly. It was now possible to determine what type of stimulus, if any, caused a particular cell to fire.

In addition to Fried, Koch, and Quiroga, the initial Los Angeles experiments also in-volved Leila Reddy and Gabriel Krieman, both from Koch's laboratory.[12] The first step was a screening session during which the subject, who had already had the recording electrodes implanted, was seated in front of a laptop computer. On the computer screen a series of images were briefly flashed, the images being those of famous and non-famous people, animals, well-known buildings, and various objects. The same images were repeated several times in random order and the recordings then analysed to deter-mine if the firing of a neuron could be correlated to a particular picture. If it could, then the same image would be part of a later testing session, though with variations—for example, different views of the same head. These 'test' images would be mixed among a greater number of randomly chosen ones unlikely to produce responses. The testing procedure would then be repeated.

The results were extraordinary. For example, in one subject a neuron was found that responded exclusively to photographs of the actress, Jennifer Aniston. In another sub-ject it was a different actress, Halle Berry, who stimulated a neuron and did so regard-less of her pose or clothing outfit; the same neuron also fired to a written spelling of the actress' name. A third neuron, in a different subject, responded to images and to the written name of the Sydney Opera House (Figure 24.3). All three neurons were said to show 'invariance' in their responsiveness, in that each was excited only by the one subject, regardless of the form in which information about the subject was presented.

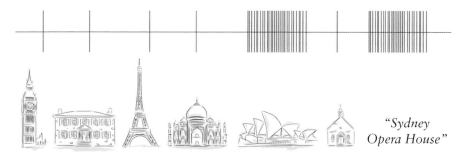

Figure 24.3 Simulation of hippocampal neuron responding to an image of the Sydney Opera House but not to those of other well-known buildings, as well as to the written name of the famous concert hall.

The authors referred to these neurons as 'concept' cells but, as noted earlier, they had been postulated to exist by previous scientists who had given them various names— grandmother cells, pontifical cells, gnostic neurons.[13] As matters now stand, however, they seem destined to be known as Jennifer Aniston neurons—a legacy that may out-live the subject's fame as an actress.

In later work, Christof Koch, Moran Cerf, and their colleagues went a step further, by showing that the very act of thinking about the subject of a concept cell would increase the number of nerve impulses fired (in one example, by a 'Marilyn Monroe' cell).[14]

The proof of the existence of concept cells was a triumph for the investigators as well as for the neurophysiological approach to the study of brain function. The results were unambiguous—the hippocampus, throughout its length, was a store of memories, memories that were encoded by single neurons. One might add that, by virtue of the nature of the testing, it was semantic memory that had been examined.[15]

At the time that single cell recordings were yielding unequivocal results, the hippo-campus became the subject of an increasingly heated debate. It concerned an important question, one that was relevant not only to the normal function of the structure but also to the consequences of aging and disease. It was a question that challenged the pre-vailing dogma.

Was it possible that new neurons were being formed in the hippocampus throughout life?

Notes

1. C. Koch, *Consciousness. Confessions of a Romantic Reductionist* (Cambridge, MA; MIT Press, 2012).
2. F.H.C. Crick, 'Thinking about the Brain' (1979) 241 *Scientific American* 219–32.
3. J.F. Delafresnaye (ed.), *Brain Mechanisms and Consciousness* (Springfield, IL: Charles C Thomas, 1954). See also Chapter 3.
4. F.H.C. Crick and C. Koch, 'Are We Aware of Neural Activity in Primary Visual Cortex?' (1995) 375 *Nature* 121–4.

5. F.H.C. Crick, 'Function of the Thalamic Reticular Complex: The Searchlight Hypothesis' (1984) 81 *Proceedings of the National Academy of Sciences, USA* 4586–90.

6. F.H.C. Crick and C. Koch, 'The Problem of Consciousness' (1992) 267 *Scientific American* 152–9.

7. See Crick, 'Function of the Thalamic Reticular Complex', see note 5.

8. F.H.C. Crick and C. Koch, 'What is the Function of the Claustrum?' (2005) 360 *Philosophical Transactions of the Royal Society of London, B* 1271–9.

9. F.H.C. Crick, *The Astonishing Hypothesis. The Scientific Search for the Soul* (New York, NY: Scribner, 1994). The reviews of the public were mixed, common complaints being (i) that the hypothesis of nerve impulses being responsible for the many properties of the brain was not astonishing at all; (ii) that to include 'Soul' in the title was misleading and, given the well-known atheism of the author, smacked of a marketing ploy to attract believers; and (iii) too much emphasis had been placed on vision as opposed to other senses and brain mechanisms. On the other hand, many readers did like the book, some finding it inspirational, and even established neuroscientists appreciated the liveliness of the writing and the intelligent mind behind it.

10. See Chapter 14.

11. Jorge Luis Borges (1899–1986) was an Argentinian writer renowned for the richness, variety, and imagination of his short stories, some of which had a dream-like, surrealistic style. At one time Borges was a Professor of Literature at the University of Buenos Aires. Prematurely blind through a familial disorder, he continued writing and, though the recipient of many awards, was considered unlucky not to have been awarded a Nobel Prize in Literature.

12. Unsurprisingly, given its importance, the first publication of the experiments appeared in *Nature*: R.Q. Quiroga, L. Reddy, G. Kreiman, C. Koch, and I. Fried, 'Invariant Visual Representation by Single Neurons in the Human Brain' (2005) 435 *Nature* 1102–7. The *Scientific American* provided an easily assimilated version: R.Q. Quiroga, I. Fried, and C. Koch, 'Brain Cells for Grandmother' (2013) February *Scientific American* 31–5. The publication with the most detailed description of the methodology as well as later (United Kingdom) results is: H.G. Rey, M.J. Ison, C. Pedreira, A. Valentin, G. Alarcon, R. Selway, M.P. Richardson, and R.Q. Quiroga, 'Single-Cell Recordings in the Human Medial Temporal Lobe' (2015) 227 *Journal of Anatomy* 394–408. Lastly, Quiroga has given an excellent overview: R.Q. Quiroga, 'Concept Cells: The Building Blocks of Declarative Memory Functions' (2012) 13 *Nature Neuroscience* 587–97.

13. There is at least one distinction between the various terms in that Konorski appeared not to envisage the possibility of gnostic units resulting from combined processing in different sensory modalities (vision and hearing, for example), as may occur for concept cells.

14. M. Cerf, N. Thiruvengadam, F. Mormann, A. Kraskov, R.Q. Quiroga, C. Koch, and I. Fried, 'Online, Voluntary Control of Human Temporal Lobe Neurons' (2010) 467 *Nature* 1104–8.

15. This work has now been taken up elsewhere. Rodrigo Quian Quiroga presently holds a Research Chair at the University of Leicester (United Kingdom) where he is Director of the Centre for Systems Neuroscience. The subjects that he studies are epileptic patients at King's College Hospital in London.

25

New Cells or Not?

(1983–present, New York, Boston, Princeton, New Haven,
La Jolla: Fernando Nottebohm, Joseph Altman, Michael Kaplan,
Elizabeth Gould, Pasko Rakic, Fred Gage)

It was birdsong that had started the debate, though the arguments might have begun much sooner.

Like Rodrigo Quian Quiroga, Fernando Nottebohm (Figure 25.1) had been born in Argentina, though in an earlier generation.[1] His father had been a rancher and it was while exploring the family pampas that young Fernando had acquired his love of birds and fascination for their songs and behaviours. After graduating from school in Buenos Aires he had left Argentina for the United States and the study of farming at the University of Nebraska. A year had been enough for Fernando Nottebohm to realize his calling was for an academic life, rather than that of a farmer or rancher. He had enrolled at the University of California at Berkeley where he had come under the influence of the enterprising biologist Peter Marler, himself a former student of the noted Cambridge (United Kingdom) ethologist, William Thorpe. Marler had been studying birdsong and, as his eventual doctoral student, Nottebohm discovered that songbirds, like humans, exhibited neural laterality; just as the left side of the human brain-controlled speech and the dominant (right) hand, so the left side of the avian brain-controlled song production by the muscles of the syrinx. It had been yet another example of a fortuitous discovery. Nottebohm had then proceeded to work out the neural circuits in the avian brain responsible for producing song, identifying one particularly important region that he termed the HVC (Higher Vocal Centre).

By now, Nottebohm was a junior professor at Rockefeller University in New York; not only was he at one of the country's most prestigious universities but it was a university that had a field centre and aviary in the country north of the city. Of particular interest to him were birds such as canaries and zebra finches, the males of which acquired new songs for the mating season each spring. He noticed that the HVC was considerably larger in the male birds than in the (non-singing) females, the enlargement developing in the spring and disappearing later in the year. However, if he injected female canaries with the male hormone, testosterone, not only did their HVCs enlarge but the birds now sang like males.[2] Though there was lengthening of dendrites and formation of additional synapses in the HVC neurons, was this enough to account for the remarkable increase in size of the structure? Was it possible that new neurons were being formed as well? With a student, Steve Goldman, Nottebohm determined to find out.

Aranzio's Seahorse and the Search for Memory and Consciousness. Alan J. McComas, Oxford University Press.
© Oxford University Press 2023. DOI: 10.1093/oso/9780192868244.003.0027

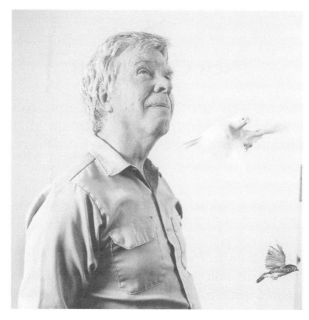

Figure 25.1 Fernando Nottebohm. Photograph courtesy of Dr Nottebohm and Rockefeller University.

The new experiments were carried out on female canaries that received injections of [³H]-thymidine, the rationale being that this base would have been incorporated in the nuclear DNA of any recently formed neurons. The radioactivity of the thymidine could then be detected using silver particles in a photographic emulsion. The results of the experiments were unambiguous––new neurons had indeed been created in female canaries, but only in those treated with testosterone.[3] It was, or so it seemed, the first time that neurogenesis had been demonstrated in an adult warm-blooded vertebrate. It was also the overturning of a well-entrenched dogma, namely, that the maximum number of neurons was established in infancy; after that nerve cells might die but none could be formed to take their place. It was at this point in his research that Fernando Nottebohm made a disconcerting discovery. Twenty years before a similar finding had been published and then forgotten.

Not in birds but in rats.

The earlier work had been carried out in Cambridge, Massachusetts, in the Psychophysiological Laboratory at MIT, where Joseph Altman would have been a colleague of Suzanne Corkin––the latter by then the lead investigator of the amnesic patient, Henry Molaison.

Altman's life story was impressive.[4] A Hungarian Jew (Figure 25.2), he had been one of the few to survive the Holocaust; after the Second World War he had emigrated with his family to the United States via Germany and Australia. Despite an interrupted education he had managed to keep himself by working as a librarian, at the same time making use of the books to study psychology, human behaviour, and brain anatomy. Having eventually gained admission to New York University, he had succeeded in

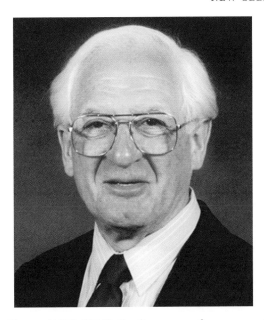

Figure 25.2 Joseph Altman (1925–2016), the discoverer of neurogenesis in the adult mammalian brain, in his later years. Photograph courtesy of Dr Shirley A Bayer.

obtaining a PhD in psychology. He had then been appointed to a faculty position in psychology at MIT and it was there that he had embarked on a study of the rat brain. Though familiar with the belief that new neurons were not formed in adult mammals, he had been aware of old literature showing that this was not the case for the cerebellum in young animals, in which small granule cells continued to be produced. Even so, it had been a bold move on Altman's part to explore the situation for the mammalian cortex––negative studies are readily forgotten, even if they are accepted for publication.

For his experiments Altman, working with Gopal Das, had employed the same approach Nottebohm would use 20 years later––the injection of a radioactive tracer, [3H]-thymidine, followed by a search for its incorporation into the DNA of dividing cells. Altman had already shown that the other type of cell found in nervous tissue, the glial cell, not only multiplied after part of the brain had been damaged but that new cells continued to form throughout life. For his new work on rats, Altman had concentrated on the dentate gyrus, the most medial part of the hippocampus. The results had been unequivocal––though there was a large number of labelled neurons in young animals, as might have been expected, a smaller but still appreciable number were found after adult rats had been injected with the tritiated thymidine. Further, the newly formed neurons appeared to have arisen immediately below the cells lining the fluid cavity (lateral ventricle) and to have then migrated into the substance of the dentate gyrus. Altman and Das found evidence of continuing neurogenesis also in the olfactory bulb and cerebellum of adult rats. In all three situations it was the small neurons (granule cells) that were newly formed; the larger neurons, those with long axons, did not appear to increase.[5]

Altman's finding that new nerve cells continued to be produced in the adult mammalian brain had been a major discovery. Moreover, his publication (with Gopal Das as co-author) had been in *Nature*, one of the two top general science journals,[6] and there would be other reports. So why had the work not received the attention it deserved? The most likely answer is that the prevailing dogma was too strong for it to be contradicted by a single study. If one were to search for a weakness in Altman's approach, it might be a failure to differentiate granule neurons from glial cells, since both types of cell were small and could be mistaken for each other with the light microscope. In 1913, eight years after winning a Nobel Prize, the great Spanish neuroanatomist Ramon y Cajal, had written: 'None of the methods used by these investigators are capable of distinguishing absolutely a multiplying neuroglia cell from a small mitotic neuron.'[7] Even within his own university department it seemed that the importance and originality of Altman's research was not recognized; denied tenure at MIT, Altman would continue his academic career at Purdue University.

Altman would not be the only one to have his work ignored, however.

In 1970 Michael Kaplan began undergraduate studies at Tulane University in New Orleans, and came under the influence of Professor J.W. Harper.[8] Harper was one of the few to have taken note of Altman's publications and to have accepted the latter's findings. Was it possible, Harper wondered, that neurogenesis would be enhanced in an enriched environment? It was an interesting question for a student to answer. Like Altman before him, Kaplan injected rats with [^{3}H]-thymidine and at the end of an experiment examined autoradiographs of excised visual cortex with the light microscope. And, indeed, not only was there evidence of neurogenesis but the latter was greatest in rats reared in an environment enriched with wheels, balls, and toys.

Unable to get the work published, Kaplan had returned to the project as a doctoral student at Boston University. Having access to an electron microscope, he was now able to use the greater magnification to identify neurons by the presence of dendrites and synapses. Kaplan was able to confirm the presence of neurogenesis in the rat visual cortex as well as demonstrating it in the olfactory bulb.[9,10] This time the work was published. Later, as a postdoctoral fellow at Florida State University, Kaplan extended his studies to the rat hippocampus, again finding evidence of neurogenesis and again publishing his findings in a reputable journal.[11] Yet again, however, there was little interest or, worse, disbelief.

Matters came to a head in 1984 at a meeting sponsored by the New York Academy of Sciences. It was then, as a contributor to the 'Hope for a New Neurology' meeting, that Kaplan came face-to-face with the world's leading authority on the development of the cerebral cortex.

Pasko Rakic (Figure 25.3) had been born in the former Yugoslavia before the Second World War and had graduated in medicine at the University of Belgrade.[12] With the intention of becoming a neurosurgeon, Rakic had gone to Harvard on a Fulbright Fellowship in order to increase his knowledge of the nervous system. It was there, in Boston, that he had fallen under the influence of the neuroanatomist Paul Yakovlev and become attracted to the study of brain development. After returning to Belgrade and

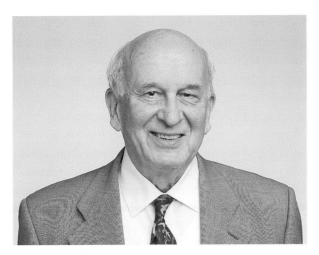

Figure 25.3 Pasko Rakic. (Royal Society photograph. Wikimedia Commons file: Professor Pasko Rakic. ForMemRS.jpg. Creative Commons Attribution-Share Alike 3.0 Unported license.)

conducting research on this subject for a PhD, Rakic was invited back to Harvard, this time as a faculty member. He had not been the first to choose a career in basic neuroscience over life as a neurosurgeon.[13] At Harvard, Rakic had embarked on an investigation of cerebral development in primates, using [^{3}H]-thymidine to detect dividing neural stem cells and to follow the fates of their progeny. It had been an ambitious study, one that had involved the preparation and examination of a huge number of brain sections. Neurons were shown to be produced by stem cells immediately under the linings of the ventricles. The same stem cells also formed glia and it was the radial processes of the glial cells that served as scaffolding along which the immature neurons moved to take up their final positions in the cerebral cortex.[14,15] It was important and elegant work and immediately recognized as such. It led to Rakic being recruited by Yale University and becoming both the founding Chair of the Department of Neurobiology and, like Edvard and May-Britt Moser in Trondheim, the director of a Kavli Institute for Neuroscience. Many honours would follow, among them the 1995–96 Presidency of the Society for Neuroscience.

Pasko Rakic and Michael Kaplan were not the only neuroscientists at the 1984 meeting 'Hope for a New Neurology', sponsored by the New York Academy of Sciences. Fernando Nottebohm had been invited to talk about neurogenesis in songbirds, and there, sitting in the audience though not presenting, was Joseph Altman. Also present was Shirley Bayer, Altman's former student and now his wife and research colleague at Purdue University. Bayer had continued Altman's work, showing that the rat hippocampus increased both in size and in the number of neurons throughout adult life. The finding of a continuing production of neurons was in agreement with the results of Michael Kaplan.

But Rakic had been dismissive about neurogenesis in the adult,[16] reminding the audience that Nottebohm's novel findings had been restricted to songbirds. As for the mammals, Rakic claimed that there was still doubt about the identities of any newly formed granule cells––most likely they were glia. Even if some were neurons, the process was almost certainly restricted to the brains of 'lower' mammals. He, Rakic, in his huge study of primate brains (10,000 slides from ten monkeys) had never observed neurogenesis in adults. Surely, he reasoned, cognition and social behaviour was best served by having a stable population of neurons. The meeting, with Rakic's strongly expressed opposition to the concept of adult neurogenesis, proved a turning point. Michael Kaplan abandoned neuroscience to become a medical student.

And yet Kaplan's position had been a strong one. He had cleverly developed a technique that enabled him to examine the ultrastructural features of any cell with radioactive evidence of having been recently created. And, sure enough, synaptic vesicles could sometimes be seen, confirming that such a cell was a neuron rather than a glia. By combining light microscopy and electron microscopy on the same cell, he had achieved something that Rakic had not. Moreover, Kaplan, despite his academic juniority, now had a series of publications in good journals. Also, he was not alone––there was Nottebohm and Altman, and now Shirley Bayer too, all of them reporting neurogenesis. But there was still Rakic's objection that, even if the process did occur in adult animals, it did not take place in humans.

The situation for humans could have been resolved if a new and powerful experiment had been allowed––to mimic the rat experiments by injecting terminally ill patient volunteers with [^{3}H]-thymidine and examining the brains post-mortem for evidence of neurogenesis. The idea had occurred to Fernando Nottebohm. He had approached the Sloan Kettering Memorial Hospital in New York only to be turned down by the hospital's ethics committee. Kaplan had had a similar thought later, his being to inject tritiated thymidine directly into brain tumours and to look for evidence of newly produced neurons at post-mortem. Though the project had received funding, it had not gained the support of the university administration. A third attempt at a similar study using patients was successful, however; remarkably, one of the lead investigators was a descendant of a famous neurological patient. That ancestor had been Phineas Gage, the young railway engineer who had survived an accident in which a large iron tamping rod had been driven through the front of his brain.[17]

It was Phineas' descendant, Fred Gage (Figure 25.4), who, more than a century later, would also think of using a labelled DNA precursor in terminally ill patients as a means of detecting any formation of new neurons in the human hippocampus. At the time Gage was at the Salk Institute in La Jolla, California, but the patient volunteers and colleagues would be in Sweden, a country that Gage knew well from an earlier collaboration. In the new study there were five cancer patients who had received an analogue of thymidine, bromodeoxyuridine (BrdU), as part of a diagnostic procedure. The advantage of BrdU over thymidine was that, unlike the latter, it could be detected by immunofluorescence. The study also made use of cell-specific molecular markers to distinguish neurons from glial cells in the post-mortem tissue. The results were unambiguous–– some 20 per cent of neurons in the dentate nucleus of the hippocampus had been recently generated, and a similar figure was obtained for glial cells.[18] Like Nottebohm's

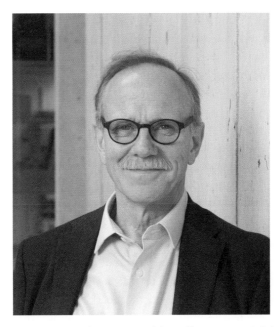

Figure 25.4 Fred Gage. Photograph courtesy of the Salk Institute, California.

canaries and the rats studied by Altman and Kaplan, humans created new neurons (in the hippocampus) throughout life. Interestingly, Gage had been at the New York Academy of Sciences Meeting in 1984, together with Nottebohm, Kaplan, Rakic, and Joseph Altman. However, rather than speak about the new studies in patients Gage had, with Anders Bjorklund, presented earlier work on grafting neural tissue into rat models of parkinsonism and Alzheimer's disease.

The publication of the results in the Swedish patients came at a fortuitous time for another researcher. Elizabeth Gould had also fallen foul of Rakic through her experiments. Her interest in the hippocampus had arisen while investigating the effect of stress on the rat brain. In the laboratory of Bruce McEwen at the Rockefeller University, Elizabeth had noticed that there was widespread death of hippocampal neurons following removal of the adrenal glands. This, by itself, was a striking finding but there was another one to follow––when she counted the neurons remaining in the hippocampus, the number was normal! The only possible explanation was that new neurons had been formed, potentially mitigating any effects of the cell death.[19]

Puzzled by her observations, Elizabeth Gould then spent long hours in the Rockefeller Library searching for any report of neurogenesis in the adult mammalian brain. And eventually she found it––Joseph Altman's publications on the use of $[^3H]$-thymidine to demonstrate the phenomenon in rats (and, later, in cats and guinea pigs). Ironically, there was someone in Elizabeth's own university who had also described neurogenesis and whose research was ongoing––Fernando Nottebohm, the discoverer of massive seasonal formation of neurons in male songbirds. Encouraged by these precedents, Elizabeth now devoted her research to the study of neurogenesis, using rats and more advanced techniques than those available to Altman. She was able to show, as others had, that neurogenesis was enhanced by an animal's exposure to an enriched environment, one that included a running wheel and various 'toys' to investigate. In the opposite direction was her finding that neurogenesis was suppressed in tree shrews subjected to stress (for example, by the presence of a rival).[20] In recognition of her research Elizabeth Gould had been appointed to Princeton in 1987, acquiring tenure and a full professorship three years later. By then she was searching for evidence of neurogenesis in different species of primate––and finding it.

Inevitably, just as had happened to Michael Kaplan, she had incurred Rakic's displeasure. There was a difference between her situation and Kaplan's, however, in that she had the support of a senior neuroscientist, one who was a close colleague. Charles Gross, before moving to Princeton, had been Chair of the Psychology Department at Harvard. Among many accomplishments he had been the first to show the presence in the primate temporal lobe of neurons responding to a visual object (in his experiment, a hand). Generous in his attitude to others, Gross had also supported the work and ideas of the Polish neuroscientist, Jerzy Konorski, including the latter's concept of 'gnostic units' in the brain. Also in Elizabeth Gould's favour was the new report, by Fred Gage and his Swedish colleagues, of neurogenesis in adult humans, those terminally ill cancer patients who had received BrdU infusions for diagnostic purposes.

The pressure was now on Rakic and a publication from his laboratory duly appeared in 1999.[21] It now appeared that there was, after all, evidence of neurogenesis in the hippocampus of the adult macaque monkey. It was a grudging admission, however, for the new cells were described as being few in number and capable of being easily overlooked. Moreover, Rakic cautioned, the finding did not necessarily apply to humans.

Further evidence on the matter was to come, however. Especially convincing were the results of a novel strategy, namely to look for incorporation of ^{14}C in the post-mortem brains of humans who were alive in 1955–63, a period when atmospheric radioactivity had sharply increased as a result of atomic bomb testing.[22] The theory behind this approach was that radioactive carbon would have been converted to carbon dioxide in the atmosphere, taken up by plants and then entered into the food chain, some ultimately appearing in the DNA of newly formed cells throughout the body. With mathematical treatment of the data, the international team of investigators estimated that the adult human hippocampus formed an average of 700 new neurons every day, a rate that continued at least into middle age; there was, in addition, evidence of a slow turnover of neurons. The authors suggested, as others had, that the new hippocampal neurons would become operational, entering neural circuits involved in learning and memory.

The radioactive carbon study was an important contribution to research on the hippocampus. When the results of all the various investigations were combined, the balance of evidence was that the hippocampus (specifically, the dentate gyrus) continued producing neurons throughout life.[23] The rate, however, was not constant. There was some decline with age and a potentially severe depression with stress; on the other hand, cell production was increased by cognitive challenge (environmental enrichments) and, perhaps more surprisingly, by physical exercise.

Despite all the findings indicative of hippocampal neurogenesis, including Rakic's own paper on the macaque monkey, the scientific issue was not totally laid to rest, however. Rakic's paper might have signalled a retreat but it was not the end of his war, as dissenting papers on neurogenesis from his laboratory or those of former colleagues continued to appear. Nevertheless, for the majority of those in the field, the intellectual struggle was over—as had happened for some of the other great controversies in neuroscience.[24]

Adding to the excitement generated by the validation of neurogenesis as a biological phenomenon in adult humans was a further thought. Not only did the findings help explain how the brain normally functioned but they offered the prospect of future treatments for neurodegenerative disorders. Parkinsonism could be one such target and even Alzheimer's disease might prove remediable.

But this supposed that the new neurons formed in adult brains were able to function.

Did they, in fact, develop normally and make synaptic connections with other neurons—especially those that were their natural destinations? And, in the case of the hippocampus, was there any evidence that the new neurons were active in learning and memory?

Not surprisingly, given his earlier work demonstrating hippocampal neurogenesis in cancer patients, these were questions of interest to Fred Gage, among others. The approach of Gage's group at the Salk Institute was to inject mouse hippocampi with the gene for a fluorescent protein, using a retrovirus as vector (to get the external gene included in the cell's genome).[25] Any newly formed neurons would then express the (green) fluorescent protein and would glow when the tissue was illuminated under the microscope. In the dentate gyrus newly formed granule cells were seen to move into position in the granular layer before growing and extending dendrites into the molecular layer. At the same time axons appeared and grew towards the pyramidal cells in the hippocampal CA3 region, with which they would form synaptic connections. Meanwhile the dendritic branches became more elaborate and, by a month, had developed most of their spines.

The new hippocampal neurons now appeared sufficiently mature to be integrated into functioning neural circuits. Though Gage and his colleagues found that the same steps occurred in the same order irrespective of the age of the mice, they took rather longer in older animals. A further observation was that mice reared in cages with a running wheel had more than double the number of new hippocampal neurons when compared with sedentary controls.

But what about behaviour—were the new hippocampal neurons operational? Forty years earlier Joseph Altman, the discoverer of neurogenesis, had explored the possibility following his move to Purdue University. With young colleagues he had irradiated the hippocampi of young rats so as to prevent further granule cell production; the effects on various behaviours were mixed, though in some tests significant differences from control animals emerged, suggestive of impaired learning in the treated ones.[26]

Since Altman's study there have been others reporting behavioural changes following interference with hippocampal neurogenesis. However, a recent investigation has suggested that newly formed hippocampal neurons may also be involved in attention. The study was initiated by Heather Cameron, Elizabeth Gould's colleague at the time they had discovered hippocampal cell death and neogenesis following adrenalectomy. Now at NIH, Cameron transfected rats with herpes simplex virus thymidine kinase gene and then, at specified times, killed the cells with an antiviral agent. She and her colleagues found that rats that had been receiving the antiviral drug for at least four weeks, and consequently had been unable to form new neurons during that time, differed from controls in at least one very obvious respect. They were less able to shift their attention. The experiments differed from previous ones in that they did not require any previous training, nor were electric shocks involved. All that was necessary was to observe whether a thirsty rat, while drinking water from a bottle, would shift its attention on hearing an unexpected sound (finger snapping, or audio clicks). Control ('wild-type') rats would cease drinking and turn their heads towards the sound. Treated rats did not.[27]

In summary, then, not only are new hippocampal neurons required for learning but they enable attention to be switched more readily. This is unlikely to be the last word on hippocampal neurogenesis for, as important as the various ablation studies have been, in terms of elegance, versatility, and investigative power they have been overtaken by a new science.

Optogenetics.

Notes

1. The story of Nottebohm's life and research, together with an extensive list of his publications, is given in: F. Nottebohm, *The History of Neuroscience in Autobiography*, L.R. Squire (ed.) (Washington, DC: Society for Neuroscience, 2014) 8: 324–60. A very readable account of his work was given by Michael Specter in *The New Yorker*, 23 July 2001 ('How the songs of canaries upset a fundamental principle of science').
2. F. Nottebohm, 'Testosterone Triggers Growth of Brain Vocal Control Nuclei in Adult Female Canaries' (1980) 189 *Brain Research* 429–36.
3. S.A. Goldman and F. Nottebohm, 'Neuronal Production, Migration and Differentiation in a Vocal Control Nucleus of the Adult Female Canary Brain' (1983) 80 *Proceedings of the National Academy of Sciences, USA* 2390–4.
4. Joseph Altman (1925–2016). Wikipedia. <en.wikipedia.org/wiki/Joseph_Altman>
5. J. Altman and G.D. Das, 'Post-Natal Origin of Microneurones in the Rat Brain' (1965) 207 *Nature* 953–6.
6. The other being *Science*.
7. S. Ramon y Cajal, *Degeneration and Regeneration of the Nervous System* (translated by R.M. Day from the 1913 Spanish edition) (London: Oxford University Press, 1928), cited by C.G. Gross, 'Neurogenesis in the Adult Brain: Death of a Dogma' (2000) 1 *Nature Reviews Neuroscience* 67–73.
8. M.S. Kaplan, 'Environment Complexity Stimulates Visual Cortex Neurogenesis; Death of a Dogma and a Research Career' (2001) 24(10) *Trends in Neurosciences* 617–20.
9. M.S. Kaplan, 'Neurogenesis in the Three Month Old Rat Visual Cortex' (1981) 195 *Journal of Comparative Anatomy* 323–38.

10. M.S. Kaplan and J.W. Hinds, 'Neurogenesis in the Adult Rat: Electronmicroscopic Analysis of Light Radiographs' (1977) 197 *Science* 1092–4.

11. M.S. Kaplan and D.H. Bell, 'Neuronal Proliferation in the Nine-Month-Old Rodent: Radioautograhic Study of Granule Cells in the Hippocampus' (1983) 52 *Experimental Brain Research* 1–5.

12. Wikipedia. <http://www.en.wikipedia.org/wiki/Pasko_Rakic> accessed 24 April 2022.

13. Other examples of neurosurgeons becoming leading neuroscientists include John Fulton, Vernon Mountcastle, and Rodolfo Llinas.

14. P. Rakic, 'Mode of Cell Migration to the Superficial Layers of Fetal Monkey Neocortex' (1972) 145(1) *Journal of Comparative Neurology* 61–83.

15. P. Rakic, 'Neurons in Rhesus Monkey Visual Cortex: Systematic Relation Between Time of Origin and Eventual Disposition' (1974) 183(4123) *Science* 425–7.

16. P. Rakic, 'DNA Synthesis and Cell Division in the Adult Primate Brain' (1985) 457 *Annals of the New York Academy of Sciences* 193–211.

17. See Chapter 4, also: A.J. McComas, *Sherrington's Loom. An Introduction to the Science of Consciousness* (New York, NY: Oxford University Press, 2019).

18. P.S. Eriksson, E. Perfilijeva, T. Björk-Eriksson, A.-M. Alborn, C. Nordborg, D.A. Peterson, and F.H. Gage, 'Neurogenesis in the Adult Human Hippocampus' (1998) 11(4) *Nature Medicine* 1313–17.

19. H.A. Cameron and E. Gould, 'Adult Neogenesis is Regulated by Adrenal Steroids in the Dentate Gyrus' (1994) 61(2) *Neuroscience* 203–9.

20. E. Gould, B.S. McEwen, P. Tanapat, L.A.M. Galea, and E. Fuchs, 'Neurogenesis in the Dentate Gyrus of the Adult Tree Shrew is Regulated by Psychosocial Stress and NMDA Receptor Activation' (1997) 17 *Journal of Neuroscience* 2492–8.

21. D.R. Kornack and P. Rakic, 'Continuation of Neogenesis in the Hippocampus of the Adult Macaque Monkey' (1999) 96 *Proceedings of the National Academy of Sciences, USA* 5768–73.

22. K.L. Spalding, O. Bergmann, K. Alkass, S. Bernard, M. Salehpour, H.B. Juttner, E. Boström, I. Westerlund, C. Vial, B.A. Buchholz, G. Possnert, D.C. Mash, H. Druid, and J. Frisén, 'Dynamics of Hippocampal Neurogenesis in Adult Humans' (2013) 153 *Cell* 1219–27.

23. Newer, more advanced, techniques continue to show the presence of substantial neurogenesis in the human hippocampus throughout life, as in the doublecortin expression study of Moreno-Jiménez and colleagues in Madrid. See: E.P. Moreno-Jiménez, M. Flor-Garcia, J. Terreros-Roncal, A. Rábano, F. Cafini, N. Pallas-Bazarra, J. Ávila, and M. Llorens-Martin, 'Adult Hippocampal Neurogenesis is Abundant in Neurologically Healthy Subjects and Drops Sharply in Patients with Alzheimer's Disease' (2019) 25 *Nature Medicine* 554–60.

24. The reality or not of hippocampal neurogenesis was but the most recent major argument in neuroscience. There had been others equally severe. At the Nobel Prize ceremony in 1905 Camillo Golgi had strongly disagreed with Ramon y Cajal, his fellow Laureate, over the latter's contention that neurons were anatomically separate rather than joined in a protoplasmic network. In 1935 there had been the heated clash at the Cambridge (United Kingdom) meeting of the Physiological Society, when a young John Eccles had argued against the existence of chemical transmission at synapses, his opponent being the Nobel Laureate, Sir Henry Dale. Then, after the Second World War, had come the rather one-sided battle between Lorente de Nó and the team of Alan Hodgkin and Andrew Huxley. Lorente, who was arguably the most brilliant of Cajal's pupils, had spent several years on a monumental study of the electrical properties of frog peripheral nerve fibres, only for his painstaking work to be overtaken and largely refuted by a brief but intensive exploration of the giant axon of the squid.

The sequels to the arguments are interesting. Eccles had recognized his error and, rather than abandon the field of synaptic transmission, had quickly become its foremost neurophysiologist. Similarly, having argued with Patrick Wall against the possible presence of presynaptic inhibition in the mammalian nervous system, he had later carried out the most thorough investigation of the very same mechanism. Lorente, however, rather than admit his mistake, had continued to fight for a lost cause. It was an unfortunate blemish on an otherwise magnificent career, one that had included detailed descriptions of the neuronal architecture of the cerebral cortex and the hippocampus. It was he, Lorente, who had been the first to describe the columns of neurons in the cortex and it was his division of the hippocampus into four regions (CA1, CA2, CA3, CA4) that is used today.

25. C. Zhao, E.M. Teng, R.G. Jr Summers, G.-I. Ming, and F.G. Gage, 'Distinct Morphological Stages of Dentate Granule Neuron Maturation in the Adult Mouse Hippocampus' (2006) 26(1) *Journal of Neuroscience* 3–11.

26. S. Bayer, R.L. Brunner, R. Hine, and J. Altman, 'Behavioural Effects of Interference with the Postnatal Acquisition of Hippocampal Granule Cells' (1973) 242 *Nature* 222–4.

27. C.S.S. Weeden, J.C. Mercurio, and H.A. Cameron, 'A Role for Hippocampal Adult Neurogenesis in Shifting Attention Towards Novel Stimuli' (2019) 376 *Behavioural Brain Research* 112152. <https//doi.org/10.1016/j.bbr.2019.112152>.

26

Neurons that Glow

(Toronto, Cambridge, Massachusetts, 2020: Sheena Josselyn, Susuma Tonegawa)

Now Canada's largest city, Toronto sits on the north shore of Lake Ontario with the CN Tower rising high above the multi-storied banks, offices, and apartment buildings (Figure 26.1). Unlike Montreal 500 kilometres to the east, Toronto has developed in a safe, cautious way, embodying the philosophy of its British founders. For many years it had been a city of business, and for the wealthy—of whom there were many—life had included the Royal Toronto Yacht Club, dinner parties, and, in the hot summers, weeks spent at cottages in Muskoka. Though possessed of a fine university and superb hospitals, Toronto had achieved little in clinical or basic neuroscience research. In contrast to the situation in Montreal there had been no Penfield, no Jasper, and no Neurological Institute, nor had there been a Donald Hebb to galvanize experimental psychology. True, there had been Oleh Hornykiewicz, recruited from Vienna after having identified the loss of dopaminergic neurons in the brainstem as the cause of parkinsonism and having instituted treatment with L-dopa, but even he had spent only half of his time in Toronto.[1]

In some ways Toronto's character and history is reflected in University Avenue, the most handsome of the city's downtown streets. Originating opposite the city's Union Station, the street makes a slight bend before heading directly north to end at the castle-like sandstone edifice of Queen's Park, the provincial legislative building. A century before it had grown into an eight-lane boulevard, the Avenue had been a narrow, tree-lined dirt road leading to the university. As it had widened so its new occupants had given it importance. Toronto General Hospital had been constructed on its east side in 1913 and, forty years later, had gathered Toronto Sick Children's Hospital as its southerly neighbour. At about the same time, on the opposite side of the boulevard, there had appeared Mount Sinai Hospital, once the professional home of Jewish doctors denied hospital appointments elsewhere in the city. Over the years, each of the three hospitals had expanded and, given their proximity to each other, clinical collaborations had ensued, the interactions made all the easier by a tunnel beneath the boulevard. Yet, despite the presence of the three world-class hospitals and the Osgoode Hall Law School, for many years the most imposing building on University Avenue had been the Canada Life Insurance Company at its north end. And that building's function seemed to epitomize the character of the city and its inhabitants—solid, safe, and rather unexciting. The presence of a nudist beach on Toronto Island was never mentioned.

Aranzio's Seahorse and the Search for Memory and Consciousness. Alan J. McComas, Oxford University Press.
© Oxford University Press 2023. DOI: 10.1093/oso/9780192868244.003.0028

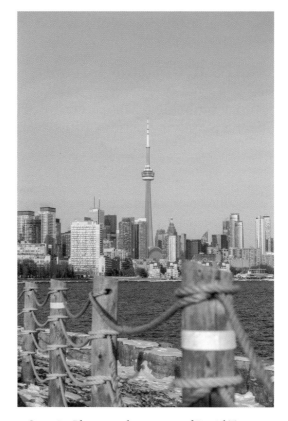

Figure 26.1 Toronto, Ontario. Photograph courtesy of David Turner.

In the latter part of the 20th century, however, there had been developments. The city had become the destination of choice for the majority of immigrants to Canada. New restaurants had opened and were offering ethnic dishes, downtown had become livelier, and the new 553-metre high CN Tower had become the visual symbol of the city. Along University Avenue there were changes too. The major hospitals had added imposing research wings to their clinical buildings and some of the new research, especially that involving molecular biology, had been outstanding.[2] But 'hard core' neuroscience was missing, an absence made all the more obvious by the creation of a department of neurosciences at McMaster University just a few miles to the west.[3] Even clinical neurology and neurosurgery had been eclipsed by developments at the University of Western Ontario (now Western University), a three-hour drive away.

And then, through a single appointment, the situation had changed. When Andres Lozano accepted a position at the city's Western General Hospital in 1991, Toronto had acquired one of the world's leading neurosurgeons.[4] Already expert on the application of deep brain stimulation to treat movement disorders, and parkinsonism in particular, Lozano would show similar stimulation in other deep structures could sometimes abolish depression and, important for memory, possibly promote neogenesis in the human hippocampus. In the most successful cases, the results in the various neuro-logical disorders were very impressive.

More neuroscience was to come. At the north end of University Avenue, at its junc-tion with College St, a massive glass-fronted building with two towers would be erected. Named the MaRS Discovery Centre, it offered accommodation for research workers in engineering, information technology, and medical science. Built in the grounds of Toronto General Hospital, the Centre stood on the very site where insulin, extracted and purified from animal pancreases in the university's Physiology Department, had been given to a diabetic patient for the first time. That had been in 1922 and the work had resulted in the following year's Nobel Prize being awarded to Frederick Banting and John Macleod.[5]

At the present time the MaRS building includes, among its many tenants, the neuro-scientists Sheena Josselyn (Figure 26.2) and her husband, Paul Frankland. A Fellow of the Royal Society of Canada, Sheena is a senior scientist at the Toronto Sick Children's Hospital and an associate professor in the departments of physiology and psychology in the university. She and Paul had met while working in the same laboratory in the University of California, Los Angeles. At the confluence of neuroscience, psychology and psychiatry, her research, like her husband's, is centred on the molecular mechan-isms and neuronal circuitry involved in the laying-down and retrieval of memory. An expert in both molecular biology and neurophysiology, Sheena has made particular use of a new and exciting experimental approach—*optogenetics*. The term describes two types of experimental activity, both of them involving the emission or absorption of light in genetically modified nervous tissue. In one instance light emission is used to demonstrate a neural structure[6] or to show its activity while in the other application it is light that initiates and controls the activity.

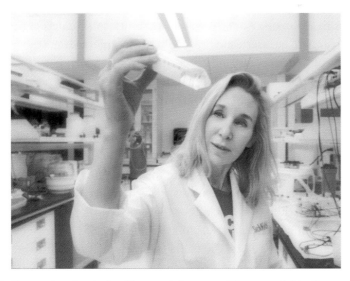

Figure 26.2 Sheena Josselyn in her Toronto laboratory. Photograph kindly supplied by Dr Josselyn.

That light should be capable of affecting nerve cells should come as no surprise since this is what happens in the rods and cones of the retina. A single photon, by combining with a light-sensitive molecule (a *chromophore*) attached to a specific membrane protein in a rod or cone, will alter the cell's electrical potential.[7] But humans and other vertebrates are not the only creatures that respond to light. Even the single-celled alga, *Chlamydomonas reinhardtii*, will use its two flagellae to swim towards or away from light. Exactly how such a simple creature could respond to light was a question that attracted the attention of curious zoologists and led to the discovery of molecular mechanisms similar to those in rods and cones—light-sensitive chromophore-protein complexes ('*channelrhodopsins*') were embedded in the *Chlamydomas* membranes. In each channelrhodopsin it was found that, in response to light, the chromophore momentarily alters the shape of a pore in the attached protein molecule. In channelrhodopsin-2, the open pore allows cations (sodium, potassium, calcium) to flow across the membrane and into the cell.

Having identified the genes coding for channelrhodopsin it was possible to modify them in such a way that the channel became selective for one particular ion species rather than several. Also, by making it responsive to light of two different wavelengths, the channel could be kept open for varying amounts of time. The next step was to introduce the modified channel into neurons. This was done by either injecting it directly into a cell or, better, instructing the organism to manufacture the channel (by transfecting cells with a virus altered to contain the channel genes). Depending on the structure of the modified channelrhodopsin, the transfected neurons would then respond to a pulse of light by firing a single impulse or a train, or they could be inhibited from firing at all. The final step in optogenetics was to devise methods for selecting the neurons for this type of study. This was achieved by inserting a suitable promoter with the channel genes so as to restrict synthesis of the channel to a particular nucleus, fibre pathway, or region of the nervous system. Alternatively one could narrow the stimulating light beam (if working with a tissue slice or cells on the brain surface). For deeper neurons, a thin fibreoptic cable could be inserted to bring light to the target area.

If asked, most contemporary neuroscientists would point to optogenetics as the most exciting branch of their discipline. It is one that is expanding rapidly and, in mice, has already proved especially useful for exploring behaviour. Many laboratories are involved[8] and Sheena Josselyn's is prominent among them. It was Sheena who, with husband Paul Frankland, demonstrated that optogenetics could be used to induce or to selectively erase memories in the mouse amygdala.[9] The experiments made ingenious use of genetic engineering. First, by causing them to overexpress the gene-regulating protein CREB, a population of neurons was selected to encode the memory of an auditory tone associated with a foot shock. Then the same neurons, which had also been engineered to make diphtheria toxin receptors, were selectively destroyed by injecting the toxin. When that had been done, the treated animals no longer 'froze' in expectation of a foot shock on hearing the auditory tone. In contrast, non-selective destruction of a small fraction of untreated amygdala neurons had no effect—the mice still froze on hearing the tone. This important study clearly showed that memories were housed in separate assemblies of neurons, in keeping with the ideas expressed by Donald Hebb in *The Organization of Behaviour*. In a very convincing manner, the Toronto neuroscientists had also confirmed that the amygdala–hippocampal complex contained the memory 'engrams', the location of which had somehow eluded Karl Lashley's determined search, using multiple cortical ablations, many years earlier.

The memory deletion work had been published in 2009. Ten years later Sheena Josselyn and her Toronto group reported another breakthrough in memory research—the use of optogenetic techniques to implant false memories.[10] As for other studies of this nature, mice had been used. In this case the mice had been genetically engineered to have fluorescent channelrhodopsin-2 molecules expressed in the olfactory bulb—but only in the one or two glomeruli known (from previous work) to respond to odours of acetophenone. When the same glomeruli were stimulated by a light pulse, it was as if the mice had smelt acetophenone. Next, the stimulating pulse to the olfactory glomeruli was combined with one that excited neurons in the ventral tegmental area (a midbrain region associated with pain sensation). That an artificial memory had now been created by simultaneous stimulation of the two brain areas, a memory that associated a particular olfactory sensation with pain, was shown by the subsequent behaviour of the animals. Despite never having been exposed to acetophenone in their lives, the experimented mice, unlike their untreated controls, now avoided an area of the training box containing that odour. In a follow-up study that involved more genetic engineering the Toronto group showed that the amygdala had been necessary for establishing the false memory.

Among the other molecular biologists employing optogenetics to study memory mechanisms is Susuma Tonegawa (Figure 26.3), a Japanese-born neuroscientist working at MIT. Like University College London and Trinity College Cambridge, MIT can claim many Nobel Laureates, indeed more than any other university or institute (95 Laureates at the 2020 count). It was at MIT that Jerry Lettvin had postulated the existence of pontifical neurons, incorporating the idea in his delightful fable of the Russian neurosurgeon and the ablated (grand)mother cells. It was at MIT, too, that Suzanne Corkin had continued the all-important study of Henry Molaison, the patient who had enabled Brenda Milner and William Scoville to identify the hippocampus as being crucial for memory.

Born in 1939, Tonegawa is older than most, if not all, of those in the new field of optogenetics and, having already won a Nobel Prize, is certainly the most distinguished. Remarkably, his 1987 Prize in Physiology or Medicine had had nothing to do with neuroscience but was awarded for work in immunology. It had been Tonegawa who had discovered the solution to the hitherto baffling problem of antibody diversity—how a modest 19,000 genes could provide instructions for the synthesis of millions of different species of antibody. Like Gerald Edelman, a previous Nobel Laureate for molecular research in immunology,[11] Tonegawa had left immunology and entered neuroscience. Before devoting himself to molecular mechanisms in memory, he had devised new technologies both for introducing new genes into mammalian embryos and for 'knocking out' existing ones.

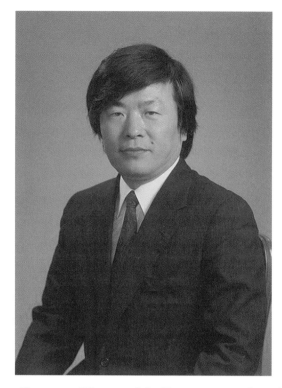

Figure 26.3 Susumu Tonegawa. (Photograph by User9131986. Wikimedia Commons file: Susumu Tonegawa Photo.jpg. Creative Commons Attribution-Share Alike 4.0 International license.)

In 2012 Tonegawa had been able to report the results of a unique memory experiment in mice. He and his colleagues had used optogenetics to identify a population of neurons in the hippocampus that became active whenever the mouse was subjected to an unpleasant electric shock. Then, using a different optogenetic method, Tonegawa's group was able to show that stimulating the same hippocampal cells artificially (with a light pulse) was sufficient in itself to evoke a fear response.[12]

Looking at the field from outside, there seems to be a great excitement among the optogeneticists, as if even the most difficult questions will yield to this technology. Anything and everything to do with the investigation of behaviour now seems possible, once the appropriate genes have been inserted into an embryo. There is a sense of fun, too, with one laboratory leapfrogging over another in technical ingenuity. To some extent that sense is reflected in the lives of the investigators outside the laboratory. It transpires that Susuma Tonegawa, the Nobel Laureate, is a keen baseball fan while Sheena Josselyn's Wikipedia entry shows her blowing bubble-gum. There is also a kinship among the investigators and a widespread appreciation of Karl Deisseroth's role in introducing channelrhodopsin-2 technology. And Tonegawa and Josselyn have collaborated in writing an extensive recent review on the use of optogenetics in memory research.

But how does all the information about the hippocampus, information gleaned not just from optogenetics but from so many other sources, most of it in the past 50 years, relate to consciousness? What role does memory play in consciousness, and how might consciousness have evolved? Are there other observations, some mostly forgotten, that might have a bearing on these issues? It is the attempt to answer these questions that forms the second part of the book. First, however, there is the need for a summary of the chapters on memory and the hippocampus.

Notes

1. Oleh Hornykiewicz (1926–2020) was born in Poland but fled to Austria with his parents, where he remained during the Second World War. He entered medical school in Vienna in 1945 and it was in that city that he carried out his seminal studies in parkinsonism. There was a strong sentiment within the neuroscience community that he should have received a Nobel Prize for his work.

2. Included among many fine achievements in molecular biology has been the work of Ronald Worton (Duchenne muscular dystrophy gene), Tak Mak (T-cell receptors in the immune system), Lap-Chee Tsui (cystic fibrosis gene), Janet Rossant (control of embryological development, pluripotent stem cells).

3. McMaster University, in Hamilton, created the world's first department of neurosciences, with Jack Diamond as the founding Chair. The highly successful department was subsequently subsumed into Biomedical Sciences before falling victim to university politics.

4. Born in Spain, Lozano had grown up in Canada, entering medical school in Ottawa and then training in neurosurgery at McGill and the Montreal Neurological Institute.

5. The first partially successful single dose treatment was that given to a 14-year old diabetic boy. The entire work had been a heroic success and the Nobel Prize a fitting reward for Banting's persistence through weeks of discouraging animal experiments in the summer's heat. Banting's determination and MacLeod's profound knowledge of carbohydrate metabolism had brought the unlikely project to its brilliant conclusion. Remarkably, Banting had not been a researcher but a general practitioner and frustrated surgeon when he had conceived the idea of ligating the pancreatic duct in an animal, so as to cause its enzyme-producing cells to atrophy while leaving intact the insulin-secreting islets of Langerhans. A riveting and well researched account of the discovery of insulin has been provided by the late historian Michael Bliss, *The Discovery of Insulin* (Toronto: McClelland & Stewart, 1982).

6. Fred Gage and his colleagues had employed optogenetics to trace the creation and development of new granule cells in the rat hippocampus (see Chapter 25).

7. The action of the photon on a rod or cone is not what might have been anticipated. Rather than exciting the receptor, it does the opposite, blocking the ongoing flow of sodium ions into the cell. If the cell had been inhibiting the next cell in the circuit (a bipolar cell in the retina), it is the latter that is now excited, firing an impulse.

8. Among the pioneers in optogenetics is Karl Deisseroth (Stanford) who developed the use of channelrhodopsin-2. Recognition should also be given to Ken Foster who was the first to identify rhodopsin in algae. Even though a Nobel Prize (in Chemistry) was awarded to Roger Tsien in 2008 for early work on the development and application of fluorescent markers in biological reactions so much has happened since that further Prizes in optogenetics seem inevitable.

9. J.-H. Han, S.A. Kushner, A.P. You, H.-L. Hsiang, T. Buch, A. Waisman, B. Bontempi, R.L. Never, P.W. Frankland, and S.A. Josselyn, 'Selective Erasure of a Fear Memory' (2009) 323 *Science* 1492–6.

10. G. Vetere, L.M. Tran, S. Moberg, P.E. Steadman, L. Restivo, F.G. Morrison, K.J. Ressler, S.A. Josselyn, and P.W. Frankland, 'Memory Formation in the Absence of Experience' (2019) 22 *Nature Neuroscience* 933–40.

11. Gerald Edelman (1929–2014) won the Nobel Prize in Physiology or Medicine in 1972 and like Tonegawa's later, the award was for research into antibody diversity—though at the level of amino acid-based structure rather than of genes. Edelman subsequently discovered cell adhesion molecules, demonstrating their importance in enabling cells to attach to one another during embryological development and especially in the shaping of the nervous system. His ideas on the generation of consciousness were based on the importance of neuron connectivity and feedback (re-entry) in neural circuits. Connectivity was enhanced by repetition of sensory inputs and therefore more likely to persist ('neural darwinism').

12. X. Liu, S. Ramirez, P.T. Pang, C.B. Puryear, A. Govindarajan, K. Deisseroth, and S. Tonegawa, 'Optogenetic Stimulation of a Hippocampal Engram Activates Fear Memory Recall' (2012) 484 *Nature* 381–5.

    S.A. Josselyn and S. Tonegawa, 'Memory Engrams: Recalling the Past and Imagining the Future' (2020) 367 *Science* eaawd4325. DOI: 10.1126/science.aaw4325.

27

Summary

The hippocampus is part of the limbic system of the mammalian brain; the limbic system itself comprises a number of interconnected neural structures situated above the brain stem and at the base of the cerebral hemispheres.

Patients with damage to both hippocampi show impairment of memory.

The impairment is for 'declarative' memory (people, places, and events) rather than for 'procedural' memory (how to do things). There is a brief period ('short-term memory') before a declarative memory becomes fully established ('long-term memory').

Studies on a simple organism (the giant sea slug, *Aplysia*) have shown that the formation of a memory involves changes at the junctions (synapses) between neurons. Short-term memory is due to increased transmitter release from nerve endings while long-term memory is achieved by the formation of new synapses and enlargement of existing ones. The switching-on of genes in the nucleus of a neuron directs the protein synthesis needed for the synaptic growth.

The patterns of synaptic connections between neurons in the hippocampus and associated entorhinal cortex enable spatial maps to be made.

Recordings from the brains of patients have shown the presence of 'concept' cells in the human hippocampus. These are memory neurons responsive to multiple features (i.e. the sight and the spoken or written name) of a person, object, or place. Such cells have also been termed 'pontifical', 'grandmother', 'gnostic', and 'Jennifer Aniston' by various workers.

New neurons are formed in the hippocampus throughout life while others are destroyed.

Aranzio's Seahorse and the Search for Memory and Consciousness. Alan J. McComas, Oxford University Press.
© Oxford University Press 2023. DOI: 10.1093/oso/9780192868244.003.0029

PART II

THE EVOLUTION OF CONSCIOUSNESS

Theses:

(a) The evolution of consciousness increased the success of movements necessary
    for survival.
(b) In mammals the hippocampal complex, part of the limbic system, is essential for
    consciousness.
(c) Consciousness is short-term memory.

A.

GENERAL ISSUES

28

Preamble

Such is the nature of consciousness, there cannot be certainty or even the prospect of a definitive answer regarding some of its aspects. For example, we cannot prove that a machine or a computer is not conscious, even though it does seem very unlikely, and the concept of consciousness as some elemental property of the universe (see below) will appear absurd to most people. Nor can we offer a scientific solution to the so-called hard problem of consciousness—that aspect of consciousness that enables one to appreciate the 'redness' of a sunset, the exquisite perfume of a flower, or the beauty of a musical cadence. How is it possible that electric impulses in nerve cells can be transformed into these sensory experiences? And, above all, how do nerve impulses give us our sense of 'self'? There is no direct experiment, at least one that is presently conceivable, that would enable a scientist to solve problems of this nature.

What we can do is provide a rational basis for two aspects of consciousness—namely, how it developed and which parts of the brain are involved. There are answers at hand and these draw heavily on the work that has already been presented. The studies of Brenda Milner, Eric Kandel, John O'Keefe, and all the others previously mentioned have relevance. The account that now follows contains additional narrative, introducing the reader to other neuroscientists and neurologists, including some who were active long before the modern story began. The account also contains some brain anatomy (optional for a lay person) and some zoology. In places the style of writing differs from that in Part I, as the reader is now asked to imagine a situation, or is addressed directly by the author. However, if the last two chapters (Recapitulation and Synthesis; Epilogue) fulfil their respective functions, they will serve to bring the many strands of the book together.

The first item of business, however, is to provide a definition of consciousness.

Aranzio's Seahorse and the Search for Memory and Consciousness. Alan J. McComas, Oxford University Press.
© Oxford University Press 2023. DOI: 10.1093/oso/9780192868244.003.0030

29

Definition of Consciousness

We all know what it is to be conscious. It is our consciousness that enables us to admire a colourful garden or the loveliness of a face, to thrill to the majestic chords of a Beethoven piano sonata or the intricacies of a Bach fugue, and to enjoy the flavours in a well-prepared meal. It is consciousness that enables us to understand a newspaper article, to appreciate the significance of something said by a friend. It is consciousness that gives an astronomer the ability to probe the universe, a scientist to explore the nature of matter, and an artist to create a work of beauty. It is consciousness that allows us to make decisions of the moment and plans for the future, and it is consciousness that guides our everyday actions. Above all, it is consciousness that gives us our sense of self, that each of us is a unique individual.

So far, so good. But if we probe a little deeper, consciousness becomes difficult to pin down. For example, in the laboratory we can deprive someone of all their external senses (sight, hearing, touch, smell, and taste) and yet he or she will remain fully conscious. And although we may feel that we are in command when we make a decision or perform an action, introspection will usually reveal that the decisions and actions were prompted by something seen, heard or remembered. More troubling still is that neurophysiological experiments have shown that the electrical activity in the brain associated with a decision begins well before we are aware of the thought—free will appears to be an illusion. Piece by piece, we can remove parts of what we had considered consciousness to be.

And so we struggle to define consciousness, a difficulty that accounts for the large number of attempts (29 in one survey).[1] In the end, it may be best to accept a simple definition that others have used and that describes what is left when all the bits and pieces have been taken away. It is that *consciousness is the sense of self*. We should note that such a definition does not restrict consciousness to human beings. There are strong arguments for consciousness in other creatures, as Darwin recognized long ago and as we have summarized elsewhere.[2] As Chapter 30 describes, some philosophers would go much further, and attribute consciousness to inanimate objects, even to particles.

Notes

1. I. Barüss, 'Metanalysis of Definitions of Consciousness' (1987) 6 *Imagination, Cognition and Personality* 321–9.
2. A.J. McComas, *Sherrington's Loom. An Introduction to the Science of Consciousness* (New York: Oxford University Press, 2019).

Aranzio's Seahorse and the Search for Memory and Consciousness. Alan J. McComas, Oxford University Press.
© Oxford University Press 2023. DOI: 10.1093/oso/9780192868244.003.0031

30

Theories of Consciousness

There are at least five types of theory (Figure 30.1):

Panpsychism. There are many forms of panpsychism. The most widely held version is that 'mind' is an elemental property of matter throughout the universe. Accordingly, while this property is strongly embedded in living creatures, and in humans particularly, miniscule traces are present in the atomic particles of which the world is made. This idea, which has roots in Ancient Greek philosophy, has undergone a renaissance, receiving support from the contemporary philosopher David Chalmers as well as from Christof Koch. An elegant description of the postulated emergence of animal consciousness from matter was given by Clifford in the late-19th century:

Mind-stuff is the reality which we perceive as matter. A moving molecule of inorganic matter does not possess mind or consciousness, but it possesses a small piece of mind-stuff. When molecules are so combined together to form the film on the underside of a jelly dish, the elements of mind-stuff which go along with them are so combined as to form the faint beginnings of Sentience. When the molecules are so combined as to form the brain and nervous system of a vertebrate, the corresponding elements of mind-stuff are so combined as to form some kind of consciousness … .[1]

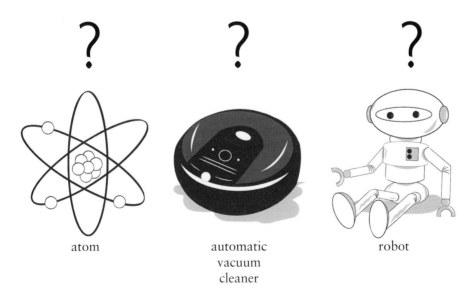

atom   automatic   robot
                              vacuum
                              cleaner

Figure 30.1 Examples of objects that would be regarded by some as having elementary consciousness.

Aranzio's Seahorse and the Search for Memory and Consciousness. Alan J. McComas, Oxford University Press.

Other forms of panpsychism are based on the fact that the only knowledge of the world is through our senses and that the true nature of reality can therefore never be known. What is perceived and brought into consciousness may thus be but one aspect of events and properties of the universe of which we have no further awareness.

Appliance consciousness. Consciousness is envisaged as a property of any physical device able to acquire information about itself and its environment, and to act on the basis of that information. Automatic vacuum cleaners and lawn mowers would be obvious candidates, but the principle could be extended to many simpler devices, for example a thermostat controlling a heating or cooling system, or a photocell switching on a lamp.

Artificial intelligence (AI). Consciousness is envisaged as emerging in a computer capable of learning (i.e. developing its own programs). The underlying logic is that the computer, in processing information without prior instruction and proceeding to recognize patterns, is learning in essentially the same way as a newborn infant. Giving strength to this proposition is the phenomenal success of AI in beating the best human players at chess and GO. Ray Kurzweill, the first to develop language recognition by computer, is a firm believer in the evolution of consciousness in AI.[2] Alan Turing was not so sure, cleverly deflecting the question into his famous test, in effect saying that it is illogical to deny consciousness to a machine that can pass all the tests of consciousness (such as answering questions correctly).[3] For those that believe, consciousness could be present in the many contemporary robots, including the 'smart' domestic ones that, with smiling faces, move around and employ AI to learn about their owners and their environments, making decisions as they go.

Information integration. Consciousness is thought to develop in any information-handling system, organic or non-organic, provided there is sufficient integration (especially through feedback). Information integration theory, or IIT, is the brainchild of Giulio Tononi, who studied the matter with the late Nobel Laureate, Gerald Edelman.[4] There is considerable mathematics involved, the end result being a value of '*phi*'; thus, the greater the feedback (and other types of connection) between the elements of an information-processing system, the larger the value of *phi* and the more likely it is for the system to have consciousness. Critics have pointed out that such criteria would mean that a physical device such as a compact disc, by virtue of its error-correcting codes, would have a much larger *phi* than a human brain and therefore should have a higher consciousness. (This would not pose a difficulty for a panpsychist, however, and Christof Koch is also a strong supporter of IIT).

Brains. Consciousness can only be generated by a brain (though possibly by other neural structures in non-vertebrates). This is the position held by most neuroscientists and by a number of philosophers. But is the whole brain involved or is there one special part? A prominent advocate for the entire brain is the philosopher Daniel Dennett. In his 'Multiple Drafts' model of consciousness,[5] Dennett proposes that during wakefulness various types of sensory information are being simultaneously processed by the brain but only one of these 'multiple drafts' will achieve consciousness at any given time; it is the processing itself which is consciousness.

The possibility that, rather than the whole brain, there is an 'observer' in some special part was raised by René Descartes, the 17th-century philosopher, anatomist, and mathematician (Figure 30.2). The pineal gland, a small midline structure in the upper brain stem, was considered by Descartes to be the locus where thoughts, previously independent of the body and brain, were translated into matter. While the concept of 'dualism' —the separation of mind and body—has been largely rejected by philosophers and scientists alike, the concept of a 'Cartesian theatre' lurking somewhere in the brain remains. Though the pineal gland was long dismissed as a contender, a number of alternatives have been put forward:

(a) **Brain stem**. One of the earliest proposals was that of the William Carpenter (1813–1885), a professor of physiology and forensic medicine at University College London. Carpenter interpreted the gross anatomy of the human brain as indicative of consciousness residing in the thalamus and sensory ganglia of the brain stem, with the cerebral hemispheres on either side acting as repositories of information.[6] The thalamus was also favoured by Henry Head (1861–1940), an experimental neurologist in London who was influenced by his observations of sensory disturbance in patients with lesions affecting the thalamus.[7] However, it was Wilder Penfield (1891–1974), the Montreal neurosurgeon, who was the most vigorous proponent of a brain stem locus for consciousness, pointing out that its connections made it well equipped to act as a 'central integrating system' where sensory information was brought together and where voluntary actions were conceived. Penfield was vague as to exactly where in the brain stem the integration was carried out, at various times describing it as 'below the cortex and above the midbrain,'[8] 'the intralaminar systems of the thalamus and the reticular formation of the brain stem,'[9] and 'the diencephalon, midbrain and pons—the higher brain stem that includes the two thalami'.[10] Though Penfield's proposal was summarily rejected by Francis Walshe,[11] Penfield had nevertheless offered evidence, all of which remains relevant to any alternative scheme. The evidence included the centrality and pathway convergence of the brain stem, the dramatic effects on consciousness of stimulation or damage to the brain stem, the primary involvement of deep brain structures during generalized epileptic seizures (with loss or alteration of consciousness), the minor consequences of large lesions involving prefrontal cortex, and the retention of voluntary movements after separation of the motor area from other cortical regions. Further observations consistent with Penfield's concept came from experiments in rats, in which learning was disrupted more readily by lesions that were made in the brain stem rather than in the cortex.[12]

(b) **Cerebral cortex**. It is natural to associate consciousness and intelligence with the great enlargement of the cerebral hemispheres that occurred during the evolution of modern humans (and Neanderthals). According to this view, consciousness would be absent or only present to a lesser extent in animals with smaller brains, though those with similar or greater brain sizes, such as whales,

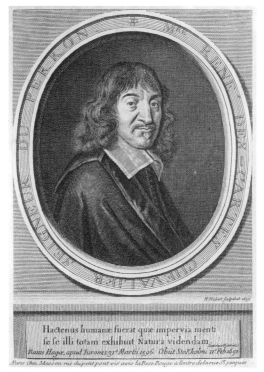

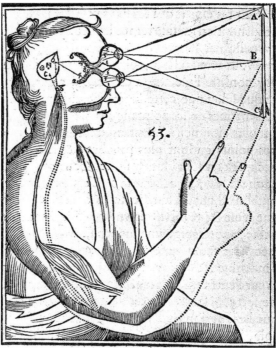

Figure 30.2 *Upper.* Renè Descartes. Line engraving by C. Ammon, 1654. *Lower.* Descartes: coordination of muscle and visual mechanisms (from *L'homme et un traitte …*). The person is looking downwards to a point, *C*, to which the right index finger points. When the biceps muscle in the upper arm contracts, under the influence of nerves connected to the pineal gland, the elbow is bent further so that the index finger now points to *A*, the new object of the person's attention. (Both figures from Wellcome Images.)

dolphins, and elephants, could possess consciousness and intelligence comparable to those of humans. Within the cerebral cortex, the anterior (prefrontal) regions were initially identified by Francis Crick and Christof Koch as the sites where visual information achieved consciousness.[13] This view was then discarded, presumably because of the continued ability of patients to see perfectly well following prefrontal lobotomies or lobectomies(!). The same authors, immediately prior to Crick's death in 2004, proposed that consciousness was generated by the claustrum, a thin sheet of neurons deep to the cortical layers.[14]

(c) **Cerebral cortex *and* brain stem**. In *Self Comes to Mind. Constructing the Conscious Brain*,[15] Antonio Damasio (Figure 30.3) has made a case for the development of a primordial consciousness in the tectum ('roof') of the midbrain. At this level of the nervous system there would be sufficient information from internal body systems (gastrointestinal, cardiovascular, respiratory, etc.), the external surface of the body and head, and from the eyes and ears for the assembly of an awareness. This basic consciousness would underlie a stronger and more versatile consciousness generated by cortical activity, with the thalamus having

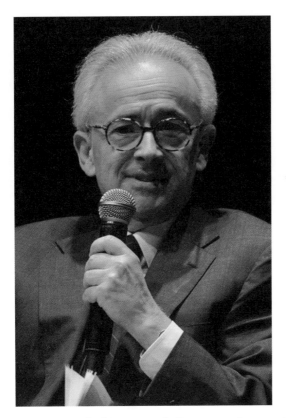

Figure 30.3 Antonio Damasio at the 'Fronteiras do Pensamento' symposium in Porto Alegre, Brazil, 2013. (Wikimedia Commons file: António Damásio no Fronteiras do Pensamento Porto Alegre 2013 cropped.png. Creative Commons Attribution-Share Alikke 2.0 Generic license.)

a key role in coordinating the two levels. Damasio's proposal is not dissimilar to that of Penfield whose 'centrencephalic system' in the brain stem was also envisaged as working in conjunction with the cortex (though the latter would have had the subsidiary role).

(d) **Limbic system**. The remainder of this book provides the logic and the evidence for regarding consciousness as essentially the product of the limbic system, with the cortex and other regions of the brain having accessory roles. Within the limbic system the hippocampus is seen as the key structure, with support from its immediate neural neighbours (amygdala, entorhinal cortex, subiculum); together these are sometimes referred to as the 'hippocampal complex' in the following chapters.

It is now time to say more about the limbic system and to identify at the anatomists and physiologists who gave us this information. We already know that one of its features, the hippocampus, was discovered almost four centuries ago by Aranzio. But where did the idea of a 'limbic system' come from?

Notes

1. W.K. Clifford, 'On the Nature Of Things-In-Themselves' (1878) 3 *Mind* 56–67.
2. R. K.urzweil, *How to Create a Mind: The Secret of Human Thought Revealed* (New York, NY: Penguin, 2012).
3. A.M. Turing, 'I. Computing Machinery and Intelligence' (1950) 59 *Mind* 433–60.
4. Gerald Edelman (1929–2014) graduated in medicine but devoted his life to research, first at the then Rockefeller Institute in New York and subsequently in San Diego, California. In 1972 he shared the Nobel Prize in Physiology or Medicine with his colleague Rodney Porter for revealing the chemical structure of antibodies. Later, Edelman became interested in the development of the animal body, discovering cell-adhesion molecules. He then switched to the origin of consciousness, espousing a neural selection process that created functional modules during brain development (akin to Darwinism in species). With Giulio Tononi, Edelman co-authored *A Universe of Consciousness: How Matter Becomes Imagination* (New York, NY: Basic Books, 2000), in which re-entry (feedback) in neural systems was emphasized as an important factor in the development of consciousness.
5. D. Dennett, *Consciousness Explained* (Boston, MA: Little Brown, 1991).
6. W.B. Carpenter, *Principles of Human Physiology*, 4th edn (London: Churchill, 1853), cited by F.M.R. Walshe (reference 11, below).xyz
7. H. Head, *Studies in Neurology*, Vols 1–2. (London: Henry Frowde, 1920).
8. W. Penfield, 'The Cerebral Cortex in Man. I. The Cerebral Cortex and Consciousness' (1938) 40 *Archives of Neurology and Psychiatry* 417–42.
9. W. Penfield, 'Mechanisms of Voluntary Movement', (1954) 77 *Brain* 1–17.
10. W. Penfield, 'Studies of the Cerebral Cortex of Man: A Review and an Interpretation' in J.F. Delafresnaye (ed.), *Brain Mechanisms and Consciousness* (Springfield, IL: Charles C. Thomas, 1954), 284–304.
11. F.M.R Walshe, 'The Brain-Stem Conceived as the "Highest Level" of Function in the Nervous System; with Particular Reference to the "Automatic Apparatus" of Carpenter (1850) and to the

"Centrencephalic Intergrating System" of Penfield' (1957) 80 *Brain* 510–39. Walshe's repudiation of Penfield's views is described in Chapter 5.

12. R. Thompson, F.M. Crinella, and J. Yu, *Brain Mechanisms in Problem Solving and Intelligence: A Lesion Survey in the Rat Brain* (New York, NY: Plenum Press, 1990).

13. F.H.C. Crick and C. Koch, 'Are We Aware of Neural Activity in Primary Visual Cortex?' (1995) 375 *Nature* 121–4.

14. F.C. Crick and C. Koch, 'What is the Function of the Claustrum?' (2005) 360(1458) *Philosophical Transactions of the Royal Society of London, B* 1271–9. According to Koch, Crick had still been working on the manuscript in his hospital bed on the day that he died.

15. A. Damasio, *Self Comes to Mind* (New York, NY: Random House, 2012).

LIMBIC SYSTEM AS LOCATION
OF CONSCIOUSNESS

31

Recognition of the 'Limbic System'

Giulio Cesare Aranzio (1530–1589) had come upon the hippocampus in the course of anatomical dissections during his time as professor at the University of Bologna. Though he had reported his discovery in a treatise published in 1579, the hippocampus and its neighbouring structures appear to have attracted little subsequent interest, other than as anatomical features in drawings of the human brain. Indeed, little attempt was made to localize function in the brain, though gross localization was implicit in the support for phrenology, a pseudoscience that linked mental traits to variations in the shape of the skull. This was to change with the curiosity of an eminent French physician and surgeon, Pierre Paul Broca (1824–1880).

Born in Bordeaux, Broca had graduated in medicine at the University of Paris unusually early.[1] First as a lecturer in anatomy and then as professor of clinical surgery and professor of pathology, he had become interested in the origins of many medical disorders and was not reticent in disseminating his thoughts and observations. Possessed of an adventurous mind and a dark, penetrating gaze (Figure 31.1) Broca had also embraced Darwinism, studied anthropology, measured human skulls (craniometry), and practised hypnosis, on occasion employing the latter as anaesthesia. Today Broca is best known for being the first to locate a function in the cerebral cortex. He had had as a patient a man who, despite his obvious intelligence and understanding, had been unable to say anything other than the same single syllable ('*Tan*'), regardless of the nature of the question or topic. At post-mortem the man had been found to have damage to the lower, posterior frontal cortex on the left side. The same location had later been identified in other patients with a similar speech disorder, causing that region of the human brain to be referred to as Broca's area (for speech).[2]

As one of the early supporters of Darwinism, Broca had sought to understand how the human brain had evolved and to this end had dissected the brains of other mammals. His range of specimens had been vast—the 30 species examined had ranged from badger and bat to horse, dolphin, and elephant. Though the brains had differed in size and shape from each other and from human and other primate brains, he was able to conclude that 'all parts of the primate brain have analogous parts in other brains and vice versa.'[3]

From P. Broca, 'Anatomie comparée des circonvolutions cérébrales: le grande lobe limbique et la scissure limbique dans la série des mammifères' (1878) 1 *Revue d'anthropologie* 385–498. This paper has been translated and republished as: P. Broca, 'Comparative Anatomy of the Cerebral Convolutions. The Great Limbic Lobe and

Aranzio's Seahorse and the Search for Memory and Consciousness. Alan J. McComas, Oxford University Press.
© Oxford University Press 2023. DOI: 10.1093/oso/9780192868244.003.0033

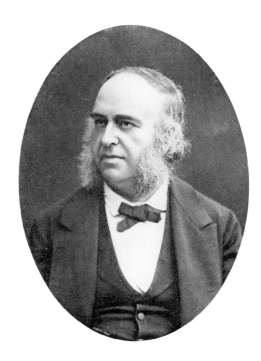

Figure 31.1 Pierre-Paul Broca (1824–1880). (Wellcome Images.)

the Limbic Fissure in the Mammalian Series' (translated by D. Furlani). Wiley Online Library 2015. DOI 10.1002/cne.23856.

One aspect of the brain that was of special interest to Broca was the medial (inner face) of a cerebral hemisphere. To his eyes, the fold of cortex immediately above the corpus callosum (the massive bridge of nerve fibres connecting the two cerebral cortices) appeared to run backwards round the central brain stem structures and continue into the top of the medial temporal lobe (Figure 31.2). He likened this cortical continuity to the head of a tennis racquet (visualizing the olfactory bulb and tract as the handle of the racquet) and termed the structure the 'great limbic lobe'. He saw the great limbic lobe as forming the basal part of the cortex, the overlying mantle of folds and fissures constituting the remainder. Broca emphasized that, even in a small brain with a smooth cortical surface ('lissencephalic') such as that of a rat or rabbit, the great limbic lobe was still present. What distinguished the human brain from the other brains he had examined, including those of other primates, was the great enlargement of the frontal lobe. He also noticed that the olfactory lobe was smaller in humans, an observation he related to the lesser importance of smell.

The next advance came half a century later, with the work of a dedicated neuroanatomist at the University of Chicago. Charles Judson Herrick (1868–1960; Figure 31.3), like Broca, had been interested in comparing the brains of various animal species and would become largely responsible for the modern recognition of comparative anatomy as a separate discipline. Herrick had been born in the American Midwest, gaining his

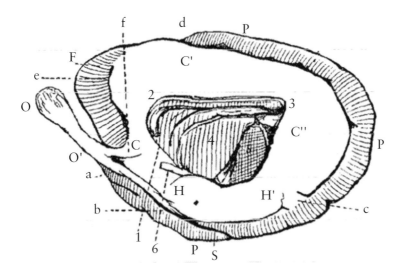

Figure 31.2 Broca's 'great limbic lobe', as revealed by his dissection of the brain of an otter. The medial aspect of the brain is shown, with *C*, *C'*, and *C"* indicating the upper part of the 'great limbic lobe' in white; the lobe is envisaged as continuing into the lower part—*H*, *H'*, also shown in white. *O*, *O'* are the olfactory bulb and tract respectively, while *F* and *P* denote the frontal and parietal lobes. In this figure a large part of the 'lobe' would actually comprise the fibres of the corpus callosum running between the two cerebral hemispheres. From Broca, P. Anatomie comparée des circonvolutions cérébrales: le grande lobe limbique et la scissure limbique dans la série des mammifères. *Revue d'anthropologie* 1878; 1: 385-498. Republished as: Broca P. Comparative anatomy of the cerebral convolutions. The great limbic lobe and the limbic fissure in the mammalian series (translated by Furlani D). Wiley Online Library 2015. DOI 10.1002/cne.23856.

baccalaureate at the University of Cincinnati.[4] Like his elder brother, Clarence,[5] who had founded the *Journal of Comparative Anatomy*, Charles had decided to devote his academic life to exploration of the mind–body relationship.

In a paper read to the American National Academy of Sciences in 1932, Charles Herrick had compared brain structure in a variety of animal species.[6] He pointed out that, in fishes and amphibia, the forerunner of the cortex (the 'pallium') was relatively small and poorly differentiated (Figure 31.4); the relatively few neurons present received their connections from the olfactory bulb, which in contrast to the pallium, was prominent. In a 'lower' mammal such as a rat or opossum, smell was still the primary sense and this was reflected in its cortical territory. As evolution proceeded in other mammalian lines, however, smell became less important than sight and hearing in navigation, feeding, mating, and interaction with the environment. Accordingly, while the olfactory cortex stayed much the same or even regressed, the cortex devoted to touch and hearing, and especially to vision, became progressively larger and more developed.

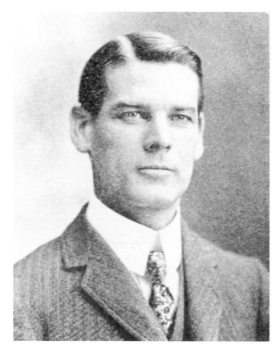

Figure 31.3 Charles Judson Herrick, 1909. (Wikimedia Commons file: PSM V74 D210 Charles Judson Herrick.png. Author unknown. Creative Commons CC0 License.)

In summary, Herrick regarded the most primitive cortex as olfactory; it, and the subcortical parts of the olfactory system, were not only responsible for the sense of smell but, as brains evolved, became 'activators' of complex behaviours involving other senses. If in his paper Herrick had not used the term 'limbic system', it was because he had not needed to; 'olfactory brain' was sufficient. Charles Judson Herrick lived to a great age (92) and, despite poor sight, was still working in his last years.

James Papez (1883–1958) had been born after Herrick and had died just before him. The two men had overlapped not only in time but in their research interests, for Papez, while working at Cornell University, had discovered a neural pathway within the limbic system that might be responsible for emotion. In a landmark paper, published in 1937, he had described what would come to be known as the 'Papez circuit':

> The central emotive process of cortical origin may then be conceived as being built up in the hippocampal formation and as being transferred to the mammillary body and thence through the anterior thalamic nuclei to the cortex of the gyrus cinguli. The cortex of the cingular gyrus may be looked on as the receptive region for the experiencing of emotion as the result of impulses coming from the thalamic region . . . .[7]

One of those attracted to Papez' work and had visited him to discuss it was Paul MacLean (Figure 31.5).

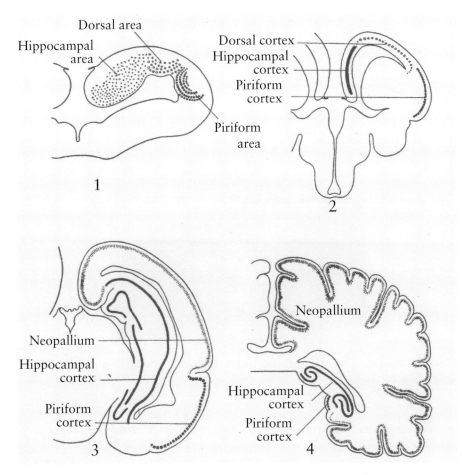

Figure 31.4 Herrick's comparison of vertebrate brains, illustrating differences in proportions of cerebral cortex/neopallium to deep brain structures. All of the neopallium is devoted to olfaction in a mud-puppy (1), and much of it in a tortoise (2), and the same is true for the cortex of an opossum (3); in human cerebral cortex (4), however, olfactory representation is much less, especially in relation to those of other senses. From: Herrick CJ. The functions of the olfactory parts of the cerebral cortex. *Proceedings of the National Academy of Sciences, USA* 1933; 19: 7-14.

Like Herrick and a surprising number of other prominent neuroscientists, MacLean was the son of a church minister and was born in the scenic Finger Lakes area of western New York State.[8] He had studied medicine at Yale and, after an internship at Johns Hopkins Hospital in Baltimore, had found himself serving as a psychiatrist in the US army in New Zealand. Following the American entry into the Second World War, there had been numerous mental illnesses among combatants, the majority of whom would now have been diagnosed as suffering from post-traumatic shock disorder. Having had no special training in psychiatry but having been intrigued by the cases, MacLean had decided to explore the relationship between brain and behaviour at the end of the war. It was while studying under Stanley Cobb at the Massachusetts General Hospital

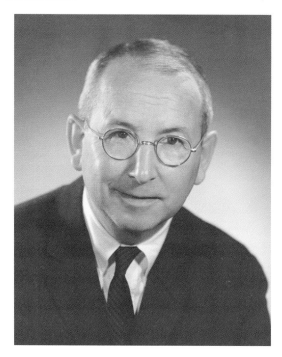

Figure 31.5 Paul MacLean. Photo by Edward A Hubbard, National Institute of Health, United States. (Wikimedia Commons file: Paul D MacLean.jpg.)

in Boston that he had undertaken EEG studies of patients with psychomotor epilepsy and found evidence of abnormal electrical activity in the base of the brain, most likely arising in the hippocampus.

Partly because of Papez's work, MacLean came to see the structures at the base of the cerebral hemispheres as a 'visceral' brain, an older part of the brain where sensory information about the outside world might overlap with that from the body itself.[9] Later, dissatisfied with his own term and mindful of Broca's earlier one, he proposed 'limbic system' instead.[10] As his career took him back to Yale (to work in John Fulton's department of physiology) and then to the National Institutes of Health, he continued to explore the newly named system. Using strychnine and, in later experiments, electrical stimulation, he was able to confirm that there were connections between wide areas of cortex and hippocampus. MacLean had further thoughts, too. He now considered the mammalian brain to comprise three interlocking parts, the whole forming a 'triune brain'.[11] In addition to a limbic system concerned with emotional behaviour there was, in the brain stem, a visceral brain that ran the various body systems (heart, lung, gut, etc.), and a more discriminative brain that occupied the bulk of the cerebral cortex and made particular use of the special senses (vision, touch, hearing) to provide information about the external world.

While the general public readily adopted the idea of a reptilian brain as an explanation for selfish or deceitful behaviour, the response of the neuroscientific community was mixed, and for some the triune brain provided an opportunity to attack the concept of the limbic system itself. Alf Brodal, a pioneer of the Norwegian school of neuroscience and one of Per Andersen's former mentors in Oslo, would go so far as to write:

> It is difficult to see that the lumping together of these different regions under one anatomical heading, 'the limbic lobe,' serves any purpose ... It is even less justifiable to speak of a 'limbic system.' ... it is the author's opinion that the use of the terms 'limbic lobe' and 'limbic system' should be abandoned.[12]

Brodal's opinion was not easily dismissed. He was sole author of the most comprehensive neuroanatomy textbook at the time and had studied the neural connections of the olfactory lobe and other structures in the base of the brain himself.[13] Others were prepared to accept the idea of a limbic system but unsure as to its territory within the brain. While accepting that structures such as the hippocampus, amygdala, fornix, and cingulate gyrus were key parts, there was doubt about the olfactory lobe. And might there not be a case for including most of the central brain stem, in view of the connections to the hypothalamus, a region intimately involved in emotive expression?

As for the triune brain, it was a concept that slowly withered after enjoying a burst of attention, and, in his later writing, MacLean himself seemed almost apologetic for having made his suggestion.[14] He should not have been. The idea of a triune brain was a natural development of the painstaking comparative neuroanatomical studies of Broca and Herrick.

But what are the anatomical features of the limbic system that, in addition to controlling various important physiological systems of the body, would be consistent with a role as the generator of consciousness? Above all, does it contain structures that have the complexity and connectivity that might enable it to fulfill such a role?

Notes

1. The Wikipedia article on Broca is excellent in covering his life and the remarkable range of his professional activities.
2. For a recent review of the history of cerebral localization, see: A.J. McComas, *Sherrington's Loom. An Introduction to the Science of Consciousness* (New York, NY: Oxford University Press, 2019) 69–102.
3. P. Broca, 'Anatomie comparée des circonvolutions cérébrales: le grande lobe limbique et la scissure limbique dans la série des mammifères' (1878) 1 *Revue d'anthropologie* 385–498. This important historical paper has been translated and republished as: P. Broca, 'Comparative Anatomy of the Cerebral Convolutions. The Great Limbic Lobe and the Limbic Fissure in the Mammalian Series' (translated by D. Furlani), (2015) Wiley Online Library. DOI 10.1002/cne.23856.
4. G.W. Bartelmez, 'Charles Judson Herrick (1868–1960)' (1973) 43 *Biographical Memoirs of the National Academy of Sciences (USA)* 77–108.
5. Clarence Luther Herrick (1858–1904) had inspired his younger brother in pursuit of natural history. Because of tuberculosis, he had finished his career in the southern United States, becoming the second president of the University of New Mexico.

6. C.J. Herrick, 'The Functions of the Olfactory Parts of the Cerebral Cortex' (1933) 19 *Proceedings of the National Academy of Sciences, USA* 7–14.

7. J.W. Papez, 'A Proposed Mechanism of Emotion' (1937) 38 *Archives of Neurology and Psychiatry* 725–43.

8. P.D. MacLean, *The History of Neuroscience in Autobiography*, L.R. Squire (ed.) (San Diego, CA: Academic Press, 1998) 2: 244–75.

9. P.D. MacLean, 'Psychosomatic Disease and the "Visceral Brain." Recent Developments Bearing on the Papez Theory of Emotion' (1949) 11(9) *Psychosomatic Medicine* 338–53.

10. P.D. MacLean, 'The Limbic System and its Hippocampal Formation. Studies in Animals and their Possible Application to Man' (1954) 11(1) *Journal of Neurophysiology* 29–44.

11. P.D. MacLean, 'The Triune Brain: Emotion and Scientific Bias' in F.O. Schmitt (ed.), *The Neurosciences: Second Study Program* (New York, NY: Rockefeller University Press 1970) 336–49.

12. A. Brodal, *Neurological Anatomy in Relation to Clinical Medicine* (New York, NY: Oxford University Press, 1981).

13. A. Brodal, 'The Hippocampus and the Sense of Smell. A Review' (1947) 70 *Brain* 179–222.

14. P.D. MacLean, *The Triune Brain in Evolution: Role in Paleocerebral Function* (New York, NY: Plenum Press, 1990).

32

Anatomy of the Limbic System

The main structures that have been considered to form the limbic system are shown in Figure 32.1. To describe them all would be beyond the scope of this book; instead, four have been selected so as to give an idea of the variety of structure and function, and of the interconnectedness, that characterizes the limbic system. Of the four, the *hippocampus* is the largest structure and its importance stems from its important role in learning and memory, as already described. Some features of the hippocampal anatomy were described in Part I but it is convenient to go over them again. The *amygdala* is also involved in memory and, though smaller, resembles the hippocampus in having a host of incoming and outgoing connections. One of the connections has a special evolutionary significance for it is the chemosensory pathway from the olfactory lobe. The *nucleus accumbens* is a key part of the brain's 'reward' ('pleasure') system and is connected to both the hippocampus and the amygdala. Through its output to the latter structures and to the 'basal ganglia' it would be able to assist in the learning of movements that would bring reward. The final structure to be described is the *olfactory bulb*. Although most authorities would not include it in the limbic system, it—or its neural forerunner—provided the original guidance for movement towards food or a mate, movement that, in the course of evolution, became associated with a primal pleasure.

(1) *Hippocampus.* While there is uncertainty as to what should be included in the 'limbic system', there is general agreement that the hippocampus is the most important element. The importance is hinted at by the central position of the hippocampus in the brain—above the brain stem and covered by the mantle of the cerebral cortex. Also pointing to the importance of the hippocampus is the richness of its connections, enabling it to communicate with almost every part of the central nervous system—the cortical lobes, the basal ganglia, the thalamus, other elements in the limbic system, the brain stem, and the spinal cord. Indeed, the hippocampus is probably the most connected structure in the entire brain. If any part of the brain has the appearance of being a command centre, it is the hippocampus.

Though the importance of the hippocampus is recognized today (not least by having a journal devoted to it), three centuries were to pass before the cellular architecture of Aranzio's 'seahorse' was examined—this by the person regarded by many as the greatest neuroscientist of all.

Aranzio's Seahorse and the Search for Memory and Consciousness. Alan J. McComas, Oxford University Press.
© Oxford University Press 2023. DOI: 10.1093/oso/9780192868244.003.0034

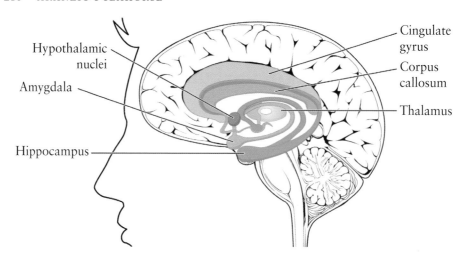

Figure 32.1 Limbic system in a human brain. Much has been added since Broca's description of a 'great limbic lobe' (see Figure 31.2) but even the present figure is greatly simplified. (Wikimedia Commons file: 1511 The Limbic Lobe. jpg. Original coloured. Author: OpenStax College.)

Ramón Santiago y Cajal (1852–1936; Figure 32.2) had been born in an impoverished region of northern Spain and after an adventurous childhood had attended medical school in Zaragoza.[1] After serious illnesses contracted while serving with the army in Cuba, Cajal had returned to Spain and become attracted to the study of the nervous system. Working alone and spending long hours looking down his microscope, Cajal made beautiful black ink sketches of what he had seen. He had insight as to the functions of the various parts of a neuron—the dendrites, through their many branches, would collect information from other neurons, while the axon would send excitation onwards to the next cell in the neural pathway. Importantly, he recognized that nerve cells, though closely apposed to one another, were nevertheless physically separate—a conclusion very much at odds with that of his illustrious contemporary, Camillo Golgi.[2] There had been irony in the argument between the two men, an argument that had lingered after their sharing of the 1905 Nobel Prize in Physiology or Medicine, for it had been Golgi's histological staining method that had set Cajal off on his neuroscientific career.

While describing the features of the cells in the hippocampus Cajal had observed a neural arrangement quite different to that of the neocortex covering the cerebral hemispheres. Though there were pyramidal cells in both situations, the cell bodies were confined to a single layer in the hippocampus while in the neocortex they were present throughout its thickness. It was Cajal's former student, Lorente de Nó (1902–1990),[3] who would later show that the neocortical cells were disposed in columns perpendicular to the surface of the hemisphere—an important clue as to how the cortex functioned. It was Lorente who also took Cajal's observations on the hippocampus further, partly in his descriptions of the various types of neuron present in addition to the

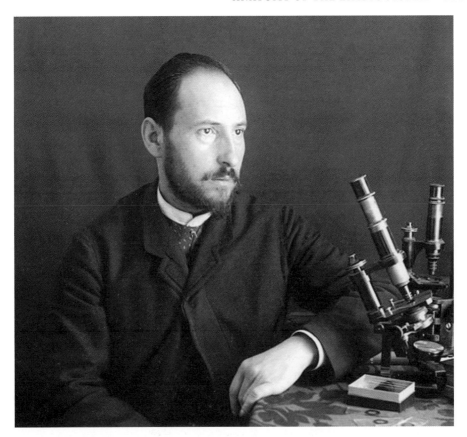

Figure 32.2 Santiago Ramón y Cajal with the Zeiss microscope presented to him by the provincial government of Zaragoza for his work during the regional cholera epidemic in 1885. Photo by Zeiss Microscopy from Germany (Wikimedia Commons CC BY-SA 2.0.)

pyramidal cells, but especially in his recognition that histological differences justified a division of the hippocampus into four areas (Figure 32.3, Upper).

Mindful that the hippocampus had also been given the name Ammon's Horn because of its resemblance to the musical instrument of Ammon, god of the ancient Egyptians, Lorente referred to the four regions as CA1, CA2, CA3, CA4 (with CA standing for Cornu Ammone).[4] The differences observed by Lorente were evident when the hippocampus was examined in cross-section as it curved around the *hippocampal fissure*. The *dentate nucleus* bulged into the fissure from above, merging into area CA3/4 which became successively areas CA2 and CA1. Below the fissure CA1 was continuous with the *subiculum* and the latter with the *entorhinal cortex*.

A remarkable feature of the hippocampus is that it is organized transversely and not in its long axis. A cross-section taken from one part closely resembles that from another, rather like two slices of a Swiss roll. By combining histology with neurophysiological recordings, Per Andersen and his Oslo colleagues were able to determine the sequence of events in the hippocampus—the direction in which information is processed (see later in this chapter).[5] The most prominent source of incoming information is the

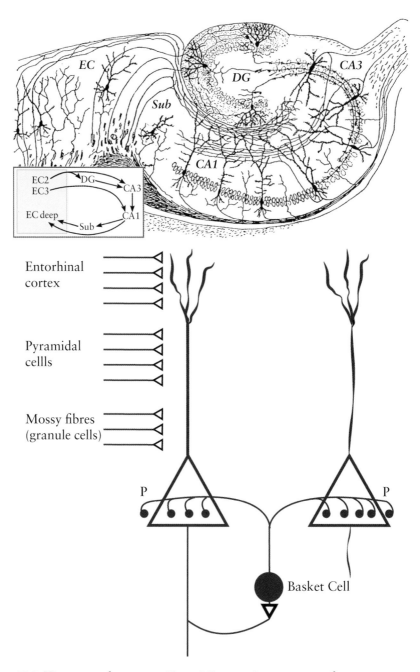

Figure 32.3 Hippocampal structure. *Upper*. Microscopic appearance of a transverse section of the hippocampus. Some typical neurons have been drawn with their axons and dendrites, others shown simply as ovals. Original by Cajal in his *Histologie du Système nerveus de l'Homme et des Vertébrés* (Paris: A Maloine, 1911) with lettering added subsequently as follows: *CA1*, *CA3*, divisions of hippocampus; *DG*, dentate gyrus; *EC*, entorhinal cortex; *Sub*, subiculum. The pyramidal cell bodies lie in a single curved layer throughout the hippocampus; two are shown below the *CA3* lettering. *Insert* shows the direction of impulse activity in the hippocampus, as determined by Per Andersen and his colleagues. (Wikimedia Commons File: CajalHippocampus (modified).png.) *Lower*. Synaptic connections on cell body and dendrites of a *CA1* pyramidal cell. Note basket cell with inhibitory synapses on cell body of pyramidal neuron (*P*). This figure appeared previously in Box 6.1.

neighbouring entorhinal cortex which sends fibres to the hippocampus in the *perforant pathway*. These fibres make synaptic connections with the dendrites of granule cells in the molecular layer of the dentate nucleus. The axons of the granule cells (the '*mossy fibres*') in turn form giant synapses with the dendrites of the CA3/4 pyramidal cells. The latter cells then synapse with the CA1 pyramids through the *Schaffer collateral branches* of their axons. After it has completed its processing, the hippocampus passes its information on to other parts of the brain through the fimbria—the other main branches of the pyramidal cell axons.

When a single pyramidal neuron is examined (Figure 32.3, Lower), its cell body is seen to be covered with synapses made with the axon terminals of *basket cells*—the cells that Per Andersen and John Eccles had shown to be inhibitory. Like major output neurons in other parts of the nervous system (cortical pyramids, Purkinje cells in the cerebellum, motoneurons in the spinal cord), the hippocampal pyramidal cells exhibit negative feedback, a powerful means of controlling their excitability and made possible by an axon branch to a basket cell. At the base of the apical dendrite of the pyramidal cell are synapses formed with the terminals of *mossy fibres*, the axons of the plentiful *granule cells* in the dentate gyrus. The granule cells, which are now known to be continually replenished during life,[6] themselves receive excitation via the *perforant path* from cells in the *entorhinal cortex*, a structure bordering the hippocampus in which Edvard and May-Britt Moser had discovered 'grid cells'.[7] The entorhinal cortex, via the perforant path, also sends information directly to the pyramidal cells throughout the length of the hippocampus, the synapses being situated on the distal branches of the apical dendrites. Among the many inputs to the hippocampus, the entorhinal cortex and its perforant path is probably the most important, bringing information from other parts of the temporal lobe and the *thalamus*, as well as from the *olfactory bulb, amygdala, occipital lobe*, and *brain stem nuclei* (the sources of acetylcholine, noradrenaline, and serotonin). The hippocampal cells are also interconnected, those in CA3 passing information on to those in CA1.

The fibres leaving the hippocampus (and, to a greater extent, the subjacent *subiculum*) are the axons of the pyramidal cells and most run in bundles in the *fornix*, whence they are distributed to the *mammillary body, septal nuclei, anterior thalamic nucleus, hypothalamus* (emotion), *nucleus accumbens* (pleasure), *amygdala*, and *periaqueductal grey matter* (pain). In addition, the two hippocampi are connected to each other by *commissural fibres*. Some fibres, mainly from the subiculum, reach the *cingulate gyrus* above the corpus callosum.

The preceding description is based on the work of a large number of neuroscientists who used a variety of techniques. Most often, especially in the earliest studies, the approach was to trace degenerating nerve fibres after sectioning them; later, the transport of horseradish peroxidase or radioactive amino acids was observed, following their incorporation into fibres at a particular site. However, it is now possible to go a step further using *tensor diffusion MRI*, a methodology based on the orientation of water molecules in nerve fibres and one that can be applied to living human brains. Though the methodology cannot indicate the direction of the nerve fibres—whether they are entering or leaving a part of the brain—it does reveal the sizes of different pathways and, by implication, their relative importance. When applied to the human hippocampus, it was found that there were especially strong connections to other parts of the ipsilateral temporal lobe, occipital lobe, thalamus, parahippocampal gyrus (a fold of grey matter adjacent to the hippocampus), amygdala, and central brain stem structures; in addition there were commissural fibres linking the hippocampi on the two sides.[8]

(2). *Amygdala (Amygdaloid nucleus)*. Named because of its resemblance to an almond, the amygdala lies immediately anterior to, and beside, the hippocampus in the medial temporal lobe (Figure 32.1). Despite its small size it contains a number of nuclei and, like its hippocampal neighbour, a host of connections to other parts of the nervous system. Among the incoming (afferent) fibres are those from the *olfactory bulb*, pointing to the importance of the amygdala (and thence the hippocampus) in the evolution of the nervous system, with its early dependence on chemosensation. Although the pathways are unclear, electrophysiological recordings have shown that, in addition to smell, other senses are represented in the amygdala—vision, hearing, and touch. The amygdala also receives fibres from the *frontal and temporal lobes, the subiculum* (below the hippocampus), *hypothalamus, thalamus, central grey matter in the brain stem* (including the nuclei secreting acetylcholine, noradrenaline, serotonin, and dopamine respectively) as well as many other structures. The outgoing (efferent) amygdaloid fibres are equally diverse, many of them going back to the various nuclei and cortical areas from which the amygdala received inputs, the hippocampus among them.

Given its complex internal structure and the number and variety of its fibre connections, it is hardly surprising that electrical stimulation of the amygdala has been observed to produce varied effects; respiration, movement, gastric secretion, bowel movement, blood pressure may all alter. In terms of behaviour, early experiments on cats by the Oslo group, and by Kaada in particular, showed that stimulation of the amygdala could reproduce all the features of an animal that was either fearful or angry.[9] Suggestive of fear were rapid glancing and searching movements, restlessness, running away, and hiding, while anger was simulated by growling, hissing, and piloerection (hair standing on end). There could also be an 'attentive' response in which the aroused animal appeared to be searching for something nearby.

As important as the control of behaviour, and related to it, is the involvement of the amygdala in memory. As in the neighbouring hippocampus, electrode recordings in the amygdalas of patients have revealed the presence of 'concept' cells.[10] In view of its ability to generate emotional behaviour, and the frequent association of emotion with important personal events, it seems likely that the amygdala is especially concerned with episodic memory and with the conversion of short-term memory to long-term. This is discussed later.

(3). *Nucleus accumbens.* The nucleus accumbens, situated anteriorly in the fore-brain, achieved prominence when James Olds and Peter Milner discovered that there was a 'pleasure' or 'reward' centre in the vicinity of the nucleus. As described earlier,[11] the McGill students observed that rats with stimulating electrodes implanted in this area would activate them repeatedly, even to the point of no longer feeding. Under more natural circumstances the nucleus has been shown to alter its firing pattern during feeding[12] and presumably during other pleasurable behaviours.

Composed of an outer shell and an inner core, the nucleus contains mostly *'spiny' neurons.* Those in the shell receive excitatory inputs from the *amygdala* and the *hippocampus,* with glutamate as the transmitter. The spiny neurons in the core, in contrast, are inhibited by dopamine released from fibres arising in the *ventral tegmental area (VTA).* It is this inhibition which appears to be associated with, and presumably responsible for, feelings of pleasure. Conversely, dislike (aversion) is accompanied by increased activity in the spiny neurons.

The nucleus accumbens projects back to the VTA, as well as to the basal ganglia, substantia nigra, and reticular formation. It is thought that, through the projection to the basal ganglia, the nucleus helps to establish motor programmes that will result in future reward.

(4). *Olfactory bulb.* In mammals an olfactory bulb is an obvious feature of the under-surface of each hemisphere, as in the accurate and beautiful 17th-century etching by Christopher Wren (Figure 32.4). The etching also shows the equally prominent *olfactory tract,* the nerve fibre bundle connecting the bulb to the rest of the hemisphere. In humans the bulb lies immediately above a thin layer of bone, the cribriform plate, that overhangs the nose and is pierced by fibres attached to sensory endings, the olfactory receptors, in the nasal epithelium. As with so much of the brain, the fine structure of the olfactory pathway was examined by Ramon Cajal. He showed that the olfactory fibres end in very fine branches that intermingle with those of the dendrites of *mitral* and *tufted cells* to form *glomeruli* (Figure 32.5, *right*). The axons of the mitral and tufted cells, in turn, project to the main brain mass via the olfactory tract; the latter also contains axons running in the reverse direction, from brain to bulb. Much of the neurophysiology of the olfactory system was worked out by Gordon Shepherd and his colleagues over the course of Shepherd's long career at Yale.[13] However, especially striking novel insights were to come from Richard Axel and Linda Buck during a 13-year span of research in the Howard Hughes Institute at Columbia University in New York.

Axel, the more senior of the two, had been a close colleague and friend of Eric Kandel in the Institute. This was at the time that Kandel was studying the intracellular pathway,

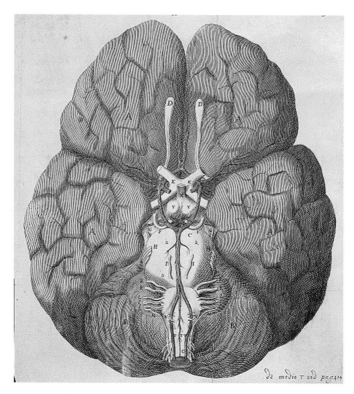

Figure 32.4 Etching of the undersurface of the human brain by the famous 17th-century English architect, Christopher Wren, (D, olfactory bulb with tract). The etching appeared as one of the illustrations in his colleague Thomas Willis' treatise: *Cerebri anatome: cui assessit nervorum descriptio et usus.* Amsterdam: G. Schagen, 1664. Wellcome Images.

from surface membrane to nucleus, that enabled *Aplysia* to switch on genes controlling the protein synthesis needed for the formation of new synapses during learning experiments. It had been a mutually beneficial interaction, Kandel's knowledge of neuroscience in exchange for Axel's expertise in molecular biology. In his memoir Kandel provides a description of Axel (Figure 32.6). 'Tall, lanky, stoop-shouldered, Axel had an intense, angular face made even more intense by the shiny steel-rimmed glasses he always wore.' Axel had already made his mark as a molecular biologist by introducing a method of transfection and then, still young, had decided to apply his knowledge and skills to solving a problem in the nervous system. With his former postdoctoral student Linda Buck as collaborator, he had eventually chosen chemosensation, recognizing its primal importance in the animal kingdom. Put simply, how do we smell things?

One of the fundamental questions that Axel and Buck had sought to answer was whether there was a small number of types of receptor in an olfactory epithelium (in ourselves, the lining of the nose) that become active in different combinations so as to cover a range of odour-generating molecules. The alternative was a large number, so that the chemical responsible for a particular odour would combine with a specific receptor. If the latter were the case, Axel argued, then there should be a host of genes

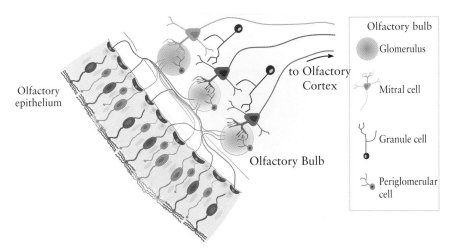

Figure 32.5 Mammalian olfactory system. The nerve fibres of the olfactory receptors in the mucosa run to synapse with mitral cells in the olfactory bulb glomeruli and are arranged so that each glomerulus can only respond to one specific odour. Reproduced from: Dibattista M, Pifferi S, Menini A, Reisert J. Alzheimer's disease: what can we learn from the peripheral olfactory system? *Frontiers in Neuroscience*: 19 May 2020 (original figure in colour; Creative Commons Attribution Licence (CC BY) A similar olfactory system, but involving chemoreceptors in antennae, is found in ants and other insects.

coding for receptors among those for the olfactory epithelium; moreover the receptor genes were likely to be part of G-protein family.

And so it proved. A human was found to have approximately 500 odorant receptors and a mouse even more—1,300. With each receptor the product of an individual gene, approximately 5 per cent of the entire mouse genome was devoted to chemoreceptors! It was an astonishing result but one in keeping with the importance of chemosensitivity in early evolution. For comparison, the mammalian retina, the product of a much later stage in evolution, has only four types of photoreceptor. Nor was the situation different in other species; a fruit fly (*Drosophila*) was found to have 80 olfactory genes, and *C. elegans*—the one millimetre-long worm with a scant 302 neurons—to have 1,000 olfactory receptor genes. Axel and Buck then showed that, although the receptor neurons appeared to have a haphazard distribution in the olfactory epithelium, the mitral cells to which they projected had specified locations within the olfactory bulb; further, there were only two mitral cells in the bulb for each of the many types of odorant receptor (Figure 32.6). Thus there was a spatial map of receptors in the bulb, corresponding to a map of odours. Axel and Buck went on to demonstrate that a topographic map was also present in the olfactory system of an insect. In the fruit fly the many members of the 80 types of chemoreceptors are distributed among the hairs of the antenna; the sensory cells for each of the 80 types then project to just one or two neurons at fixed locations in the antennal lobe.[14]

It was brilliant work and recognized as such by the award of the 2004 Nobel Prize in Physiology or Medicine to Richard Axel and Linda Buck. It had been an elegant

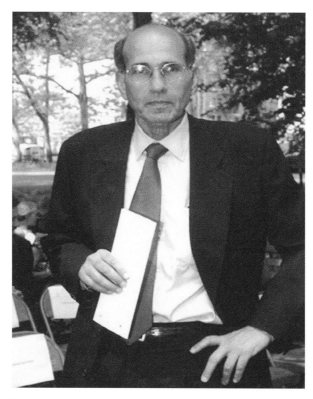

Figure 32.6 Richard Axel. A molecular biologist who collaborated with Eric Kandel in the latter's *Aplysia* research and then went on to study the genetic and neural basis of olfaction, winning the Nobel Prize with his colleague, Linda Buck. (NIH photograph. Wikimedia Commons file: Richard Axel.jpg.)

demonstration of the power of molecular biology in solving a difficult problem in neuroscience, though it left unanswered the question that had so baffled Francis Crick—how does the brain read a neural map? Or, as Axel put it at the end of his Nobel Lecture, 'the old problem of the ghost in the machine'.

Notes

1. Santiago Ramon y Cajal (1852–1936) wrote his autobiography, *Recuerdos de mi Vida*, before he had been awarded the Nobel Prize. It is an extraordinary life history, one that succeeds in capturing a brilliant but humble mind, Spanish academia, and the evolution of neurohistology. Fortunately an English translation by E.H. Craigie was republished in 1989 by MIT Press. Like the original, it includes some of Cajal's superb pen-and-ink sketches of stained nerve tissue.

2. Camillo Golgi (1843–1926), like Cajal, trained in medicine before becoming fascinated by research. His initial histological experiments were performed in a former hospital kitchen near Milan, but it was to Pavia, in present-day Italy, that he would return and make his academic career. His great achievement was the discovery of a method of staining nerve cells individually with a deposit of silver nitrate that enabled their fine structure to be seen. His dispute with Cajal is

described in the latter's autobiography and more recently in: A.J. McComas, *Galvani's Spark. The Story of the Nerve Impulse* (New York, NY: Oxford University Press, 2011).

3. Rafael Lorente de Nó spent the greater part of his life and scientific career in the United States, first at Washington University in St Louis and then at the Rockefeller Institute in New York. At the time Lorente was unique in being able to combine expertise in brain histology with electrophysiology and to deduce how neurons might interact at synapses. A fine record was marred when he became the loser in a dispute with Alan Hodgkin and Andrew Huxley over the mechanism of the resting and action potentials of nerve fibres (see: McComas, *Galvani's Spark*, see note 2).

4. R. Lorente de Nó, 'Studies on the Structure of the Cerebral Cortex. II. Continuation of the Study of Ammonic System' (1934) 46 *Journal für Psychologie und Neurologie* 113–77.

5. P. Andersen, T.V.P. Bliss, and K.K. Skrede, 'Lamellar Organization of Hippocampal Excitatory Pathways' (1971) 13 *Experimental Brain Research* 222–38.

6. See Chapter 25.

7. See Chapter 21.

8. J.J. Maller, T. Welton, M. Middione, F.H. Callaghan, J.V. Rosenfeld, and S.M. Grieve, 'Revealing the Hippocampal Connectome through Super-Resolution 1150-Direction Diffusion MRI' (2019) 9 *Nature Scientific Reports* article number 2418.

9. B.R. Kaada, Jr J. Jansen, and P. Andersen, 'Stimulation of the Amygdaloid Nuclear Complex in Unanesthetized Cats' (1953) 3 *Neurology* 844–57.

10. See Chapter 24.

11. See Chapter 3.

12. S. Ahn and A.G. Phillips, 'Modulation by Central and Basolateral Amygdalar Nuclei of Dompaminergic Correlates of Feeding to Satiety in the Rat Nucleus Accumbens and Medial Prefrontal Cortex' (2002) 22(24) *Journal of Neuroscience* 10958–65.

13. G.M. Shepherd, W.R. Chen, D. Willhite, M. Migliore, and C.A. Greer, 'The Olfactory Granule Cells: From Classical Enigma to Central Role in Olfactory Processing' (2007) 55(2) *Brain Research Reviews* 373–82. This is an example of the many pioneering studies on olfaction from Shepherd's laboratory. Shepherd has used the olfactory system as a model for neural computations; one of his many laboratory findings is of synaptic interactions between dendrites of mitral cells in the olfactory bulb.

14. R. Axel, 'Scents and Sensibility. A Molecular Logic of Olfactory Perception' Nobel Lecture, 2004. <http://www.nobelprize.org/uploads/2018/06/axel-lecture.pdf> accessed 24 April 2022.

33

Clinical Evidence of Hippocampal (Limbic) Involvement in Consciousness

(a) Brain stimulation during surgery

As described earlier, the effect of stimulating the amygdala in animals is to produce behaviours that are highly suggestive of an alteration in consciousness, and of fear or anger in particular. Though the opportunities have been fewer, the results of stimulating the amygdala and other parts of the limbic system in patients have been still more rewarding. The first report would come not from a university hospital but from Hartford in Connecticut and this at a time when William Scoville, Henry Molaison's future surgeon, was performing his many orbital undercuttings of the prefrontal lobe in psychiatric patients at the state hospital. With Wladimir Liberson acting as the electrophysiologist, Scoville found that electrical stimulation of the exposed parts of the frontal lobe produced little effect. In contrast, stimulation of the uncus (anterior region of the medial temporal lobe that includes the amygdala) caused a marked reduction in consciousness, with the patients no longer responding to the examiner or else doing so with difficulty and with no recollection afterwards.[1]

Not surprisingly, Wilder Penfield and his colleagues at the Montreal Neurological Institute would also investigate the temporal lobe in this way. Penfield's initial stimulation studies of the human brain had been made with small repetitive electrical pulses delivered through a twin-wire (bipolar) electrode touching the surface of the cerebral hemispheres, a technique similar to that employed by physiologists on animal brains a half-century earlier. When Herbert Jasper's electroencephalography (EEG) studies on the Institute's patients indicated that the epileptic focus was often at the base of the temporal lobe, Penfield had begun to use a stimulating needle electrode that he or William Feindel, another of the Institute's neurosurgeons, would push deeply into the lobe through one of the fissures on the surface. Herbert Jasper would have been present in the operating theatre gallery to make EEG recordings from the temporal lobe surface and Oslo's Birger Kaada, during his year in Montreal, would also have attended, interacting with the patients in the operating theatre. By 1954 Penfield and William Feindel had accumulated results on 155 patients with temporal lobe epilepsy, of whom 121 had histories suggestive of automatism—behaviours of which they seemed unaware at the time and were unable to recall afterwards.[2]

Penfield and Feindel found that deep stimulation within the temporal lobe often reproduced the patient's seizure pattern. In addition to confusion there might be licking and smacking of the lips, unusual postures of an arm or leg, grasping and plucking

Aranzio's Seahorse and the Search for Memory and Consciousness. Alan J. McComas, Oxford University Press.
© Oxford University Press 2023. DOI: 10.1093/oso/9780192868244.003.0035

movements of the hand, and staring of the eyes. Sometimes the patients could answer questions, but more often they were unable to; any spontaneous remarks could be nonsensical in content and language. During this time Herbert Jasper would often note that the EEG had altered, the larger waves being replaced by lower amplitude fast activity. At the end of the stimulation, the patient would usually have no awareness of what had transpired. Though they could not be certain of the exact position of the tip of the stimulating electrode during the sessions, Penfield and Feindel identified the amygdala and the surrounding structures as having been the likeliest sites.

(b) Psychomotor epilepsy (Hughlings Jackson's 'dreamy states')

In addition to the information from electrical stimulation studies, there is a rich supply from nature's own experiment, the patient with epilepsy. Rather than an experimenter applying the stimulation, it is the damaged brain itself that produces the abnormal electrical discharges. Though epilepsy had been known since antiquity, it was the French physicians of the 18th and 19th centuries who made careful studies and provided good descriptions of their patients. It was the French who gave the term 'grand mal' (major illness) to the most severe seizures, those in which the patients would lose consciousness, fall to the ground, stiffen and then jerk their limbs, and soil their clothes. 'Petit mal' (minor illness) was used to describe brief episodes, lasting a few seconds or possibly a minute or so, when the patient would cease whatever he or she had been doing, appear unaware of his or her surroundings and stare vacantly—before resuming activity as though nothing had happened. It was the latter form of epilepsy that Henry Molaison had first exhibited before progressing to grand mal attacks a few years later.

Later, French neurologists would recognize another, less frequent, form of seizure. It was one in which the patient would appear detached from their surroundings, usually for some minutes. As with petit mal, he or she would not fall or jerk; instead the patient would engage in some repetitive motor activity. Any speech would be nonsensical and there would be no awareness of the episode afterward. In less severe attacks, however, the patient might recall having had an unusual sensation immediately beforehand: tingling, a buzzing sound, or—especially suggestive of hippocampal involvement— an unpleasant smell. Alternatively, rather than loss of awareness, there might be 'déjà vu', a feeling of intense familiarity with the surroundings. Sometimes, too, surrounding objects were distorted, appearing unusually small or large or else misshapen.

One might hastily add that an episode in a patient with this third form of epilepsy is very different to the everyday experience in which a healthy person may walk a familiar route without any awareness of his surroundings—the houses, the people, the gardens, the new patch of sidewalk. When questioned afterwards, he or she will say that they were deep in thought at the time and simply had not noticed these things. (And, if challenged, will be able to recount their thoughts.)

Though the French had provided the first descriptions, the fullest accounts of altered consciousness with automatism were those of the British neurologist, John Hughlings

Jackson (1835–1911; Figure 33.1), who termed them '*dreamy states*'. Jackson—who had added 'Hughlings' to give his name more substance—was revered by his fellow neurologists. A bearded, patriarchal figure, Jackson was practising at a time when others were competing among themselves in the rapidly developing fields of clinical and basic neuroscience. At least two of the disputes had become public—Charles Sherrington and Victor Horsley's over publications concerning the descending fibres from the motor cortex into the spinal cord, and David Ferrier and Edward Schäfer's over the effects of temporal lobectomy.[3,4] In contrast, Jackson's reputation as a neurologist, indeed as the leading British neurologist, was unchallenged.

Jackson's eminence was due, in part, to his ideas as to how the nervous system might be organized and how it might be disturbed by disease. He had suggested that different levels of organization had evolved, with the higher, more recent level controlling the lower. He had also made an especially thorough study of patients with epilepsy, noting how involuntary shaking could begin in the hand, for example, and then successively involve the muscles of the forearm, upper arm, and shoulder before loss of consciousness supervened. From this 'march' Jackson had deduced that there was an orderly representation of movements in the human brain, though he had not immediately placed

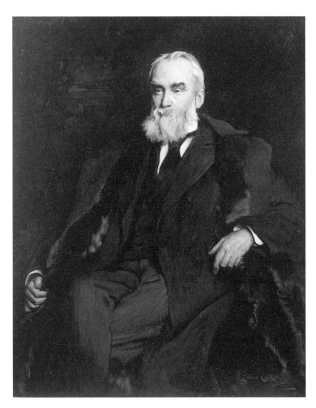

Figure 33.1 John Hughlings Jackson (1835–1911). The great pioneering British neurologist is pictured in 1895, towards the end of his career. (Photogravure after L. Calkin, cropped.) Wellcome Library, London. Wellcome images.

it in the cortex. Even to his contemporaries, however, Jackson had difficulty in articulating his thoughts clearly and his philosophical and physiological writings still make demands on the reader today. Nevertheless, at a time before EEGs and magnetic resonance imaging (MRI) scans were available, a successful neurological diagnosis depended largely on the taking of a detailed history and the carrying out of a careful physical examination—tasks in which Hughlings Jackson and his fellow neurologists excelled. The following is Jackson's description of a patient suffering from a 'dreamy state', an account that includes Jackson's insights as to what might be happening inside the patient's brain:

A.B., a man 37 years of age, was sent from the out-patient room to George Ward, London Hospital, to see me, November 7, 1884 ... The first attack was in 1882; it only lasted about 5 minutes. He had no more until May 1884; since which date he had had many, sometimes three or four a week. The attacks began by smells, which he declared to be horrible, but he could give no particular description of them; his wife said that he had likened them to the smell of phosphorus. There was no loss of smell (tested November 17) as there sometimes is in epileptics who have paroxysms beginning with such so-called 'subjective' smells. (There was no organic disease of the nose.) The patient had another preluding sensation—one seeming to him to start from the epigastric region. No doubt both these crude sensations were concomitant with the onset of the central discharges causing the fits—of the cells of that part of the cortex risen into that high degree of instability that I call a 'discharging lesion.' ... in the attacks the patient would become "vacant" and would sometimes lose consciousness for a short time. But besides negative affection of consciousness ... there was at the same time the diametrically opposite, the super-positive state, 'increase of consciousness,' that is, there was the so-called 'intellectual aura,' what I call the 'dreamy state.' ... He said that he 'began to think of things years gone by, ... things from boyhood's days.'[5]

Another of Jackson's patients was a doctor himself, a man who was able to give a very detailed history of his attacks. In some there had been an intense sense of familiarity (the déjà vu phenomenon), in one he had done something foolish (running over the surface of a glacier oblivious of possible crevasses), on another occasion he had returned home without any recollection of having completed the journey on the London Underground and of then leaving the station and walking to his house. Even more remarkable had been the time when he had not been aware of taking a history from a patient, examining him with a stethoscope, making a diagnosis of pneumonia at the base of the left lung, writing appropriate notes, and recommending that the patient 'take to his bed at once' (all of which he was able to piece together afterwards).

Unfortunately, at the end of the 19th century, the time when Jackson was practising, neurosurgery was still in its infancy, though it had a brilliant proponent in Victor Horsley[6] at the National Hospital for the Relief and Cure of Paralysis and Epilepsy (the future National Hospital for Nervous Diseases in London's Queen Square). All too often, however, the neurological patient would die without having had surgery, nor would there be an autopsy. In the case of Jackson's medical practitioner, however, an autopsy had been carried out and had revealed the presence of a cyst in the uncus of the left medial temporal lobe. In another of Jackson's patients, a female cook who had had feelings of suffocation accompanied by a 'horrid' smell, there had been a tumour in the right temporal lobe that had involved the amygdala. So convinced was Jackson of the location of the lesions causing the dreamy states that he would frequently refer to the clinical condition as 'uncinate fits'. Nevertheless, the proof that Jackson's 'dreamy states' were caused by abnormal electrical discharges in the uncus, amygdala, and general hippocampal area had to await the invention of EEG.

(c) EEG recordings during psychomotor epilepsy

The discovery of ongoing electrical activity in the brain had been made at the time Jackson was achieving his fame. Richard Caton (1842–1926; Figure 33.2), like Jackson, was a Yorkshireman. After training in medicine in Edinburgh, Caton had moved to Liverpool, working first as a children's physician and then as a lecturer in physiology. Using a mirror galvanometer to amplify and record any electrical potentials, he had put

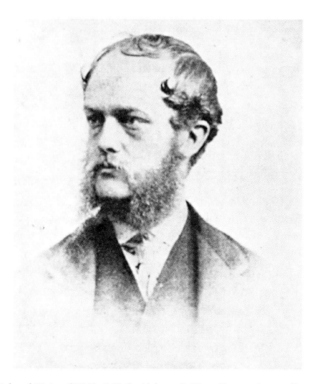

Figure 33.2 Richard Caton (1842–1926). Although Hans Berger is usually credited with the discovery of the EEG, Caton preceded him, though his recordings were of the brain activity in rabbits rather than in humans and his study lacked the depth of Berger's. An early neurophysiologist, Caton later became Lord Mayor of Liverpool, United Kingdom.

electrodes on the exposed brain of a rabbit and shown that there were continuing oscillations. It had been the first known EEG, and Caton had been able to repeat his novel finding at a meeting of physicians in Edinburgh in 1875.[7]

Despite Caton's success there seemed little interest in his discovery, at least in his own country, though his results would be confirmed independently by investigators in Poland and Russia. In 1925, however, there had been a report of spontaneous electrical activity in the human brain, activity that could even be detected with electrodes placed on the scalp. Though the author, Hans Berger, was the head of neurology and psychiatry at the University of Jena in Germany, the reported findings had not been immediately accepted by the medical and scientific communities. Once they had been confirmed by Edgar Adrian and Bryan Matthews in Cambridge, however, other workers were quick to move into this new field. One of them had been Herbert Jasper,[8] then in the Psychology Department at Brown University on Rhode Island, who would demonstrate to Wilder Penfield the usefulness of EEG in pinpointing the location of a cortical tumour. Later, after his recruitment to Montreal, Jasper would standardize the scalp electrode placements for future generations of electroencephalographers.

However, even before Jasper, and possibly before Adrian and Matthews too, there had been an EEG recording in the United States. Hallowell Davis, then in the Physiology Department at Harvard, had designed a valve amplifier and ink-recording unit, which he used on himself in the winter of 1933–34 with the help of two graduate students.[9] He would later jest that his alpha rhythm had been the first to be recognized as such in the western hemisphere. Davis had then had Frederic Gibbs and William Lennox join him in applying the new technology to the study of epileptic patients attending Boston City Hospital. They had used a needle electrode inserted into the scalp at the top of the head as the 'active' electrode and, with this simple recording system, had been able to detect relatively large 'wave and spike' discharges (Figure 33.3) during the momentary unawareness characteristic of petit mal attacks. In grand mal seizures, by contrast, there had been runs of spike activity.[10]

A second paper had followed three years later, this time by Gibbs, Lennox, and Gibbs' wife, Erna.[11] By then they were using multiple electrodes on the scalp and better recording equipment, the latter having been designed and built by Albert Grass, the founder of the future Grass Instrument Company. This time the Harvard physiologists had included investigation of patients whose disordered consciousness was associated with very abnormal behaviour— for example, there was a woman who began to tear her clothes and a man who started to eat a letter. Though these behaviours corresponded to Hughlings Jackson's 'dreamy states' or 'uncinate fits', the Gibbses and Lennox applied a different name to them—'*psychomotor epilepsy*'. With their electrode array the Harvard group discovered widely dispersed, flat-topped slow waves in the EEG at the time of the seizures. But in which region of the brain were the abnormal discharges arising? Since the epileptic activity could appear simultaneously across the head, might there be a subcortical source? The latter possibility was certainly in the mind of Herbert Jasper.

Having completed his move from the United States to the Montreal Neurological Institute, Jasper had also pressed on with his EEG research and in 1941 would publish

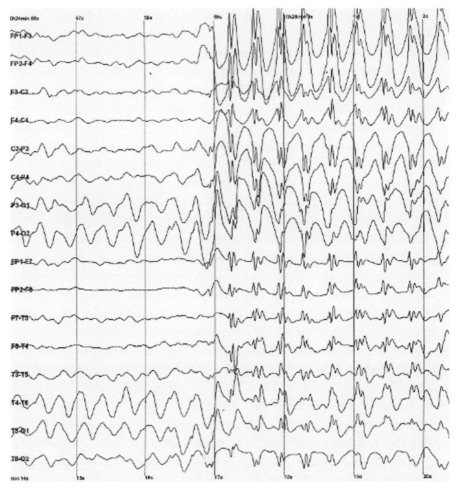

Figure 33.3 EEG recording of spike-and-wave activity in a child with absence epilepsy. The recording runs from left to right. Initially there is synchronized slow-wave activity towards the back of the head (Traces 7,8,14,15 from the top) that is suddenly replaced by large spike-and-waves on both sides. (Image created by Der Lange in 2005; Wikimedia Commons file: Spike-waves.png. Creative Commons Attribution-Share Alike 2.0 Generic license.)

an extensive review. As Jasper had no medical degree he had depended on the collaboration of a young neurologist, John Kershman, and the two had analysed the clinical features and recordings from almost 500 patients.[12] Part of the importance of the review was that it had demonstrated that there could be little correlation between the clinical features of a seizure and the type of EEG abnormality. For example, wave and spike discharges, though typical of petit mal, could also be observed in grand mal or psychomotor epilepsy. Moreover the same patient could display the various types of EEG abnormality at different times. Important, too, had been the use of a long electrode inserted through the nose so as to lie immediately below the bone separating it from the medial temporal lobe. With this electrode it had been possible to show that the generalized wave and spike activity accompanying petit mal or psychomotor attacks was indeed being generated deep within the temporal lobe. Later, similar findings would come from someone else extremely interested in whatever electrical activity might be going on in the medial temporal lobe— Paul MacLean.

MacLean was then at the point in his career when he had gone to Massachusetts General Hospital to learn neurophysiology from Stanley Cobb, and had found himself in the EEG department of the hospital working under Robert Schwab. In addition to using a nasopharyngeal lead, MacLean had thought of getting closer to the undersurface of the temporal lobe by placing an electrode deep in the external canal of the ear. With these additional electrodes and with a reference on the neck, MacLean was able to show, for the first time, that abnormal spike discharges arising in the deep temporal lobes could also initiate psychomotor epilepsy.[13]

The inference of these early EEG investigations, together with the results of intraoperative temporal lobe stimulation, seems as obvious now as it must have been 80 or more years ago. *Structures in the base of the brain, presumably parts of the limbic system, control consciousness.*

(d) Concept cell activity during thought

In the first part of the book the remarkable findings of Rodrigo Quian Quiroga, Christof Koch, Itzhak Fried, and their collaborators in Los Angeles were described.[14] They had used very fine wire electrodes to record from single neurons in the hippocampi of patients undergoing investigation of their epilepsy. Quian Quiroga had continued this work after moving to the University of Leicester in the United Kingdom. The investigators had found neurons that increased their firing when the patient was briefly shown a picture of a person or building, or when either was named. Examples had been former president Bill Clinton, the actresses Jennifer Aniston and Halle Berry, and the Sydney Opera House. Quiroga and his colleagues had further observed that the neural representation was 'invariant', in the sense that it did not matter which clothes the subject was wearing, whether she was seated or standing, looking at the camera or to the side, and so on. Though the investigators had used the term 'concept cell' (the 'concept' of Jennifer Aniston, for example), such neurons had been postulated to exist long before, first by William James (as 'pontifical' cells), and then by Jerry Lettvin and Horace Barlow (as 'grandmother' cells), and by Jerzy Konorski (as 'gnostic' units). The alternative idea for storing information in the brain, one that had previously enjoyed the greater support, was that bits and pieces of the person or place were represented in various parts of the brain and then combined into consciousness by synchronized impulse firing.

Perhaps not surprisingly, the chances of finding a responsive cell are a function of the relevance of the person, place, or object to the subject being examined. Thus cells responsive to family members or to the research staff were more frequently encountered than those firing to celebrities, and the latter, in turn, outnumbered those responsive to unfamiliar faces. A proportion of the cells, however, were excited by more than one stimulus, though within the same class (e.g. two female actresses or two famous buildings).

Although the mere existence of concept cells might suggest that consciousness is a result of their activity, the evidence for such a relationship would be strengthened if impulse firing was shown to be affected by thought. In another study from Los Angeles, this was demonstrated—for example by the imagining of a still picture, or by giving a verbal description of a video, both of which had just been viewed.[15] Further evidence correlating hippocampal activity with consciousness comes from another type of study, one in which the recognition of a face was affected by showing that of another person immediately beforehand (a 'forward masking' experiment). It was found that impulse firing by a hippocampal 'concept' cell correlated strongly with what the subject actually 'saw'.[16] Another approach was to show a known face so briefly (33 milliseconds, for example) that the subject had difficulty recognizing the person; it was only on the successful occasions that the corresponding concept cell increased its firing.[17]

Notes

1. W.T. Liberson, W.B. Scoville, and R.H. Dunsmore, 'Stimulation Studies of the Prefrontal Lobe and Uncus in Man' (1951) 3 *Electroencephalography and Clinical Neurophysiology* 1–8.
2. W. Feindel and W. Penfield, 'Localization of Discharge in Temporal Lobe Automatism' (1954) 72(5) *AMA Archives of Neurology and Psychiatry* 605–30.
3. J.A. Vilensky, J.L. Stone, and S. Gilman, 'Feud and Fable: The Sherrington–Horsley Polemic and the Delayed Publication' (2003) 12(4) *Journal of the History of the Neurosciences* 368–75.
4. P.S.SV. Vannemreddy and J.L. Stone, 'Sanger Brown and Edward Schäfer before Heinrich Klüver and Paul Bucy: Their Observations on Bilateral Temporal Lobe Ablations' (2017) 43(3) *Neurological Focus* 1–7.
5. H. Jackson, 'On a Particular Variety of Epilepsy ("Intellectual Aura"), One Case with Symptoms of Organic Brain Disease' (1888) 11 *Brain* 179–207.
6. Sir Victor Horsley (1856–1916) was a man of many talents, best remembered for having been the world's first true neurosurgeon, operating at University College Hospital in London and also at the nearby National Hospital for Paralysis and Epilepsy (later the National Hospital for Nervous Diseases). As a surgeon, Horsley introduced the use of large skin flaps to access the skull, and beeswax to stop bleeding from the bone. He was an accomplished neurophysiologist as well, not only experimenting on animals but preceding Feodor Krause, Otfrid Foerster, and Wilder Penfield in stimulating exposed human brains during surgery. Horsley, with Robert Clark, invented a stereotaxic instrument for locating and stimulating deep structures in animal brains. He, with his cousin Francis Gotch, appear to have been the first to record, with a galvanometer, a compound action potential in peripheral nerve (see: A.J. McComas, *Galvani's Spark. The Story of the Nerve Impulse* (New York, NY: Oxford University Press, 2011)). Horsley was also an authority on diseases of the thyroid gland. Volunteering for active duty in the First World War, Horsley died of heat stroke in what is now Iraq.
7. For more on Caton, Berger, and the discovery of the EEG see A.J. McComas, *Sherrington's Loom. An Introduction to the Science of Consciousness* (New York, NY: Oxford University Press, 2019).

8. H.H. Jasper and L. Carmichael, 'Electrical Potentials from the Intact Human Brain' (1935) 81 *Science* 51–3.

9. Hallowell Davis (1896–1992) was one of the giants of American neurophysiology and, in his time, the world's foremost authority on hearing. Born in New York, where his father practiced law, Davis later attended Harvard Medical School, graduating with honours. A Quaker, he drove an ambulance in France in the First World War. In 1922–23 he spent a year at Cambridge University (United Kingdom) in the laboratory of Edgar Adrian before returning to join the physiology department at Harvard and investigating hearing. He carried out pioneering studies on the cochlear mechanics and potentials, demonstrated the relationship between sound frequency and site of cochlear response, and recorded impulses in auditory nerve fibres and in cells in the cortical receiving area. In 1947, still without tenure despite 24 years at Harvard and his eminence as a physiologist, Davis moved to the Central Institute for the Deaf in St Louis. Davis had met his first wife, Pauline, when they were both serving at a refugee camp in Istanbul in 1922; an accomplished neurophysiologist herself, Pauline would become the first to record auditory potentials from the human brain.

10. F.A. Gibbs, H. Davis, and W.G. Lennox, 'The Electroencephalogram in Epilepsy and in Conditions of Impaired Consciousness' (1935) 34 *AMA Archives of Neurology and Psychiatry* 1133–48.

11. F.A. Gibbs, E.L. Gibbs, and W.G. Lennox, 'Cerebral Dysrhythmias of Epilepsy' (1938) 39 *AMA Archives of Neurology and Psychiatry* 298–314.

12. H. Jasper and J. Kershman, 'Electroencephalographic Classification of the Epilepsies' (1941) 45(6) *AMA Archives of Neurology and Psychiatry* 903–29.

13. P.D. MacLean and Z.A.P. Arellano, 'Basal Lead Studies in Epileptic Automatisms' (1950) 2 *Electroencephalography and Clinical Neurophysiology* 1–16.

14. See Chapter 24.

15. M. Cerf, N. Thiruvengadam, F. Mormann, A. Kraskov, R.Q. Quiroga, C. Koch, and I. Fried, 'Online, Voluntary Control of Human Temporal Lobe Neurons' (2010) 467 *Nature* 1104–8.

16. R.Q. Quiroga, A. Kraskov, F. Mormann, I. Fried, and C. Koch, 'Single-Cell Responses to Face Adaptation in the Human Medial Temporal Lobe' (2014) 84(2) *Neuron* 363–9.

17. R.Q. Quiroga, R. Mukamel, E.A. Isham, R. Malach, and I. Fried, 'Human Single-Neuron Responses at the Threshold of Consciousness' (2008) 105(9) *Proceedings of the National Academy of Sciences, USA* 3599–604.

34

Animal Evidence Consistent with Consciousness Generation in Limbic System (rather than Cortex)

Charles Darwin (Figure 34.1) had no hesitation in accepting that human beings were not the only living creatures to possess consciousness. In *The Descent of Man* (1871), he had written:

> Nevertheless the difference in mind between man and the higher animals, great as it is, certainly is one of degree and not of kind. We have seen that the senses and intuitions, the various emotions and faculties, such as love, memory, attention, curiosity, imitation, reason etc., of which man boasts, may be found in an incipient, or even in a well-developed condition, in the lower animals.

As he had stated, Darwin's conviction arose from his many observations of animal behaviour, not only those apparently associated with emotion but those activities suggestive of thought. However, Darwin's certainty did not extend to the stage in evolution at which consciousness had first appeared and the latter remained a mystery that would be a concern to him for the remainder of his long life.

Had he been alive and present to hear them, Darwin would have been fascinated by the remarks made by a certain Alex who, on the night before he died, had said to Irene: 'You be good. See you tomorrow. I love you.' While similar sentiments are often expressed in a loving relationship, these particular ones, given the circumstances, were quite remarkable. They had been spoken by a parrot.

Dr Irene Pepperberg, a university scientist, had raised her African Grey parrot, Alex, since his infancy. It would be easy to dismiss Alex's nocturnal blessing as an example of the bird's vocal mimicry. But was it? Alex had not only mastered the rudiments of a foreign language but used them to utter three short but perfectly appropriate sentences to his life companion. While students of animal behaviour are normally frustrated by inability to communicate with their subjects, was it not possible that, in the case of Alex, the subject was actually informing the professor of his thoughts?

That certain bird species are capable of intelligent behaviour is not in doubt. Crows, for example, have been observed to bend a wire into a hook in order to lift a miniature bucket of food by its handle, to drop stones into a container so as to raise the water level and a wriggling worm, and to retrieve the edible contents of shells placed on pedestrian

Aranzio's Seahorse and the Search for Memory and Consciousness. Alan J. McComas, Oxford University Press.
© Oxford University Press 2023. DOI: 10.1093/oso/9780192868244.003.0036

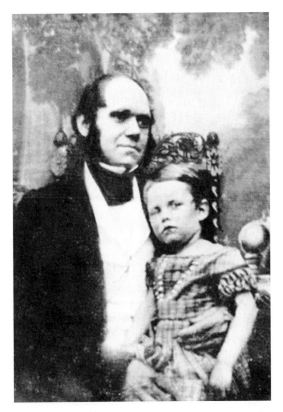

Figure 34.1 Charles Darwin (1809–1892) at age 33 with his son, William. Daguerrotype original.

(Wikimedia Commons file: Charles and William Darwin. Jpg.)

crossings to be broken by traffic. Chickadees show remarkable ability in storing and re-trieving food from their numerous caches, and homing pigeons exhibit superb naviga-tional skills. Indeed, in some of these cognitive skills, birds far surpass humans. Nor are birds alone. There are many examples of intelligent behaviour in other animals, some of which have been described elsewhere.[1] However, the concern of the present section is to answer the question:

Do those animals with brains containing a limbic system but little cortex exhibit be-haviours suggestive of consciousness?

Unfortunately, Alex and all other birds have to be excluded from consideration since they possess a well-developed pallium—the avian counterpart to the mammalian cerebral cortex. Also excluded is another strong example of animal intelligence—the octopus—though for a different reason, namely, the totally dissimilar structure of its nervous system compared to those of vertebrates. Mammals other than humans will not be considered either, since all possess a cortex, even though in many cases it is modest and lacking convolutions. Instead, attention will be restricted to three other classes of vertebrate: fish, amphibia, and reptiles. In every instance the motor component of the behaviour is limited by what is anatomically feasible—approaching, retreating, hiding,

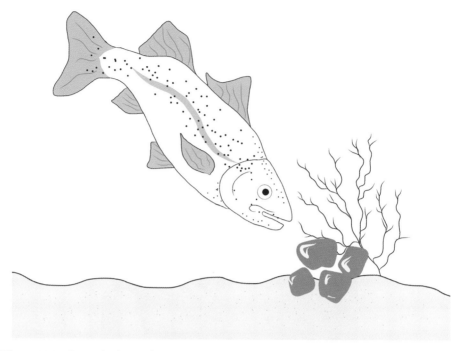

Figure 34.2 Given the limited motor activities possible, fish can display complex behaviours.

digging, eating, and so on. Rather, the intelligence lies in the circumstances in which these simple motor acts are called upon.

Fish. With the exception of those species that use electric currents in the water to navigate and detect prey, fish have notably small brains in proportion to their body size. Nevertheless, all fish contain a region within the (small) forebrain that, through its structure, fibre connections, and histochemistry, appears to correspond to the hippocampus of land vertebrates.[2] Though the observed behaviours of fish all depend on swimming or feeding, some are indicative of impressive memories. In the natural world, as opposed to the laboratory, one of the best examples is the spawning salmon. As young fish, the salmon are exposed to the odours of the stream in which they live. They then swim out to sea and after several years return to the stream of their youth in order to spawn. Evidently a unique pattern of smells was learned during their youth that provided the guidance necessary for the return. This extraordinary ability was explored by Arthur Hasler at the University of Wisconsin, who showed that it is lost if the noses of the young fish are plugged. In contrast, adding an artificial chemical to a stream causes fish to return to that same stream rather than to another nearby.

Evidence of a different kind of memory in fish has been provided by Charles Eriksen, another professor in the American Midwest. Eriksen observed that the catfish in the pond at his farm would swim to the surface whenever he called to them before feeding them pellets. After a lapse of five years, Eriksen once again called 'Fish-fish' and the auditory memories in the surviving catfish prompted their immediate reappearance.[3]

Another example of intelligent behaviour has been observed in Malaysian mudskippers, a fish found in estuaries. When the tide goes out the mudskippers retreat into burrows; consisting of a vertical shaft leading into a horizontal one, each mud burrow also contains an air chamber that enables the fish to breathe while waiting for the next tide; the chamber is filled beforehand by releasing air gulped at the surface.[4]

Laboratory examples of intelligent behaviour in fish include their ability to acquire food rewards by solving mazes, recognizing colours and shapes, or by pressing a lever. Impressive, and rather surprising, behaviours in the wild include the ability of fish to recognize individuals, to learn by observing other fish, to hunt together and to establish mutually beneficial working partnerships with other fish (as when 'cleaner fish' remove parasites from larger, 'client fish').[5]

Amphibians. The amphibian brain is of particular interest because of the relatively small size and poor development of its pallium. Also, as Charles Herrick pointed out, the little pallial tissue present is only innervated by fibres from the olfactory bulb, there being no contribution from the eye or ear. In contrast, the limbic system, represented by the hippocampus (with fornix and commissure) is substantial and, in addition to fibres from the olfactory bulb, receives visual and somatosensory inputs via the thalamus. These features suggest that, compared with those of reptiles, the amphibian brain is the product of an earlier stage of evolution. Is it capable of generating intelligent behaviour?

A number of field observations suggest 'yes'. In the first place, it is well known that a frog or toad can find its way back to a favourable location, and can do so even if moved a considerable distance.[6] In addition to having a good spatial memory, frogs may exhibit evidence of planning, as in the case of giant bullfrogs studied in South Africa. In anticipation of mating the large male bullfrogs first make depressions in the ground that, after rain, become shallow puddles. Using their strong hindlegs the males then dig narrow channels from the puddles to a large pond nearby. Mating takes place in the

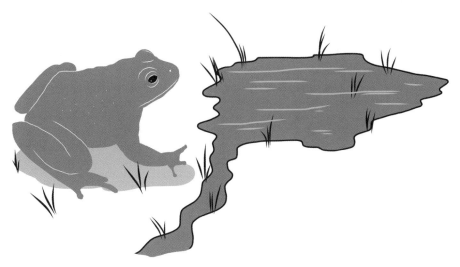

Figure 34.3 Frog with excavated puddle and channel (see text).

puddles, into which the eggs are deposited; the newly dug channels, with their communication to the pond, ensure that the water temperature in the puddle never rises so
high during daylight as to kill the eggs. After hatching, the tadpoles use the channels to
swim to the pond.[7] Other species of male frog, faced with a similar rearing problem, are
known to carry tadpoles to water in their mouths. Finally, the courtship behaviour of
some frog species may be elaborate, involving an hour-long sequence of physical and
distant interactions before mating occurs.[8]

Reptiles. The reptilian brain, like the brains of birds, fishes, and amphibians, also
contains a hippocampal structure, though one that differs from the amphibian version in being layered. While, for obvious reasons, snakes and crocodiles are not well
suited for cognitive experiments, tortoises have recently emerged as suitable candidates, largely through the work of Anna Wilkinson at the University of Lincoln (United
Kingdom). Wilkinson first demonstrated navigational ability and memory in her
own pet tortoise after challenging it with a radial maze.[9] Then, in collaboration with
Austrian researchers, she showed that tortoises were capable of learning how to operate
a computer touch screen for food and to apply their new knowledge to a field situation
with real objects (Figure 34.4).[10]

Learning of a different kind, an 'imprinting', is that of sea turtles. No less remarkable
for having been long known, the turtles return to lay eggs in the same beach where
they hatched, or in one close by, despite having been absent for a quarter of a century.
Various observations indicate that this achievement results from imprinting the local
coordinates of the Earth's magnetic field at the time of hatching.[11] Finally, further evidence of cognitive ability is the apparent appreciation of certain objects as playthings,
a behaviour observed not only in turtles and other reptiles, but in fish, amphibians,
and birds.

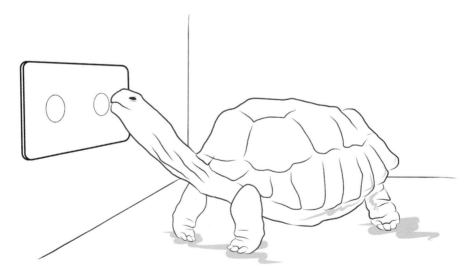

Figure 34.4 Tortoise participating in choice task.

Notes

1. A.J. McComas, *Sherrington's Loom. An Introduction to the Science of Consciousness* (New York, NY: Oxford University Press, 2019).

2. V.P. Bingman, F. Rodriguez, and C. Salas, 'The Hippocampus of Nonmammalian Vertebrates' in J. Kaas (ed.), *Evolution of Nervous Systems*, 2nd edn, vol 1 (Oxford: Elsevier, 2017), 479–89..

3. Stéphan Reebs, at the Université de Moncton, has documented these and other examples of fish memory. See: S.G. Reebs, 'Long-term memory in fishes' <http://www.howfishbehave.ca> accessed 24 April 2022.

4. A. Ishimatsu, Y. Hishada, T. Takita, T. Kanda, S. Oikawa, T. Takeda, and K.K. Huat, 'Mudskippers Store Air in Their Burrows' (1998) 391 *Nature* 237–8.

5. R. Bashary, W. Wickler, and H. Fricke, 'Fish Cognition: A Primate's Eye' (2002) 5 *Animal Cognition* 5:1–13.

6. When I lived in the country I would find a large toad lurking in shadows at the back of my house during the summer nights; during the day, however, it was never to be seen. See also: A. Pašukonis, I. Warrington, M. Ringler, and W. Hödl, 'Poison Frogs Rely on Experience to Find the Way Home in the Rainforest' (2014) 10 *Biology Letters* 20140642. <http://dx.org/10.1098/rsbl.2014.0642> accessed 24 April 2022.

7. C.L. Cook, J.W.H. Ferguson, and S.R. Telford, 'Adaptive Male Parental Care in the Giant Bullfrog Pyxicephalus adspersus' (2001) 35(2) *Journal of Herpetology* 310–15.

8. P.A. Silverstone, 'Observations on the Behavior and Ecology of a Colombian Poison-Arrow Frog, the Kõkoé-Pá (Dendrobates histrionicus berthold)' (1973) 29(4) *Herpetologica* 295–301.

9. A. Wilkinson, H.M. Chan, and G. Hall, 'A Study of Spatial Learning and Memory in the Tortoise (Geochelone Carbonaria)' (2007) 12 *Animal Cognition* 779–87.

10. J. Mueller-Paul, A. Wilkinson, U. Aust, M. Steurer, G. Hall, and L. Huber, 'Touchscreen Performance and Knowledge Transfer in the Red-Footed Tortoise (Geochelone carbonaria)' (2014) 106 *Behavioural Processes* 187–92.

11. J.R. Brothers and K.J. Lohmann, 'Evidence for Geomagnetic Imprinting and Magnetic Navigation in the Natal Homing of Sea Turtles' (2015) 25 *Current Biology* 392–6. Note: Exactly how the magnetic signal is stored and accessed, and whether or not the hippocampus is involved, is not known at present.

35

Additional Evidence against the Cerebral Cortex as Alternative

Notwithstanding the observations on various animal species in the previous chapter, it is difficult, given the proportions of a human brain, to avoid attributing consciousness to a function of its largest part—the lobes of the cerebral cortex, and of the frontal lobe in particular. After all, was it not this enlargement that, in the course of evolution, came to distinguish the brains of humans from those of other primates and 'lower' mammals? That was evidently the view of Francis Walshe in his forceful dismissal of Wilder Penfield's claim for a 'centrencephalic centre' in the brain stem.[1] But Walshe did not offer an alternative explanation for some of the clinical observations that Penfield, a curious and innovative neurosurgeon, had been able to make. One of them, and a very powerful one at that, was that a large amount of prefrontal cortex could be removed in the operating theatre without affecting consciousness and with little change in subsequent behaviour. It was a discovery Penfield had made after resecting his sister's glioma, a surgery he had been obliged to undertake soon after his move to Montreal. And then, long before Penfield, there had been the extraordinary case of the tamping rod driven through the front of Phineas Gage's brain, completely destroying the left prefrontal lobe.[2] Finally, there is the fact that, though thousands of psychiatric patients had undergone prefrontal leucotomies when that procedure had been in vogue,[3] they had not exhibited any dimming of consciousness either. It is difficult to account for these negative observations other than by proposing that, in the course of evolution, a genetic mutation suddenly gave the hominids bigger brains, parts of which (the prefrontal lobes) have yet to be fully exploited.

The following sections explore other evidence that the cerebral cortex may play a secondary, adjunctive, role to the limbic system in consciousness.

(a) **'Voluntary' movements.** In the morning of 12 April 1972, a sixty-two-year-old Norwegian professor turned over in bed, became dizzy, began to see double, and developed weakness on the left side of his body.

Alf Brodal (Figure 35.1), the neuroanatomist and a former mentor of Per Andersen, had just suffered a stroke. After being flown back to Oslo from Portugal, where he had been travelling, Brodal had been investigated and found to have partial blockage of the right internal carotid artery in the neck. Most likely a piece of the blockage had broken off and the resulting embolus had come to lodge in a branch of the middle cerebral artery supplying the internal capsule—the thick fan of nerve fibres connecting the

Aranzio's Seahorse and the Search for Memory and Consciousness. Alan J. McComas, Oxford University Press.
© Oxford University Press 2023. DOI: 10.1093/oso/9780192868244.003.0037

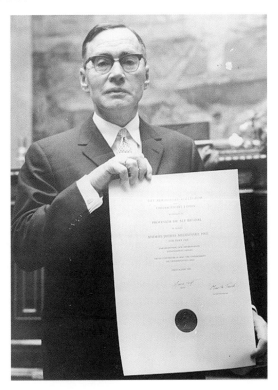

Figure 35.1 Alf Brodal, receiving an award in 1966. (Author unknown. Wikimedia Commons file: Alf Brodal OB.F13322b.jpg. Creative Commons Attribution-Share Alike 4.0 international license.)

cortex to the brain stem and spinal cord. The embolus had evidently occluded the blood supply to the fibres from the motor cortex. At least that was Brodal's diagnosis, and who could argue with the author of *Neurological Anatomy in Relation to Clinical Medicine*?[4]

Brodal did more than simply make a diagnosis. He kept a careful record of his symptoms over the following year, both before and after undergoing surgery on the partially blocked internal carotid artery, and reported his own case in *Brain*.[5] One of his observations was that the effort—the mental 'energy'—required to move the weakened left arm or leg was greatly increased, such that he would soon tire. Though Brodal's embolus had originally affected only nerve fibres, the cell bodies in the motor cortex from which they arose would have undergone retrograde degeneration. Further, direct damage to the motor cortex by tumour or a penetrating wound, would, in other patients, produce a similar situation to Brodal's—weakness despite the presence of a strong 'will' to move.

That the command for a voluntary movement originated outside the motor cortex was a conclusion that Penfield had reached, though for a different reason. In one of his patients he had been obliged to sever the fibres reaching the motor area from other regions of the cortex; despite the loss of cortical input, the patient had had little impairment of movement. The preservation of function, Penfield argued, implied that the voluntary act began in a deeper part of the brain, the fibres of which had remained intact in his patient.[6]

Konorski, the proposer of 'gnostic' units in sensory systems, speculated that movements began with a special type of unit, one that he termed 'kinesthetic'. These units had been formed by patterns of sensory input from muscle and joint receptors during passive or reflex movements, but ultimately became capable of initiating movement themselves.[7] It was a bold idea and consistent with the later finding of some unusual neurons in the parietal lobe. These were cells that responded to the combination of a certain direction of the head and position of the arm, for example. Further, in monkeys such cells began discharging before those in the motor cortex, suggestive of their having a primary role.[8] Other evidence of parietal involvement in producing movement was that stimulation of the lobe during surgery would cause a conscious patient to feel that a movement was taking place, even though it was not. In contrast stimulation of the motor cortex produced a movement but without any accompanying sensation.[9]

There is something appealing in the idea of gnostic units being created for particular movements, or series of movements. Such a mechanism would have explained Brodal's difficulty in tying a bow tie after his stroke; it was something he had been doing almost daily for 40 years. Referring to himself in the third person, Brodal would write:

> Under normal circumstances the necessary numerous small delicate movements had followed each other automatically, and the act of tying when first started had proceeded without much conscious attention. Subjectively the patient felt as if he had to stop because 'his fingers did not know the next move.' He had the same feeling as when one recites a poem or sings a song and gets lost. The only way is to start from the beginning. It was felt as if the delay in the succession of movements (due to pareses and spasticity) interrupted a chain of more or less automatic movements. Consciously directing attention to the finger movements did not improve the performance; on the contrary it made it quite impossible.

Brodal went on to cite the Swedish neurophysiologist and Nobel Laureate, Ragnar Granit:

> Even those movements which we regard as voluntary are largely automatic. Most of them intrude upon consciousness only at the moment when they are triggered off into action.

Or, as in the case of Alf Brodal, when they can no longer be performed properly.

But do the kinesthetic gnostic units (most likely situated in the parietal lobe) actually initiate a movement? Do they supply the necessary 'will'? Indeed, is there really such a phenomenon as 'will' which, in its purest form, would be an action or thought independent of our immediate circumstances?

Elsewhere it has been proposed that our 'voluntary' movements are usually triggered by something we are presently looking at, or have just seen, or are now imagining.[10] Though this is the usual case, and a reflection of the large amount of human brain devoted to vision, 'voluntary' movements could also follow an auditory cue (an unexpected noise or something said by another person), a touch (someone's hand on our shoulder), or a smell (an appetizing aroma from the kitchen). We regard our movements as voluntary because we are conscious at the time they are made and they are more complex than a simple reflex. However, in a famous experiment, Benjamin Libet was able to show that task-related electrical activity in the brain precedes any awareness of a 'desire' to move.[11]

In accepting that 'voluntary' movements are usually, if not always, triggered by something experienced at the moment or else imagined, there are reasons for thinking that subcortical activity may precede involvement of the parietal lobe (and motor cortex). Thus, although tying a bow tie or rapidly playing a complex run on the piano require practice and skill, many 'voluntary' acts do not. We may be conscious of walking on the sidewalk or of chewing a piece of chicken during a meal, but neurophysiological experiments have shown that these repetitive motor activities, walking and chewing (as well as breathing), are automatically programmed in the spinal cord and brainstem. That is, there are neural circuits ('central pattern generators'), formed in the foetus as part of a genetic blueprint, that simply need to be switched on. On receipt of a 'start' signal from a higher level, the synaptic connections between interneurons and motoneurons ensure that alternating movements will start and continue until a 'stop' signal appears. There is no need for commands from the brain to move first the left leg, then the right leg, then the left again and so on (or, in chewing, to open the jaw, close it, open it again, and so on).

The existence of circuits in the brain stem and spinal cord for repetitive movements was an inference from the pioneering experiments of Jean Pierre Flourens in the early 19th century. Flourens (1794–1867; Figure 35.2), born near the historic southern French city of Béziers, studied medicine at Montpellier and then moved to Paris where he became interested in physiology.[12] Still only 21, he began experiments of his own devising, studying the effects on behaviour of removing parts of the brains of animals and birds. Flourens observed that pigeons that had undergone ablation of the pallium (the avian analogue of the mammalian cortex) were still able to fly when tossed in the air and to swallow when food was placed in the mouth.[13] These very original experiments, ones that had involved considerable dexterity, indicated that the cortex (or, rather, the pallium) was not essential for executing certain repetitive movements—a deduction that preceded the discovery of central pattern generators in the spinal cord and brain stem.

However, when it comes to Brodal's bow tie and musical performance, the cortex certainly *is* involved—as is the cerebellum, the repository of procedural memories. Indeed, it was the evolution of the cerebral cortex that made these and other skilled manoeuvres possible. The importance of the cortical contribution is reflected in the large size of the pyramidal tract, the fibres of which leave the cortex, pass through the

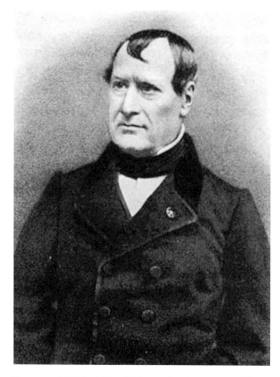

Figure 35.2 Pierre Flourens (1794–1867; Wikimedia Commons file: Pierre Flourens.jpeg).

internal capsule (site of Brodal's lesion), occupy the front of the lower brain stem and proceed down the spinal cord to summon interneurons and motoneurons into action. Just as the evolution of the occipital, parietal and temporal lobes enabled ever more detailed analysis of the external world, so the motor cortex permitted ever more complex movements of the hands. However, for the reasons given above, the neural command to start these complex movements, like the command for automatic movements, evidently arises outside the cortex.

Could the hippocampus be the initiator of the movements we refer to as 'voluntary'? On theoretical grounds, there is certainly a case for this, given that such movements naturally follow a sensory input (something just seen or heard, for example), or something remembered, or a future action that we appear to have imagined. All three instances are the concern of the hippocampus, given that the structure is involved in the interpretation of a new sensory input, retrieves memories, and provides the information required for an imagined movement. The converse of these situations is the absence of movement, as on the occasions when a rabbit will pause while nibbling grass and remain motionless for a minute or more. Or perhaps in a nursing home where an elderly patient, seated in a wheelchair, may continue to stare ahead seemingly oblivious of what may be happening around him or her. Is it possible that in both situations, the hippocampus has formed a spatial map that lingers—and thereby fails to produce a 'trigger' (impulse signal) for movement?

This is theory, however. To strengthen the case for the hippocampus as the initiator of 'voluntary' movements requires physical evidence, an obvious source being the presence of electrical activity consistently associated with movements. Perhaps the most thorough studies in this area have been those of Cornelius ('Case') Vanderwolf (Figure 35.3), another graduate of the McGill Psychology Department prior to his faculty appointment at Western University in London, Ontario. With wire electrodes implanted in the hippocampi of rats, Vanderwolf studied the interaction of rats with their surroundings just as John O'Keefe would do at University College in London, England. Vanderwolf was able to recognize three types of electrical discharge in the hippocampus related to movement, the most striking being repetitive slow waves with a frequency of 6–12 Hz.[14] These waves could appear several seconds before a movement, gradually increasing in their frequency until the moment of action. The type of movement did not seem to matter—the rhythm would appear before whole body activities such as walking, running, jumping, and struggling as well as before the pressing of a lever or the manipulation of a food pellet. Further, the amplitude of the rhythmic electric activity was found to correlate with the size and extent of the movements, and, once established, the rhythm would continue until movement ceased. John O'Keefe and other workers had also observed the same EEG activity, referring to it, somewhat confusingly, as the hippocampal 'theta' rhythm.[15]

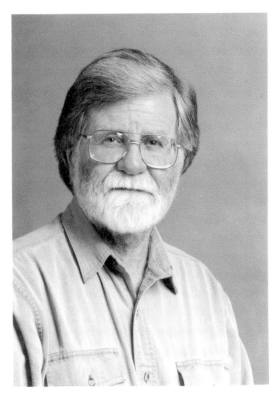

Figure 35.3 Cornelius (Case) Vanderwolf. Photo kindly supplied by György Buzsáki.

An obvious question regarding the possible role of the hippocampus is whether Clive Wearing, following the destruction of this structure on both sides by viral infection, was capable of voluntary movements. The answer is inconclusive. The former musicologist's periods of consciousness were so brief that, prompted by the solitary memory of Deborah, his wife and self-trained therapist, he barely had time to seize a pen or pencil and write a short statement (e.g. '3.14 p.m. AWAKE FIRST TIME' immediately followed by '3.15 p.m. FIRST REAL AWAKENESS DARLING, FIRST CARDS SEEN, PATIENCE').[16] In contrast, more automatic actions—walking, eating, sitting, standing, manipulating a knife and fork, holding a pen—were little, if at all, affected.

More instructive, perhaps, are the patients with psychomotor epilepsy, considered earlier.[17] During a 'dreamy state' the person may perform complex movements, or sequences of movements, that would normally be regarded as 'voluntary.' A striking example was the physician patient studied by Hughlings Jackson who, in one episode, was able to take a history, perform a physical examination, and then write a prescription for one of his patients—all without any awareness of his actions at the time. Related observations come from 'split brain' experiments, which have shown that the dominant left cortex can improvise an explanation for otherwise puzzling actions undertaken by the right hemisphere.[18] Both types of observation suggest that the brain normally initiates and supervises movements and that the impression of 'voluntariness' is something that is added on, an illusion.

If the hippocampus does initiate movement, as Cornelius Vanderwolf believed, the circuits have yet to be identified, though several possibilities exist. Most likely the circuits depend on the nature of the movement, being different for basic repetitive activities that employ a neural central pattern generator (walking, chewing, etc.) as opposed to skilled manipulations, such as those involved in constructing or repairing an object or learning to play a musical instrument.[19]

Related to bodily movement are the movements associated with speech—not only those of the vocal cords but those of the lips, tongue, jaws, and chest. We express many, though not all, of our thoughts in speech, and if the hippocampus is responsible is responsible for thought, then there must be strong neural connections to speech cortex. Indeed, the interruption of these fibres was the mostly likely explanation for the torrent of nonsense that Clive Wearing would speak during the early days of his illness. Deborah, his wife, recounts Clive talking to a taxi driver: 'in the most imperfect way, the chickens are all you would think, possibly in the local systems these are effortlessly mine, you see. It's peculiar, isn't it?' and so on.[20] To a neurologist or speech pathologist, Clive's speech problem was a perfect example of Wernicke's aphasia, a condition in which damage to the posterior part of the superior temporal gyrus ('Wernicke's area') results in speech that is fluent but abnormal in content and in the use of words. The distance between the hippocampus and Wernicke's area is relatively short, at least in comparison with other regions of the ipsilateral cerebral hemisphere and the fibre connections between the two are well developed.

Presumably it is the loss of input from the hippocampal 'concept' cells that is responsible for the aphasia, since these are the neurons that associate names with objects, places, and persons—as shown by the electrode recordings in epileptic patients studied by Itzhak Fried and his colleagues in Los Angeles.[21]

(b) **Sensory deprivation**. Migraine. Putting the situation for speech to one side, what is the relation of other cortical areas to consciousness? Again, it is convenient to begin with Penfield who, while proposing the existence of a subcortical site where information was brought together, envisioned the site operating in conjunction with the cortical areas. This is borne out by clinical observation. If, for example, a haemorrhage destroys nerve cells and fibres in the occipital lobe, there is blindness in the opposite visual field. Similarly touch sensation is affected on the opposite side of the body to a lesion affecting the parietal lobe. Consciousness of what is seen, heard, and touched depends on the normal functioning of the respective cortical receiving and processing areas. Further back in time, the very development of 'self' in an infant must have been a consequence of the information gained through its special senses and fledgling motor system—what was seen and heard, the turning of the head to see and hear more, the touching of surfaces and the grasping of objects, the bringing of things to the mouth for examination, the taste of food, and so on.

Suppose an older child or adult were to be deprived of the different senses, however—would there still be consciousness? In practice, it is impossible to get rid of all sensation, since there is always information arriving in the brain from mechanoreceptors in the stomach, intestines, heart, chest wall, nose, and throat that we can become aware of. However, it is not difficult to remove all the sensory information coming from *outside* the body. We could, for example, lie on a very soft mattress wearing frosted goggles to prevent the seeing of shapes, ear plugs to supply white noise, and gloves to interfere with touch; tubes over the arms would reduce movements and attendant sensations. Sensory deprivation experiments of this kind were carried out in the psychology department at McGill during the early years of Donald Hebb's tenure as Head. The subjects, mostly university students, remained conscious in between periods of sleep, though their unstimulated brains conjured up various forms of hallucination.[22] There is also the case of Helen Keller (1880–1968). Totally blind and deaf from infancy, this extraordinary woman not only mastered Braille but led a very active intellectual and political life that included writing and lecturing. The conclusion from these various observations is that the brain remains capable of generating consciousness in the absence, or near absence, of information from the outside world.

But what about the contribution of sensory information from *inside* the body—might this be sufficient to produce consciousness? The British neurologist, Sir Henry Head (1861–1940), argued that the brain maintains a 'schema' or map of the body with information provided by the various sensory pathways, especially those from joints and muscles.[23] In this way there is knowledge of the existence and the relative positions of our various body parts even though we are not consciously attending to them. As an example, my brain 'knows' that, while sitting at my desk, my right foot is drawn back under my chair and that I am leaning forward towards my laptop; my brain also contains a neural representation of the way my body parts are related to each other. This 'schema' is not something I am normally aware of, and I certainly don't have to consult it before I change my position, but it exists nevertheless.

Observations from the neurology clinic suggest that the body schema is housed in the temporoparietal cortex. Thus, a patient with a tumour or stroke affecting this area in the right hemisphere becomes unaware of the left side of her body, even if there is some injury, disease or weakness on that side. This hemispatial neglect ('*agnosia*') may extend to the surroundings on the left side—the furniture and any other occupants of the room or, if outside, the buildings, traffic, and sidewalks.[24]

I had previously imagined that impulse activity in these cortical areas, one on each side of the brain, was the likely basis for consciousness but an unusual situation caused me to change my mind. A close relative developed a very severe form of familial migraine. It had begun in her 20s with sudden attacks of headache, dizziness, photophobia, nausea, and vomiting. As the years passed, the attacks became associated with severe pains in other parts of the body.[25] Later still, the episodes would be complicated by transient hemiplegia and then, in still later attacks, by quadriplegia and loss of consciousness. There had also been distorted perceptions of the body, a symptom known to occur in some patients with migraine and attributed to hyperactivity in the temporoparietal area. When this would happen, she would call out in anguish that her legs might be twisted backwards, or her fingers and thumbs shortened, for example.[26] However, there was one occasion when the illusion had been the progressive loss of her entire body. Exclaiming 'All of me is gone!', she had then fallen unconscious. The logical conclusion from this unusual illusion was that the body schema, and the region of temporoparietal cortex responsible for its creation, was not essential for consciousness.

(c) **Children** with cortical **agenesis.** There is another line of evidence that at least some form of consciousness can exist without involvement of the cerebral cortex, and this comes from the study of children born with hydranencephaly. In this unfortunate condition the cerebral hemispheres either fail to develop or are destroyed in the foetus by a stroke or viral infection. A diagnosis can be readily made by the ability to shine a light through the head, cerebrospinal fluid having replaced the missing brain tissue. In his book *Self Comes to Mind*, Antonio Damasio describes these children:

[T]hey move their heads and eyes freely, they have expressions of emotion in their faces, they can smile at stimuli that one would expect a normal child to smile to— a toy, a certain sound—and they even laugh and express normal joy when they are tickled … they tend to be fearful of strangers and appear happiest near their habitual mother/caregiver. Likes and dislikes are apparent, none so striking as in examples of music....

And goes on to write: 'That these children give some evidence of mind process is not in doubt.'[27]

Damasio uses these striking observations as evidence for the presence of a primordial consciousness elsewhere than in the cortex, selecting the upper brain stem, and specifically the nuclei of the midbrain, as the likeliest site. As to be expected of the author, the case is well argued but it omits the possibility of neural structures at a rather higher level also being involved. The omission is important since autopsy reports on previously affected children have sometimes mentioned preservation of the thalami, basal ganglia, and diencephalon, as well as the cerebellum.[28] As Damasio states, the hypothalamus must have been left, but the fact that a child could remember his or her mother, or a certain toy, and show fear in the presence of an unfamiliar person, and at times exhibit absence seizures, all suggest that there was some residual function in the hippocampus and amygdala also.

(d) **Cortical structure and 'time-chunking'.** The last piece of evidence against a cortical generator for consciousness comes from the structure and operating mechanism of the cortex itself. As noted previously, in the hippocampus the pyramidal cells are concentrated in a single layer. In the neocortex, by contrast, the pyramidal cell bodies, together with the axons and dendrites, form columns perpendicular to the surface of the brain. That a cortical column is the fundamental functional unit of the sensory receiving areas is shown by the similar properties of its cells. In the somatosensory cortex, for example, the cells in a column are responsive to touching the same small area of skin on the body or head;[29] in the primary visual cortex it is the orientation of a linear slit of light or shade falling on the same part of the retina that binds the cells of a column together.[30] Within a single column the deepest pyramidal cells appear to control the more superficial cells, partly through recurrent axon branches and partly by exciting inhibitory neurons. In addition to receiving inputs from neurons at an earlier point in a sensory pathway, the cells in a cortical column are excited by feedback from later points and from the temporal lobe in particular. The combination of the columnar structure and the feedback causes the sensory cortical areas to operate in 'chunks' of time, each chunk lasting some 50–100 milliseconds (ms). Evidence that this is so comes from backward masking experiments.

Discovered in the mid-19th century by the German psychologist Sigmund Exner, 'backward masking' is the suppression of an evoked sensation by a later, stronger stimulus.[31] The phenomenon is a property of the main sensory systems (it would be difficult to test for smell and taste). Thus a bright flash of light will prevent recognition of a fainter flash, a loud tone will obscure a softer one, a forceful touch (or electric shock) on the skin will hide a lighter one. An especially dramatic illustration of the phenomenon comes from the use of coloured lights—a red flash quickly followed by a green flash produces neither the sensation or red or green but that of yellow.[32]

Since the longest permissible interval between the weak and strong stimuli in these experiments is 50–100 ms, it follows that the sensory cortex operates in time-chunks of this duration. One might then argue that, if sensory consciousness depended solely on the cortex, it would be intermittent—100 ms of nothing, then sensation, then another 100 ms of nothing, and so on. Pursuing the argument, somewhere in the brain there must be a part that integrates the intermittent information coming from the cortex so as to give the illusion of continuity. The hippocampus, with its non-columnar neural structure and its lingering excitation, is equipped to do this.

This line of thought is consistent with the thesis put forward earlier and to be discussed next, that the various sensory systems evolved because they provided better guidance for movements used for feeding, mating, and escaping predators. In mammals the development of a large cerebral cortex packed with cortical columns made possible the creation of huge numbers of 'gnostic units' coding for increasingly discriminative features of the environment (the principle that Jerzy Konorski, Horace Barlow, and Jerry Lettvin had postulated 50 years ago). Movements became ever more skilled and successful.

Notes

1. See Chapter 5.
2. See Chapter 4.
3. See Chapter 4.
4. A. Brodal, *Neurological Anatomy in Relation to Clinical Medicine*, 3rd edn (New York, NY: Oxford University Press, 1981) (the first edition was published in 1948 by the Clarendon Press, Oxford).
5. A. Brodal, 'Self-Observations and Neuro-Anatomical Considerations after a Stroke' (1973) 96(4) *Brain* 675–94.
6. W. Penfield, 'Mechanisms of Voluntary Movement' (1954) 77 *Brain* 1–17.
7. J. Konorski, *The Integrative Activity of the Brain: An Interdisciplinary Approach* (Chicago, IL: Chicago University Press, 1967).
8. V. Mountcastle, 'Brain Mechanisms for Directed Attention' (1978) 71 *Journal of the Royal Society of Medicine* 14–28.
9. M. Demurget, K.T. Reilly, N. Richard, A. Szathmari, C. Mottolese, and A. Sirigu, 'Movement Intention after Parietal Cortex Stimulation in Humans' (2009) 324 *Science* 811–13.
10. See Chapter 12 in A.J. McComas, *Sherrington's Loom. An Introduction to the Science of Consciousness* (New York, NY: Oxford University Press, 2019).
11. B. Libet, C.A. Gleason, E.W. Wright, and D.K. Pearl, 'Time of Conscious Intention to Act in Relation to Onset of Cerebral Activity (Readiness Potential). The Unconscious Initiation of a Freely Voluntary Act' (1983) 106 *Brain* 623–42. See Chapter 45 for a description of the experiment.
12. <en.wikipedia.org/wiki/Jean_Pierre_Flourens> accessed 24 April 2022.
13. For an account of early physiological studies on motor representation in the brain, see: F. Fritsch and E. Hitzig, 'Ueber die elektrische Erregbarkeit des Grosshirns' (1870) 37 *Archiv für Anatomie, Physiologie und Wissenschaftliche medezin* 300–32 translated by R.H. Wilkins, 'Neurosurgical Classic—XII' (1963) 20 *Journal of Neurosurgery* 904–16.
14. C.H. Vanderwolf, 'Limbic-Diencephalic Mechanisms of Voluntary Movement' (1971) 78 *Psychology Review* 83–113.

15. <http://www.nobelprize.org/uploads/2018/06/okeefe-lectures.pdf> accessed 24 April 2022. In clinical EEG, the theta frequency is 4–7.5 Hz, and it would have been more appropriate to describe the hippocampal rhythm as 'alpha' (7.5–13 Hz).

16. See Chapter 20.

17. See Chapter 33(b).

18. M.S. Gazzinaga, 'Cerebral Specialization and Interhemispheric Communication: Does the Corpus Callosum Enable the Human Condition?' (2000) 123 *Brain* 1293–326.

19. As noted earlier, central pattern generators are neural circuits in the brain stem and spinal cord responsible for continued alternating motor activity as in breathing, chewing, walking, and running in humans and other vertebrates. Similar circuits are found in insects and invertebrates for other activities such as flying and swimming. Although the circuitry runs by itself, it may require stop and start signals from the brain and may also be modified by incoming sensory information.

    The strong projection from the basal and lateral amygdaloid nuclei to the brainstem nuclei and from there to the spinal cord via the reticulospinal pathway would provide a possible route for activating central pattern generators. However, Vanderwolf has suggested other neural routes for initiating movements, such as one via the mammillary bodies to the pontine nuclei and cerebellum, one via the medial frontal cortex, and one via the nucleus accumbens. In contrast, relatively skilful movements, such as a rat's manipulation of a food pellet or the fingering of a musical instrument by a human (or removing a splinter from a finger, fitting parts together in a puzzle, etc.) would presumably depend on (multisynaptic) connections between the hippocampus and the motor cortex together with continuing information from vision, touch, and joint receptors.

20. See Chapter 20.

21. See Chapter 24.

22. W. Heron, 'The Pathology of Boredom' (1957) 196(1) *Scientific American* 52–6. Note that these experiments were performed on subjects who had previously been in full possession of their sensory mechanisms and therefore had a sense of self, including memory, to draw upon. This caveat would also have applied to Helen Keller, who had had vision and hearing in early childhood before the illness that destroyed them.

    In contrast, we can never know the degree of consciousness achievable in a human being congenitally deprived of sight, hearing, taste, smell, and touch.

23. H. Head, *Studies in Neurology*, Vols 1 and 2 (London: Henry Frowde, 1920).

24. E. Bisiach and C. Luzzati, 'Unilateral Neglect of Representational Space' (1978) 14 *Cortex* 129–33.

25. A. McComas and A. Upton, 'Therapeutic Transcranial Magnetic Stimulation in Migraine and its Implications for a Neuroinflammatory Hypothesis' (2009) 17 *Inflammopharmacology* 68–75.

26. A.J. McComas, *Sherrington's Loom. An Introduction to the Science of Consciousness* (New York, NY: Oxford University Press, 2019), 88–9..

27. A. Damasio, *Self Comes to Mind. Constructing the Conscious Brain.* (New York, NY: Random House, 2010).

28. N. McAbee, A. Chan, and E.L. Erde, 'Prolonged Survival with Hydranencephaly: Report of Two Patients and Literature Review' (2000) 23(1) *Pediatric Neurology* 80–4.

29. T.P. Powell and V.B. Mountcastle, 'Some Aspects of the Functional Organization of the Cortex of the Postcentral Gyrus of the Monkey: A Correlation of Findings Obtained in a Single Unit Analysis with Cytoarchitecture' (1959) 105 *Bulletin of the Johns Hopkins Hospital* 133–62.

30. D.H. Hubel and T.N. Wiesel, 'Receptive Fields and Functional Architecture of Monkey Striate Cortex' (1968) 195 *Journal of Physiology* 215–43.

31. S. Macknik and S. Martinez-Conde, 'The Role of Feedback in Visual Masking and Visual Processing' (2007) 3(1,2) *Advances in Cognitive Psychology* 125–52.

32. R. Efron, 'The Duration of the Present' (1967) 138 *Annals of the New York Academy of Sciences* 713–29.

C.

SHORT-TERM MEMORY AS THE MECHANISM OF CONSCIOUSNESS

36

The Evolutionary Argument

We have now come to the crux of the matter, the nature of consciousness. But if the identification of the hippocampal complex as the location of consciousness is correct then the problem is already half solved—since the hippocampus is concerned with memory it is therefore likely that consciousness is a function of memory. There are two strong arguments that help to make the case, however, and the first is an evolutionary one that can be summarized as follows:

(1) In order for an animal species to survive, its members must be able to feed, mate, and escape danger.
(2) Feeding, mating, and escaping require movement.
(3) In multicellular creatures, nerve and muscle cells evolved to produce such movements.
(4) For the simplest multicellular creatures, reflex movements in response to environmental cues were adequate.
(5) In more advanced creatures the evolution of sensory receptors, initially chemoreceptors and then photoreceptors and mechanoreceptors, enabled movements to be guided.
(6) However, guided movements were only advantageous if the targets were appropriate.
(7) The evolution of primal 'pleasure' on acquiring a target (i.e. food, fluid, sex) indicated the target's suitability for future occasions. Likewise primal 'pain' identified an object or act to be avoided.
(8) However, a primal sensation only had evolutionary value if a record (memory) was created of its association with a particular target.

The above statements are logical and consistent with what is known of evolution whereas the next statements are supposition, namely:

(9) When a neural system acquired memory it automatically achieved awareness (consciousness). **Consciousness is a property of memory**.
(10) Memory, and consciousness with it, evolved gradually.

The word 'property', though the best that can be found at this moment, nonetheless falls short of what is intended. While consciousness is envisaged as a property of memory, it is the 'coming alive', the 'realization' of memory, that makes consciousness happen.

Aranzio's Seahorse and the Search for Memory and Consciousness. Alan J. McComas, Oxford University Press.
© Oxford University Press 2023. DOI: 10.1093/oso/9780192868244.003.0038

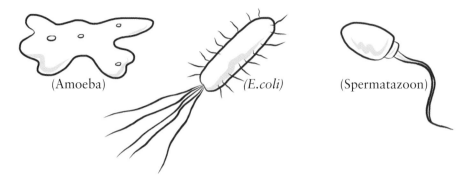

(Amoeba)   (E.coli)   (Spermatazoon)

Figure 36.1 Amoeba, *E. coli*, spermatozoon—three single cell organisms capable of directed self-propulsion.

For philosophical reasons it is important to add that not all 'memory' in the universe is considered to have the potential for 'consciousness'. If consciousness was simply the unveiling of stored information, a potential for consciousness could be attributed to CDs, DVDs, and memory sticks as well as to such natural phenomena as tree rings and glacial deposits. The analysis of a series of tree rings, for example, provides information not only about the age of a tree but also the climatic conditions that prevailed during the life of that tree. Rather, in the present view, consciousness is restricted to living biological organisms with neurons; the impulse activity of the neurons has enabled them to acquire, store, and replay information about their environments and themselves.

The memory-generated concept of consciousness can now be considered in more detail.

In order for an animal species to survive, its members must be able to feed, mate, and avoid danger. Each of these functions requires movement and the effectiveness of the movement depends on appropriate guidance.

Even unicellular organisms need movement (Figure 36.1). The many kinds of amoeba, for instance, move by forming transient bulges, the pseudopodia (false feet), and withdrawing protoplasm elsewhere. In this way they can approach and surround a source of food, either bacteria or decomposing organic matter. A wide variety of other organisms have achieved more effective propulsion with the evolution of one or more tails, each driven by a molecular motor at its base. The motor, a rotary one, turns the tail clockwise or anticlockwise, and is powered by an ion pump. This very effective form of propulsion is frequent in bacteria (*E. coli*, for example) and algae, and is also found in spermatozoa, though there are differences in composition and powering between the bacterial 'cilium' and the larger and more powerful spermatozoal 'flagellum'.

As Einstein pointed out, all motion in the universe is relative and the energy-saving alternative to active movement is to remain still and let the environment do the work—which is what sea anemones and certain shellfish do. Thus a mussel (*Mytilus*; Figure 36.2) relies on the movement of water to provide the plankton on which it feeds, drawing the minute organisms into its siphon. A mussel also uses water as a conduit for reproduction, the male releasing sperm into the water, some of which find their way

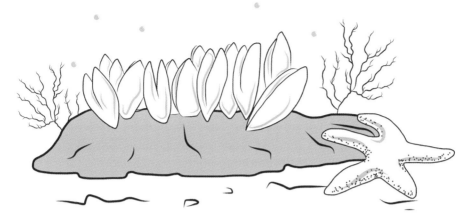

Figure 36.2 A starfish approaching its prey, a firmly anchored mussel (*Mytilus*) bed.

into the siphon of a nearby female. But even in the case of a sedentary mussel, movement of the whole organism had been essential earlier when it had been approaching a rock upon which to settle. It had done so by means of a large foot which it had repeatedly extended and transiently anchored, pulling the remainder of the body behind it; once a suitable space had been reached, the mussel had secreted a viscous fluid that hardened into strong threads permanently attaching the mussel to the rock.

But to be efficient, movement cannot be random, and this is true not only of a relatively complex creature such a mussel (in finding its eventual resting place) but even of unicellular organisms. Ciliated bacteria, amoeboid white blood cells, and flagellated spermatozoa all benefit from the guidance provided by chemical attractants released into their neighbourhood. In the case of sperm, for example, it is the combination of the progesterone secreted by the ovum with receptors in the base of the flagellum that enables sperm to swim ever closer to their target.

As evolution progressed, with the arrival of ever more complex organisms, so other movement guidance systems developed in addition to those sensing chemical attractants. But the latter still dominated. *Caenorhabditis elegans*, the one millimetre-long nematode beloved of molecular biologists and possessed of exactly 302 neurons, still depends on chemoattraction for finding food, though it has touch receptors on the body surface that affect its motility. *Aplysia*, the giant sea slug examined to such good effect by Eric Kandel, includes photoreceptors, able to detect variations in light intensity, as well as touch receptors among its 20,000 neurons. Nevertheless *Aplysia* depends on two special raised structures, the rhinophores,[1] to sense chemicals in the seawater indicative of food or a prospective mate. Similarly the chief predator of the marine mussel, the starfish, still relies on chemical clues to find its way during high tide to the mussel bed, though it also has mechanoreceptors in the tiny 'tube feet' to assist in prizing open mussel shells so that the exposed soft bodies can be devoured.

As in *Aplysia*, the starfish has evolved a primitive nervous system, the nerve cell bodies clumping together to form distinct nuclei. A ring of neurons surrounds the mouth and a single peripheral nerve runs down each of the five limbs. Connections between the sensory receptors and muscle-controlling neurons allow the starfish to move by repeatedly extending one of its limbs and dragging the rest of the body after it.

In the insect world also, there is an especially heavy reliance on chemical attractants, the *pheromones*. These compounds show considerable variety in their molecular structure and in the uses to which they are put. Ants, for example, have different pheromones for marking a trail and for alarming the colony in the event of an intruder. Though an ant has eyes on either side of its head, these are compound eyes; consisting of a few hundred small lenses, they have poor resolution and are probably only useful for detecting relatively large objects nearby. In contrast, the chemoreceptors in the ant antennae (Figure 36.3) can sense pheromones on the ground that, through its primitive nervous system, enable the ant to follow a marked trail for 100 metres or more.[2] In the case of the honeybee, a male 'drone' will be attracted by pheromones to a virgin queen and will fertilize her, the queen then altering her pheromones to prevent other queens from developing and to render female workers infertile.

The importance of pheromones in guiding behaviour (and therefore movements) has also been demonstrated in lizards, salamanders, snakes, frogs, and toads, mostly in connection with courtship and mating. In these species the attractant is picked up by the tongue and promptly transferred to a special structure in the snout, the *vomeronasal*

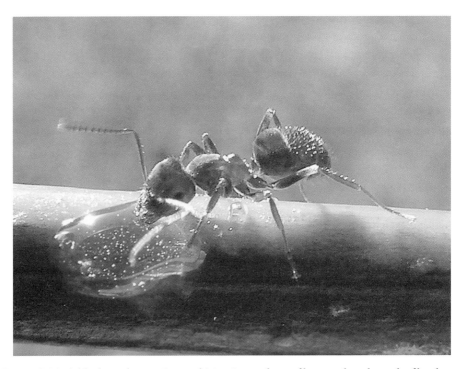

Figure 36.3 A black garden ant is seen biting into a drop of honey placed on a leaf by the photographer. The raised right antenna, with internal chemoreceptors, is clearly visible. (Coloured original photo by Jens Buurgaard Nielsen. Wikimedia Commons file: Lasius Niger.jpg. Creative Commons Attribution-Share Alike 2.5 Generic license.)

organ, where the attractant combines with chemoreceptors in the mucosa. Though lacking a vomeronasal organ, birds also respond to chemicals, as shown by the ability of crows, vultures, hawks, and eagles to detect the odours of rotting flesh.

Mammals, too, employ chemical signalling, a well-known example being the marking of territory by dogs and cats with their urine. 'Signal' pheromones cause a cat or a rat to bunch up its back (*lordosis*), signifying a readiness for mating. In all these examples, and in most mammals, the chemoreceptors in the vomeronasal organ complement those in the olfactory epithelium of the nose. In humans, however, the vomeronasal organ is vestigial; a small structure on either side of the nasal septum, it is present in the foetus but atrophies soon after birth. Though the sensitivity of the human nose to detect scents, odours, and pheromones is much less than that of a dog, it is impressive, nonetheless.

According to the present hypothesis, behaviour initiated by the combination of a chemical attractant with its receptor may or may not be associated with consciousness. On the one hand, it is very likely that, in a dog or cat, such activities as eating, mating, or detecting territorial boundaries are indeed conscious ones. On the other hand, though one can never be certain, it is much less likely that an ant is aware of its actions. Once an activity has been initiated, an ant may continue it tirelessly until daylight ends or there is a major interruption. Further, it has been shown that artificial intelligence, employing very few rules in operating a robotic ant, is fully capable of mimicking the ability of natural ants to climb, bulldoze, and build nests and bridges.[3] The activity in an ant appears as automatic as does a reflex in an animal with a highly developed nervous system—we humans promptly withdraw a hand after touching a thorn, we cough when there is a tickle in the throat, and we instinctively duck when about to pass through a low entrance. Though we are aware of these behaviours at the time, their execution has been programmed by the nervous system.

There is, however, an important distinction to be made, and it has to do with learning. The ant does not learn to follow a chemical trail, it does it instinctively by means of a genetically programmed neural circuit. A human infant, in contrast, has to learn to withdraw the hand from a sharp object or a hot surface and it is the conscious appreciation of pain that brings about the learning. In those children born with congenital insensitivity to pain or with hereditary dysfunction of the thin autonomic nerve fibres, pain is absent; it is not there to be memorized and the physical consequences are severe. Finger ends are chewed to the bone, joints are dislocated and bones broken; cuts, burns, and scalds are ignored. All of this is a way of saying that, for a movement to be effective, there must be guidance. In the child with congenital insensitivity, there was no pain to be remembered and no guidance for the future.

In mammals it is the hippocampus that remembers the nature and the location of the object that provided pleasure or pain. Other parts of the limbic system connected to the hippocampus generate the sensations—the nucleus accumbens producing pleasure and the periaqueductal grey matter pain.

But back to the rat. The experiments by Cornelius Vanderwolf showing that the hippocampus appeared to be involved in the initiation of movement have already been mentioned.[4] In other experiments, however, Vanderwolf gathered evidence that the hippocampus also took part in olfaction (smell). That the hippocampus might have a role in chemosensation was something that had been lost sight of, given all the excitement of discovering the structure's role in memory. Further, there had been Alf Brodal's authoritative dismissal of the hippocampus as part of the olfactory system. However, the hippocampus had originally been identified by Ramon y Cajal and other neuro-anatomists as part of the rhinencephalon ('smell brain'), partly on account of its location and partly because, like other sensory areas of brain, it contained a large proportion of small granule cells. Having implanted wire recording electrodes in the hippocampi of rats, Vanderwolf observed high frequency 'gamma' oscillations (*ca.* 80 hertz (Hz)) in the dentate nucleus whenever the rat sniffed, even if it was only room air.[5] However, there was another type of rhythm, a slower one in the 'beta' range (*ca.* 20 Hz), that was contingent on the nature of the odour. It would occur on exposure to organic solvent odours (e.g. benzene, toluene) and, more importantly, to chemicals normally secreted by the anal scent glands of a natural predator, such as a weasel. In making a case for the hippocampus as an olfactory organ Vanderwolf pointed out that the structure receives a projection from the ipsilateral olfactory bulb, both directly and via the pyriform cortex. He also stressed that the hippocampal gamma and beta rhythms were peculiar to olfactory stimuli, not being observed after visual or auditory ones.

Vanderwolf's experiments on the rat hippocampus, in conjunction with O'Keefe's finding of place cells, help to make the case for the evolutionary development of consciousness since they link together chemosensation, memory, and movement.

Notes

1. See Figure 10.2 of *Aplysia*.
2. I have observed ants follow a trail across a patio, up the outside wall of a house, into the kitchen, across a floor, up the side of a countertop before reaching a few drops of spilt sugary fluid on the top.
3. Several research teams are currently developing ant robotics, one of them the Self-Organizing Systems Research Group at Harvard University.
4. See Chapter 35(a).
5. C.H. Vanderwolf, 'The Hippocampus as an Olfacto-Motor Mechanism: Were the Classical Anatomists Right After All?' (2001) 127 (1–2) *Behavioural Brain Research* 25–47.

37

The 'Minimum Time' Argument
for Consciousness

There is another way of looking at the relationship between memory and consciousness and this is the observation that there can be no such thing as 'instant' consciousness. Every sensation and every thought is dependent on the brain having a certain minimum time to complete a function. I cannot have a thought, for example, unless there is sufficient time for the words to flow in my internal speech. But during those few seconds my brain has to remain aware of the beginning of the unspoken sentence in order for the thought to be completed.

'his back lawn' means only that a man has a back lawn.

'cutting his back lawn' indicates that someone, a man, is cutting his back lawn. But who is this man?

'my next-door neighbour is cutting his back lawn.' With the additional time, the thought is complete. I have heard a gas mower start up and, from experience, I know that the particular sound is coming from activity next door.

Similarly I cannot be conscious of what I am seeing unless there has been time for my eye to scan my surroundings,[1] or, in the case of recognizing a movement, to compare the present scene with that of the immediate past. As with the generation of a thought, the necessary time durations are brief, but they are nevertheless real and represent transient 'mini' memories.

Now imagine a process that requires rather more time, the waking-up after sleep. We open our eyes and, if we are on vacation, we may have no sense as to where we are. For the first moments we may still be captive to a dream, desperate because—in the dream—a train has left without us or perhaps our wallet has been stolen. And, as the journey into consciousness begins, we may become momentarily bewildered if our surroundings are unfamiliar. The hotel room is nothing like the bedroom at home; it is smaller, there is no ceiling light, and the window and door are in the wrong places. And then, as the first few seconds pass, we remember that we left home the previous morning and drove a few hundred kilometres on the highway to attend a meeting. And with that recollection comes the realization, the reassurance, as to who we are. The 'I' is now fully present.

This assembling of consciousness through memory is a phenomenon that we all experience. It seems such a natural process that we never consider its implications for the nature of consciousness. One person who did, however, was Marcel Proust. In *The Way by Swann's* the narrator in the novel, Marcel, describes his awakening from sleep:

Aranzio's Seahorse and the Search for Memory and Consciousness. Alan J. McComas, Oxford University Press.
© Oxford University Press 2023. DOI: 10.1093/oso/9780192868244.003.0039

[W]hen I woke in the middle of the night, since I did not know where I was, I did not even understand in the first moment who I was; all I had, in its original simplicity, was the sense of existence as it may quiver in the depths of an animal; I was more bereft than a caveman; but then the memory—not yet of the place where I was, but several of those where I had lived and where I might have been—would come to me like help from on high to pull me out of the void from which I could not have got out on my own....[2]

Though Proust's literary gifts enabled him to create many memorable characters, even Proust could not have imagined the existence of a person like Clive Wearing. Rather than waking once and starting the day, Clive would wake up every few seconds, with no recollection of the previous few seconds or, indeed, of any part his former life. Suddenly awake, he would not know where he was, who he was, or what had happened to him. The only person he would recognize was Deborah, his wife and constant companion in his illness.

Towards the end of the video made by Jonathan Miller, Clive is seen sitting on a couch next to Deborah. After demonstrating that he had not remembered several family events that Deborah had told him about only moments before, Clive exclaims:

> I don't know. I've never seen a human being before. I've never had a dream or a thought. The brain has been totally inactive, day and night the same ....

This is surely one of the most important statements about consciousness ever made by a patient, especially the brief sentence: 'I've never had a dream or a thought.' With understandable anger in his voice, Clive Wearing was telling the world that, with only a vestige of short-term memory, it is not possible to have thoughts or to know who you are—the very essence of consciousness. Clive's predicament suggests that, to get any further in an understanding of the neural mechanisms underlying consciousness, we must consider memory again.

We begin by comparing Clive with his more famous counterpart, Henry Molaison.

Notes

1. And to create a spatial map in the hippocampus; see Chapters 43 and 45.
2. M. Proust, *The Way by Swann's. In Search of Lost Time*, Vol. 1, translated from the French by Lydia Davis (London: Penguin Books, 2002). I became aware of Proust's passage, in a different translation, in D. Wearing, *Forever Today. A True Story of Lost Memory and Never-Ending Love* (London: Doubleday, 2005).

D.

NEURAL MECHANISMS INVOLVED

38

Clive Wearing and Henry Molaison Reconsidered

The magnitude of Clive Wearing's memory loss raises a further matter. Why was Clive's disability so much more severe than Henry Molaison's, given that both were considered to have had severe damage to both hippocampi? And, as a follow-up question, why is it always Henry who continues to be cited as *the* clinical example of amnesia following hippocampal damage—or, in Henry's case, hippocampal removal. Clive's illness had occurred in 1985 and there had been no mention of it in Suzanne Corkin's otherwise excellent *Permanent Present Tense. The Unforgettable Life of the Amnesic Patient, H.M.* The book had been published in 2013, three years before Suzanne's death from cancer.

Had the failure to mention Clive been because there was seemingly no explanation for his disability having been so much worse than Henry's?

Consider the two cases.

In her book, Suzanne describes Henry in this way:

> No one would doubt that Henry's experience was a tragedy, but he rarely seemed to suffer and was not continuously lost and frightened—quite the contrary. He always lived in the moment, fully accepting the events of daily life. From the time of his operation, every new person he met was forever a stranger, yet he approached each one with openness and trust. He remained as good-natured and pleasant as the polite, quiet person his high-schoolmates knew.[1]

In contrast, Deborah Wearing would write about her husband:

> As the months wore on, Clive's behaviour became increasingly volatile and explosive. He existed in a blinkered moment with no past to anchor it, and not enough present to be able to breathe. His panic at having no past blotted out even the few moments of present remaining in him.[2]

At Deborah's suggestion, Clive would later make a written record of events for each day, an activity that he maintained for years. As already noted, there would be a series of entries on each page, each one full of brief exclamatory statements, such as: 'I WAKE FOR THE FIRST TIME' or 'NOW I AM PERFECTLY AWAKE' or 'I AM SUPERLATIVELY COMPLETELY AWAKE'. The entries would be separated by only a few minutes and, as each was added, the previous one would be crossed out.

Aranzio's Seahorse and the Search for Memory and Consciousness. Alan J. McComas, Oxford University Press.
© Oxford University Press 2023. DOI: 10.1093/oso/9780192868244.003.0040

The immediate explanation for the different behaviour in the two men was that, whereas Henry could retain new information for 30 seconds or so, Clive's ability was restricted to a brief moment. On the cover of the paperback edition of Deborah Wearing's book, tucked into a corner, is the statement 'The Man with the Seven Second Memory'.

So while Henry had 30 seconds of memory, Clive had been reduced to seven. Henry still had short-term memory while Clive had been left with a snippet that had only lasted long enough for him to make a brief entry in his diary, or to wonder where he was and what had happened to him. Strangely, his quick-wittedness had persisted, at least to some degree. He could still play with words, pronouncing them backwards, making puns, or creating acronyms from the letters on a car licence plate. He would confabulate at times, too, inventing extraordinary reasons on the spur of the moment to explain his situation. Once he had told the nursing staff at St Mary's Hospital that, in his earlier life, he had been in charge of that very hospital. These were all thoughts but the briefest possible ones. It was impossible for Clive to have a train of thought or to recapture an identity for himself.

But this explanation raises the question as to why the severity of the memory loss should have been so different in the two men. To discover the explanation, one has to look more closely at their hippocampal lesions.

In Clive as in other patients with herpes simplex encephalitis, it was the medial temporal lobes that were initially affected and sustained the greatest damage in the brain.

But how much damage? At the time of writing, Clive is—astonishingly—still alive and so we are dependent on the results of brain imaging. At the time of his first, urgent admission to hospital Clive had a computed tomography (CT) scan of his brain which 'indicated areas of low density particularly in the left temporal lobe extending into the inferior and posterior frontal lobe and into the right medial temporal lobe'.[3] The abnormal scan had helped to confirm the clinical suspicion of herpes simplex encephalitis. That had been in 1985. Six years later, in July 1991, magnetic resonance imaging (MRI) was performed and this time the results were examined independently by three experts. Marked abnormality was reported in 'both hippocampal formations and both amygdalas' as well as in other limbic structures; there was also some involvement of other regions of the left temporal lobe in addition to the severe changes in the medial lobe. The changes on the right side of the brain were less extensive. The report concluded: 'It is of note that both the left and right thalamus were rated as being intact, and that no other frontal lobe abnormality was found apart from the left medial frontal abnormality . . .'.

The fact that, in addition to the hippocampus and amygdala, other parts of Clive's left temporal lobe had been affected had been evident from his speech in the first few months after his admission to hospital. Despite speaking fluently and clearly, the words had made no sense. Deborah would write:

> His phrases sounded almost plausible, as though the framework for conversation were there but the content wasn't ... Friends and colleagues listened, struggled to

make sense of it, and answered as best they could, catching any phrase that gave them an entry.

Chapter 35 provides an example of Clive's nonsensical speech when he attempted conversation with the driver of a taxicab. At an earlier stage of his illness, Clive's aberration had been even worse. Every object—a pen, a tie—was referred to as 'a chicken'.

Clive's inability to speak sensibly indicated that the viral inflammation had extended into Wernicke's area, a part of the left superior temporal gyrus, immediately posterior to the auditory cortex. No doubt the auditory cortex had been involved too, but its sparing on the opposite, right, side would have prevented deafness. In contrast, the fluency and excellent articulation of Clive's speech was evidence that any initial loss of function in the 'motor' speech area in the left frontal lobe had fully recovered. Nor did Clive exhibit any weakness or clumsiness of his arms or legs—further evidence of the normality of the frontal lobes.

In contrast to Clive's varied lesions, with more involvement on the left than on the right side of the brain, Henry's defects were more straightforward. Or so it might have appeared.

When Dr William Beecher Scoville came to treat Henry, he had already performed partial bilateral temporal lobotomies on other patients, all of them inmates of Connecticut's mental hospitals and suffering from schizophrenia. As described previously,[4] Scoville had first made two circular openings in the skull, each 3.8 centimetre (cm) in diameter, above the eyes. Metal retractors were then inserted through the openings so as to gently raise the frontal lobes and give access to the temporal lobes. Using a scalpel, Scoville had cut away the most anterior parts of the two medial temporal lobes before inserting a tube and applying suction to remove deeper brain tissue. This latter procedure would have been more difficult to control; nevertheless Scoville estimated that he had removed 8 cm of medial temporal lobe on each side of Henry's brain. If true, not only would much of the hippocampus have been taken away but so would the amygdala and the parahippocampal gyrus (lying below the hippocampus). While under Suzanne Corkin's supervision, however, Henry had had MRI scans performed and these indicated that the surgical ablation had been less extensive than Scoville had thought. As always when there is doubt concerning the size and nature of a pathological lesion, the final word is provided by the pathologist or, in Henry's case, by the accomplished neuroanatomist, Jacopo Annese.

Before examining stained sections of nervous tissue under the microscope, Annese had photographed the surface of Henry's brain after each thinly cut slice had been removed. The cutting had taken 53 hours and produced 2,401 slices and the same number of digital photographs. From the latter Annese had been able to make a three-dimensional (3D) reconstruction of Henry's brain.[5] The most important finding was that more of Henry's hippocampi had been spared than the MRI scans had indicated. Rather than 8 cm of medial temporal lobe[6] being removed on each side as Scoville had thought, only 5.5 cm had been taken on the left and 4.4 cm on the right. Taking into account their normal curvature, the lengths of the remaining hippocampi were 3.6 cm and 4.0 cm respectively on the left and right sides. The residual hippocampal volume was estimated as approximately 2 cm^3 on each side, a value suggesting that more than half the original neural tissue had been preserved.[7]

But could the anatomical findings in the two cases, Clive and Henry, explain their different behaviours? As a first step one could construct a table containing the respective anatomical lesions and memory defects of the two patients.

	Control	HM	CW
Amygdala	+	—	—
Hippocampi	100%	50%	?5%
Short-term memory	+	+	—
Long-term memory	+	—	—
Consciousness	Continuous	Continuous	Fragmented

Such a simple table requires explanation. Regarding the inclusion of the amygdala, this is necessary since the amygdala, lying in front and to the side of the hippocampus, would be expected to have been removed in Scoville's operation on Henry. In fact, though Annese found some residual amygdala on the two sides, it appeared that the basolateral nuclei (the nuclei projecting to the hippocampi) had indeed been removed. Regarding the two hippocampi, would 50 per cent of the normal structure be sufficient for normal function? The absence of memory loss in Penfield's epileptic patients subjected to unilateral temporal lobectomy indicate that one does not normally require two fully functional hippocampi. However, as Corkin had realized from Henry's MRI scans, the residual hippocampal tissue had been deprived of most of its main input, that from the neighbouring entorhinal cortex. This had been confirmed in Annese's 3D reconstruction of Henry's brain, which had shown only a few percent of the entorhinal fibres remaining. On the other hand, this small residuum could still have had an effect, especially as there would likely have been compensatory sprouting of the fibres. Suzanne Corkin's observation that Henry had possessed some sense of smell, even though he had had difficulty identifying particular odours, indicated that some sensory input was still reaching the hippocampus.[8] Also relevant is that, in addition to that from the entorhinal cortex, there are inputs to the hippocampus from the cingulate gyrus, septal nuclei and brain stem respectively and these would have been spared by Scoville's surgery. Finally, the appearance of the surviving hippocampal tissue suggests that it was likely to have been functioning, since there was no suggestion of the wasting that, elsewhere in the body and brain, normally accompanies the loss of a nerve supply (denervation atrophy).

The figure of 5% for the amount of Clive's residual hippocampal tissue is a guess, but one based on the MRI report of 'marked abnormality in both hippocampal formations'. Clive's few seconds of awareness, endlessly repeated, might suggest that his viral infection had spared a very small fraction of the original cell and fibre population.

Leaving aside the issue of consciousness for the moment, the comparison of Henry's and Clive's features in the table raises two interesting possibilities. The first is that the hippocampus is essential for short-term memory. This was not the view of Suzanne Corkin nor of other memory researchers, including contemporary ones.[9] Under the impression that almost all of Henry's hippocampi had been removed, they had been obliged to find another part of the brain responsible for short-term memory, and had settled on the frontal lobe. But there are arguments against the frontal lobe, the strongest being the relatively good preservation of memory in patients who have had damage to their frontal lobes, the conclusion of Brenda Milner among others. Further, though fMRI scans have been interpreted as indicative of short-term memory function in the frontal lobes, it is increasingly obvious that this type of investigation can be misleading.[10]

The second possibility raised by the two cases is that long-term memory is dependent on the amygdala, since in Henry the critical basolateral nuclei had been removed by the surgeon, while in Clive both amygdalas would have been destroyed by the virus.

What part, then, does the amygdala play in memory?

Notes

1. In this chapter all references to Suzanne Corkin's findings in Henry Molaison are taken from her monograph: S. Corkin, *Permanent Present Tense. The Unforgettable Life of the Amnesic Patient*, H.M. (New York, NY: Basic Books, 2013).
2. All references to Deborah Wearing's observations on her husband are taken from her monograph: D. Wearing, *Forever Today. A True Story of Lost Memory and Never-Ending Love* (London: Doubleday, 2005).
3. B.A. Wilson, A.D. Baddeley, N. Kapur, 'Dense Amnesia in a Professional Musician following Herpes Simplex Virus Encephalitis' (1995) 17(5) *Journal of Clinical and Experimental Neuropsychology* 668–681. This paper contains the results of the 1985 CT scan and the 1991 MRI scan in addition to the findings on psychological testing.
4. See Chapter 4.
5. The extreme care taken in the anatomical and histological examinations and the results, including photographs of Henry's brain, are described in: J. Annese, N.M. Schenker-Ahmed, H. Bartsch, P. Maechler, C. Sheh, N. Thomas, J. Kayano, A. Ghatan, N. Bresler, M.P. Frosch, R. Klaming, and S. Corkin, 'Postmortem Examination of Patient H.M.'s Brain Based on Histological Sectioning and Digital 3D Reconstruction' (2014) 5 *Nature Communications* 3122 <https://doi.org/10.1038/ncomms4122> accessed 24 April 2022.
6. Measurements taken from the anterior tip of the medial temporal lobe.
7. Annese and colleagues ('Postmortem Examination of Patient H.M.'s Brain ...', see note 4) did not give values for the normal volume of the hippocampus. However, control data points appear in Figure 2 of: J.A. Cobb, J. Simpson, G.J. Mahajan, J.C. Overholser, G.H. Jurjus, L. Dieter, N. Herbst. W. May, G. Rajkowska, and C.A. Stockmeier, 'Hippocampal Volume and Total Cell Numbers in Major Depressive Disorder' (2013) 47(3) *Journal of Psychiatric Research* 299–306.
8. Suzanne Corkin interpreted the results of Henry's olfactory testing differently, citing them as evidence for separate brain sites dealing with the intensity and the identity of an odour respectively.
9. See note 1 in Introduction.
10. C.M. Bennett, A.A. Baird, M.B. Miller, and G.L. Wolford, 'Neural Correlates of Interspecies Perspective Taking in the Post-Mortem Atlantic Salmon: An Argument for Proper Multiple Comparisons Correction' (2009) 1(1) *Journal of Serendipitous and Unexpected Results* 1–5. This

tongue-in-cheek paper reported the results of presenting photographs of human faces to a dead salmon, the task for the salmon being to identify the emotions portrayed. Embarrassingly, two 'hot spots' for this mental activity were found in the brain and spinal cord respectively! The point of the paper was serious, however, in drawing attention to false positive results with fMRI caused by improper statistical processing of data. The same point was subsequently made when 72 imaging laboratories were given the same fMRI data to process, with very different interpretations. See: R. Botvinnik-Nezer, F. Holzmeister, C.F. Camerer, A. Dreber, J. Huber, M. Johannesson, M. Kirchler, R. Iwanir, J.A. Mumford, R.A. Adcock, P. Avesani, B.M. Baczkowski…[T. Schonberg,] 'Variability in the Analysis of a Single Neuroimaging Data Set by Many Teams' (2020) 582 *Nature* 84–8.

39

Role of the Amygdala

The amygdala, as described earlier, is not only a part of the brain's limbic system but one likely to have a strong influence on the hippocampus.[1] For one thing, the two structures are neighbours with strong fibre connections to each other. Early in the evolution of vertebrate brain the cells that would later develop into the amygdala were responsible for conveying the all-important chemosensory information to the future hippocampus. As the vertebrate brain became larger and more complex, with well-developed visual and auditory systems, so the amygdala became informed of these other types of information too. But, in the intricate workings of the brain, what does the amygdala actually *do* with this information?

The first clue comes from its structure. Although relatively small, the amygdala has several parts, each part made up of one or more nuclei. The most anterior part appears to be related to emotional behaviour, accounting for Birger Kaada's early finding that stimulation of the amygdala in an awake animal caused it to exhibit physiological signs of fear or anger. But is it possible that the amygdala, especially the basolateral nuclei, also has a role in converting short-term memory to long-term? And there is a clue. Is it not those incidents with strong emotional content that are most likely to be remembered? How could one forget falling into a swimming pool and being unable to swim or being unexpectedly confronted by a black bear during a camping holiday? Or the delight of a first kiss?

There had been another clue, a faint one, from the much-cited study of Heinrich Klüver and Paul Bucy in Chicago.[2] After they had excised the entire temporal lobes in monkeys, the animals not only became more docile but appeared not to recognize objects with which they had previously been familiar. But the temporal lobe is a large structure, containing many parts. In an attempt to discover the role of the amygdala, Lawrence Weiskrantz removed only the amygdala; again, the experiments had been performed in monkeys but this time at the extraordinary research centre that the enterprising Dr Burlingame had established in the Institute for the Living in Hartford, Connecticut. Weiskrantz, who would continue his career in the Experimental Psychology Laboratory at Cambridge (United Kingdom), was meticulous in his testing of the animals and in the examination of their brains at post-mortem.[3] The results of the bilateral amygdalectomies were not dramatic, however––more suggestive than conclusive. The treated animals took longer to learn new behaviours and were quicker to forget them. That had been in 1956.

Forgotten by most workers in the field were the findings of William Scoville and Brenda Milner relating to the amygdala in their classic 1957 paper.[4] Brenda Milner had

Aranzio's Seahorse and the Search for Memory and Consciousness. Alan J. McComas, Oxford University Press.
© Oxford University Press 2023. DOI: 10.1093/oso/9780192868244.003.0041

carried out careful psychological testing of ten patients in whom Scoville had removed varying amounts of the medial temporal lobe. In all but one the surgery had been bilateral and in each case the tip and anterior part of the medial lobe had been taken out. Although the amount of hippocampus removed had varied among the patients, Scoville had been confident that the surgery had always included the amygdala. Yet in the one patient in whom the hippocampi had been spared there had not been any detectable memory loss. 'Removal of only the uncus and amygdala bilaterally does not appear to cause memory impairment', the authors had stated.

But had both amygdalas been removed in that patient? As described in the previous chapter, in Henry Molaison both the magnetic resonance imaging (MRI) scan and Jacopo Annese's post-mortem findings had revealed that substantial hippocampal tissue and some amygdala had been left despite the claim of an extensive resection. Such an error could have been easily made, even by a skillful and innovate neurosurgeon. Scoville had had to work in the small space created by raising the frontal lobe, dealing with leaking blood and cerebrospinal fluid as he did so, his instruments often obscuring the illumination of the exposed brain. And he could not have identified the amygdala for it was simply grey matter amongst other grey matter.

Given the circumstances, Scoville's bold assertion that the amygdalas had been removed in all ten patients is questionable. However, surgeons, by nature of their profession, are accustomed to reaching conclusions and making definitive statements (an operation is to be performed or rejected, a tumour must be completely excised, a bleeding vessel has to be ligated, etc.). In their decisiveness surgeons are unlike physicians who can usually temporize, make provisional rather than certain diagnoses, and can try one course of treatment before substituting another. In the light of what is now known about the importance of the amygdala in memory, it seems likely that less tissue had been sucked out in some of the ten patients than had been thought, and that this was responsible for the variable interference with memory.

The next advance regarding the amygdala had come in 1964 and, as with so much of the early research on memory, it had been Donald Hebb's Department of Psychology at McGill that had been the source.

Graham Goddard (Figure 39.1) had come to Montreal to work for his PhD in psychology.[5] The young man had been born in the United Kingdom but educated in Saskatchewan, Canada, where he had already obtained a Master's degree on the basis of experimental work on memory. The PhD studies at McGill were a continuation of this earlier work. The move had enabled Goddard to be supervised by Peter Milner, an expert on focal stimulation of the rat brain and the co-discoverer, with James Olds, of a pleasure ('reward') centre in the brain.[6] Goddard's experimental programme was complex, with the rats subjected to several training programmes and the electric stimuli being delivered to the amygdala through a needle electrode.[7] The switch from monkeys to rats for memory experiments had obvious advantages; despite the comparatively small size of the rat brain, Goddard and those who followed him would show that it was possible not only to stimulate the amygdala selectively but to perfuse the structure with neurotransmitters and their antagonists, and even to collect transmitter released in the

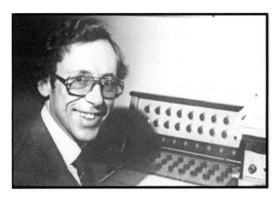

Figure 39.1 Graham Goddard (minus characteristic beard) at the time of his professorship at Dalhousie University, Halifax, Canada. Photograph kindly provided by the Department of Psychology & Neuroscience, Dalhousie University.

amygdala for analysis. In Goddard's case, the experimental intervention had been continuous electrical stimulation of the amygdala.

Graham Goddard had observed an effect in his experiments––the stimulation appeared to interfere with various learning tasks. In the conclusion of his publication of the McGill work, Goddard speculated that the stimulation had blocked the normal consolidation of memory.

Goddard had not been the only young researcher at McGill to study the amygdala. No sooner had he left to take up a junior position at the University of Waterloo than John O'Keefe had arrived from New York to start his own PhD studies under the guidance of Ronald Melzack.[8] Rather than stimulate the amygdala the future Nobel Laureate had decided to record from it, improving on the techniques previously employed in the McGill psychology department by Peter Milner and James Olds. It had been low-yield work but the few neurons that he had been able to identify successfully in the cat amygdala were intriguing in their properties, each responding to a single, very specific stimulus–– the sight of a mouse for one cell, the song of a bird for another, and a particular item of food for a third. The results had been further evidence that the amygdala was somehow involved in memory, containing a smattering of the 'grandmother neurons' postulated to exist by Lettvin and Barlow (the 'gnostic units' of Konorski).

The work of Goddard and of O'Keefe had been followed by a wealth of experiments in other laboratories, using a variety of techniques, including perfusion of the amygdala with drugs and transmitters.[9] Inevitably, details of the amygdala's activities emerged. It was shown the basolateral nuclei in the amygdala were those involved in memory and that the neurotransmitter, *norepinephrine*, was released at synapses within the nuclei; another ubiquitous neurotransmitter, *acetylcholine*, was also involved, but at a later stage in the pathway.

The picture that emerges from the disparate studies of the amygdala is of a structure that works hand-in-hand with its immediate neighbour, the hippocampus. While the entorhinal cortex is constantly presenting the hippocampus with immediate information about the body and its surroundings, it is the amygdala, with its complex structure and host of connections, that determines whether any of that information is to be retained.[10] As Henry Molaison had shown so consistently throughout his many years of being studied, without synaptic reinforcement from the amygdala there can only be short-term awareness of the world. Long-term memory is impossible.

Notes

1. See Chapter 32.
2. H. Klüver and P.C. Bucy, 'An Analysis of Certain Effects of Bilateral Temporal Lobectomy in the Rhesus Monkey, with Special Reference to "Psychic Blindness"' (1939) 5 *Journal of Psychology* 33–54.
3. L. Weiskrantz, 'Behavioral Changes Associated with Ablation of the Amygdaloid Complex in Monkeys' (1956) 49 *Journal of Comparative Physiology and Psychology* 381–91.
4. W.B. Scoville and B. Milner, 'Loss of Recent Memory after Bilateral Hippocampal Lesions' (1957) 20 *Journal of Neurology, Neurosurgery and Psychiatry* 11–21.
5. See: F. Morell, 'Graham Goddard: An Appreciation' (1987) 28(6) *Epilepsia* 717–20.
    Goddard (1938–1987) died prematurely, drowning while attempting to cross a river in New Zealand, where he was Professor of Psychology. His experiments at McGill led him to the important discovery of the '*kindling*' phenomenon later—the induction of epilepsy by repeatedly stimulating the amygdala.
6. See Chapter 3.
7. G.V. Goddard, 'Amygdaloid Stimulation and Learning in the Rat' (1956) 49 *Journal of Comparative Physiology and Psychology* 381–91.
8. See Chapter 12.
9. J.L. McGaugh, 'The Amygdala Modulates the Consolidation of Memories of Emotionally Arousing Experiences' (2004) 27 *Annual Review of Neuroscience* 1–28. Curiously, in this otherwise excellent review there is no reference to the highly relevant classic paper by Scoville and Milner ('Loss of Recent Memory after Bilateral Hippocampal Lesions' see note 4).
10. It is difficult to think of an analogy that embraces not only the hippocampus itself but the closely related amygdala and entorhinal cortex. The best I could manage was one in which the hippocampus is represented by a university lecture theatre in which all presentations are delivered in the presence of a Chairperson (amygdala). In the back row of the theatre are seated the senior professors (CA1 pyramidal neurons) while in front of them are several rows of junior faculty (granule cells and other neurons). At the front of the theatre is a whiteboard with felt pens (entorhinal cortex) that are used by a series of graduate students (sensory neurons). Each graduate student has to report on some aspect of the university campus—visiting lecturers, student residences, playing fields, science laboratories, art gallery, student protests, etc. After only 30 seconds the report is terminated and if the Chair (amygdala) decided it was important, she takes a Polaroid photograph of the display on the white board and passes it to one of the Professors (CA1 neurons) sitting in the back row. The volume of applause by the Junior Faculty (granule cells) has aided the Chair in her decision, at the same time stressing its importance to the recipient Professor.

40

Role of the Non-Hippocampal Cortex

Previously, on the basis of the animal experiments, the amygdala had been envisaged as consolidating memory by strengthening synapses in the cortex through its widespread projections to the latter; it was the neocortex that was considered to store long-term memory. The lifetime observations on Henry Molaison had been interpreted in favour of the cortex accounting for short-term memory as well. The hippocampus, in contrast, was thought to have a subservient role, organizing information for its storage and retrieval in the cortex. In David Marr's computational scheme, the transfer of information from the hippocampus to the cortex for the creation of long-term memory, would occur during sleep.[1]

In one sense, the above interpretation is true. Regions of the neocortex, especially in the temporal lobe, are able to store information that has arrived through the various sensory pathways (vision, hearing, touch, smell, and taste). It had been Edmund Rolls and his team at Oxford who had first shown the presence of neurons in the temporal lobe that were responsive to faces and objects.[2] Later, Doris T'sao and her colleagues at Harvard had explored the matter in more detail, demonstrating several closely related regions in the inferior temporal lobes of monkeys that were involved in the recognition of faces—not just faces in general but specific human (and monkey) faces.[3]

At the time of their discovery, these responsive neurons caused considerable excitement, even though their existence could have been predicted, and indeed *was* predicted, as parts of schemes for the way sensory pathways worked. Thus, starting with the receptors in the retina or ear (or skin, nose, and tongue), cells at successive stages in a sensory pathway were likely to become ever more selective in their responses. For example, in the visual pathway cells might fire in response to any round object, whether it be the wheel of a car, the face of a clock on the wall, or the face of a person. At the next stage in the pathway neurons might only respond to human faces and, at a later stage still, only to a particular human face. Such neurons corresponded to the 'gnostic units' that had been hypothesized by Jerzy Konorski half a century earlier.[4]

But we are not aware of the activity in these cells of the sensory pathway. We do not see isolated circles or heads free of bodies and so on, but only the final, complete picture. So, although there *is* memory in the neocortex, most of it—the preparatory stages—is not accessible to consciousness. Most likely it is the time-chunking behaviour of the cortical columns in the sensory neocortex that is the limitation. However, without a fully functioning hippocampus it is still possible to see and hear, as Clive Wearing demonstrated even in the earliest days after the destruction of his hippocampi. The problem for Clive was that he was unable to recognize what he saw. Faces, buildings,

Aranzio's Seahorse and the Search for Memory and Consciousness. Alan J. McComas, Oxford University Press.

books, pictures, and—in the most acute stage of his illness—even words, had lost their meaning. Only the everyday objects that formed part of his procedural memory—table cutlery, clothing, and the piano—retained their significance. Similarly, an epileptic patient in a dreamy state appears to be capable of seeing their surroundings and even of using objects appropriately, though without any awareness of doing so.

Notes

1. See Chapter 17.
2. M.K. Sanghera, E.T. Rolls, and A. Roper-Hall, 'Visual Responses of Neurons in the Dorsolateral Amygdala of the Alert Monkey' (1979) 63 *Experimental Neurology* 610–26.
3. E.M. Meyers, M. Borzello, W.A. Freiwald, and D. Tsao, 'Intelligent Information Loss: The Coding of Facial Identity, Head Pose, and Non-Face Information in the Macaque Face Patch System' (2015) 35 *Journal of Neuroscience* 7069–81.
4. J. Konorski, *The Integrative Activity of the Brain* (Chicago, IL: University of Chicago Press, 1967).

41

Back to the Hippocampus

The debate as to where memory is stored might have gone on for much longer, had it not been for the single neuron recordings from the human hippocampus by Itzhak Fried and his collaborators in Los Angeles. As described earlier,[1] the busy jumble of impulse activity picked up by the fine wire recording electrodes could be processed so as to reveal the responses of individual neurons. It was an experimental approach infinitely more powerful than functional magnetic resonance imaging (fMRI) or, indeed, anything that had gone before. And what a rich harvest it had yielded—and continues to yield, in the expert hands of Rodrigo Quian Quiroga and his colleagues in the United Kingdom!

In the first place the recordings revealed that the hippocampal cells (and cells in adjacent structures) stored all kinds of information, not just about people but about places as well. And the information was comprehensive. A neuron would respond to a photograph of a well-known actress (Jennifer Aniston or Halle Berry, for example) irrespective of the circumstances in which it was taken—from near or far, from the front or from the side, the person wearing one set of clothes or another, with sunglasses or without, and so on. Further, it was not just the sight of a person that caused a cell to fire, for their spoken or written name could be just as effective. And it was the same with famous buildings such as the Sydney Opera House or the Eiffel Tower—the picture and the words were both effective. The investigators termed these responsive neurons 'concept cells' since they were concerned with every aspect of the person or object; they were, in fact, the 'grandmother cells' that Jerry Lettvin had conceived of many years previously and closely related to the 'gnostic units' of Jerzy Konorski.

So here was incontrovertible evidence that whatever else it might do, the hippocampus was a repository for long-term memory, both visual and auditory. The recordings may have done more, however. The experiments, in which subjects were shown a succession of images on a computer screen, had tested the 'semantic' component of long-term memory, that is, the recognition of places, people, and objects. But it seemed likely that the hippocampus was also storing 'episodic' memories too—those of significant events in the life of the subject. A strong hint had come from Quian Quiroga's UK studies. To have come into a hospital to have needles and wires inserted into the brain would surely have been a major event in one's life, and in one of Quian Quiroga's subjects, a cell was encountered that was responsive to the photograph of a member of the medical staff.[2] Quian Quiroga has gone further; in demonstrating how two previously unrelated images can be combined to form a new family of concept cells (the Josh

Aranzio's Seahorse and the Search for Memory and Consciousness. Alan J. McComas, Oxford University Press.
© Oxford University Press 2023. DOI: 10.1093/oso/9780192868244.003.0043

Brolin–Eiffel Tower experiment)[3] he has raised the possibility that episodic memories are actually reconstructions from semantic ones.

If the earlier distinction between the respective lesions in Henry Molaison and Clive Wearing is valid,[4] that conclusion together with the results of recording from the hippocampus in surgical patients would indicate that the hippocampus is responsible not only for the creation of short-term memories but also for retaining some as long-term ones. And in the previous chapter it was shown that the amygdala was crucial for the transformation from short-term to long-term. But what about the details? What was happening at the synapses? As Donald Hebb had insisted in *The Organization of Behaviour*, it is not enough to be satisfied with a psychological outcome, it is necessary to explain the underlying neurophysiological processes that brought it about. In the end psychology, like everything else to do with the brain, is a matter of neurons, synapses, and impulses.

Fortunately, in the case of memory, there are important clues from Eric Kandel's experiments on the giant sea slug, *Aplysia*. Kandel had shown that 'sensitization'—the strengthening of synaptic connections in one of the slug's reflex circuits—was achieved initially by the release of increased amounts of neurotransmitter from the nerve endings and subsequently by the enlargement of existing synapses and the growth of new ones.[5] The initial potentiation was brought about by the intervention of a third neuron (an 'interneuron') in the simple circuit. As Kandel proposed, the two phases of enhanced synaptic activity could be viewed as short-term and long-term memory in the giant sea slug. The important point was that the same neurons were involved in both cases.

This situation is very different to some of the current thinking concerning memory in more highly evolved brains, especially those of humans. Perhaps through misinformation concerning the extent of Henry Molaison's surgery, short-term memory has been attributed to frontal cortex and long-term memory to still wider areas of cortex. In this view, which was also that of the late David Marr, the hippocampus is envisaged as acting as a kind of intermediary, preparing memories for storage elsewhere and also assisting in their temporary retrievals.

But why should the situation in more highly evolved brains differ in its essentials from that worked out so elegantly by Kandel in *Aplysia*? Why should it not be the same in the hippocampus, with local cells acting as the potentiating interneurons responsible for short-term memory and with structural synaptic changes responsible for long-term memory? Rather than memories being dispersed throughout the cortex, why should they not be retained in the hippocampus? Not only would this be in keeping with the finding of 'concept' cells in the human hippocampus and with the results of recent optogenetic studies in rodents, but it would be the simplest, and therefore the likeliest, arrangement. As described earlier, the perforant pathway, the main route for delivering information from sensory cortex (via the lateral entorhinal cortex), was found to initiate lingering tetanic potentiation in the hippocampus by Terje Lømo and Timothy Bliss as long ago as 1973.[6] If that potentiation accounted for short-term memory, then an input from the amygdala during an emotional event (a threat, an unexpected joy etc) could provide a stimulus for still stronger reinforcement of new synaptic connections in the hippocampus—the enlargement and creation of new axon endings and dendritic knobs, just as Kandel had shown to occur in *Aplysia*. And this would provide long-term memory.

There is another point to be made, one concerning the classification of memories. There is convenience as well as scientific evidence for dividing memory into compartments such as 'declarative' and 'procedural', 'semantic' and 'episodic', and so on. But there are aspects of memory that defy simple classification—a particular way of smiling, the hint of an accent in the voice, the rub of the forehead when perplexed. Yet all of these attributes, no less than the names of US presidents or the recollection of a childhood birthday party, are coded for by permanent structural synaptic connections in sensory and motor areas of the brain.

One of the most striking illustrations of this conclusion has come recently from an unusual accident, one involving a near-fatal experience in a snowstorm. The facts were these. Audrey Mash and her husband had been mountain hiking in the Pyrenees when they were caught in a sudden, severe snowstorm. Unable to proceed, they had tried to shelter in the snow but the storm had continued. Eventually, as conditions eased, Audrey's husband had discovered his 34 year-old wife to be ice-cold and pulseless. Alarmed, he had set off and succeeded in finding help. By the time Audrey was admitted to hospital in Barcelona, some two and a half hours later, not only was she without a heartbeat but her body temperature had fallen to 18° Celsius. With considerable skill the medical staff were able to slowly warm her while oxygenating her blood by machine, and only then to restart her heart. Miraculously, when Audrey was interviewed on television some days later, not only was her memory intact but by thought, word, smile, and gesture it was evident that her full personality had been restored. Despite the abolition of electrical activity in her brain for so many hours, the strong synaptic connections had been able to preserve all her 'Audrey-ness'.[7]

Notes

1. See Chapter 24.
2. R. Quian Quiroga, 'Concept Cells: The Building Blocks of Declarative Memory Functions' (2012) 13 *Nature Reviews Neuroscience* 587–97.
3. R. Quian Quiroga, 'No Pattern Separation in the Human Hippocampus' (2020) 24(12) *Trends in Cognitive Sciences* 994–1007. doi:10.1016/j.tics.2020.09.012. Epub 2020 Nov 5. PMID: 33162337.
4. See Chapter 38.
5. See Chapter 19.
6. See Chapter 15.
7. The *Daily Mail* (United Kingdom), British woman's heart stops for SIX HOURS but she survives: Teacher reveals extraordinary ordeal after her body temperature dropped to 18C when she was lost in a snowstorm in Spain 5 December 2019. <dailymail.co.uk/news/article-7760029/British-womans-heart-stops-six-hours-SURVIVES.html>

42

The Numbers Game

Almost every topic in science involves numbers, and the question as to how the hippo-campus functions to create and store memories is no exception. Fortunately, we have many of the numbers for the hippocampus—the numbers of cells in its different parts, the firing rates of the hippocampal neurons, and, most likely, the memory storage capacity of the entire system. We do, of course, know more than the mere numbers. We know there are hippocampal neurons (the place cells) that remember the position of a rat in its environment, while in humans there are neurons (the concept cells) that have collected different types of information about particular persons, buildings, objects, and, probably, events. What we do not know is how many neurons are involved in storing a memory ('concept') and whether those neurons are specific for that memory or whether they take part in other memories as well.

The approach adopted here is a simple one. It makes an assumption as to the numbers of memories ('concepts') stored in a 'regular' adult human hippocampus and then determines the odds of a recording electrode encountering one of the cells forming a concept during one of the Los Angeles experiments on patients with temporal lobe epilepsy—the work of Itzhak Fried, Rodrigo Quian Quiroga, Christof Koch and others described in Chapter 24. Not surprisingly, the Los Angeles group have already done this themselves; with the collaboration of Stephen Waydo they have employed Bayesian mathematics to calculate concept cell 'sparseness'.[1] In Oxford, Edmund Rolls, who has investigated the primate hippocampus extensively and was the first to report the presence of neurons in the temporal lobe responsive to faces, has used his own data to determine cell numbers.[2] The present approach is, as stated, simple, the sort that a gambler might use when playing cards.

The starting point is the number of long-term memories that the hippocampus stores during life. This is a minimum number since the total long-term memory storage capacity for a healthy brain is unknown. We do know, however, that a patient suffering from Alzheimer's disease may be left with only a handful of memories, barely enough to recognize a close relative. On the other hand there are 'savants' capable of memorizing π to 20,000 decimal places or able to recall every word on every page of a large number of books. How a brain could manage such feats is beyond comprehension; there must be some neuronal 'trickery' involved that is outside the normal process for laying down memories.

What about a 'normal' human brain, though? In my own case, I can remember the faces of my parents, aunts, uncles, children, and grandchildren, a few of those I went to school with, and probably all those in the same year at medical school. Then there are my wife, her family, my present friends, and many university faculty. All told,

Aranzio's Seahorse and the Search for Memory and Consciousness. Alan J. McComas, Oxford University Press.
© Oxford University Press 2023. DOI: 10.1093/oso/9780192868244.003.0044

however, those I presently know or have known, and whose faces I can conjure up in my mind, probably number no more than 500. If to this number, are added the celebrities I have seen pictures of, the total is still probably no more than 1,000. Then there are the scenes of my life—the houses in which I have lived; the river, seaside, and harbour of the East Anglian town I grew up in, places I have visited on holiday or at scientific meetings, and so on. Again, if the scenes are added up, probably no more than a few hundred. To these estimates are added a rather larger one for the images of various objects—everything from hammers and nails to books, cars, pianos, and elephants, and various buildings around the world. To these semantic memories must be added those for notable events in one's life—the episodic memories. When all the semantic and episodic memories are considered, however, it is still doubtful if they amount to more than a few thousand.

Though some people have much larger memory 'banks' that others, suppose that 20,000 is an average number of memories for an individual. It is likely that the pyramidal cells in the CA1 region represent the final stage of memory processing in the hippocampus, an assumption based on the histological appearance of the hippocampus and the electrophysiological studies of Per Andersen and his group in Oslo.[3] It is important to add that the majority of hippocampal recordings, those made in animal brains by Kandel and Spencer and then by Andersen and Eccles, O'Keefe and Dostrovsky, Vanderwolf, and a literal host of other investigators, have most likely been made from pyramidal cells in the CA1 region of the hippocampus; there is less information about the electrophysiology of the abundant but much smaller granule cells in the dentate nucleus.

Proceeding with the calculation, a human hippocampal CA1 region will have as many as eight million pyramidal cells available for 20,000 memories, for an average of $8 \times 10^6 \div 20 \times 10^3 = 400$ pyramidal cells for a single memory.[4] The chance that a neuron encountered by an exploring electrode is one of the 400 cells coding for a particular memory (e.g. the face of a friend) will only be 1:20,000. The chance would be higher, however, if each pyramidal cell participated in more than one memory. We can calculate the extent of this convergence from the results of a typical concept cell recording session performed on epileptic patients in Los Angeles. On average each of 42 neurons was tested with 88 visual stimuli, giving $42 \times 88 = 3596$ opportunities for a 'hit'; an average of eight responsive neurons were found.[5] The recordings were not from the hippocampus alone, however, but included neighbouring structures (amygdala, entorhinal cortex, parahippocampal cortex). Suppose that the incidences of responsive cells among the various populations were similar. Since there are possibly 20,000 memories in the hippocampus, a positive result in a recording session would indicate that there is a 43-fold overlap (i.e. number of memories × number of hits ÷ number of opportunities = $20,000 \times 8 \div 3596 = 43$). That is, rather than a single memory being coded for by 400 cells, as in the initial calculation, the memory is contained within approximately $400 \times 43 = 17,200$ cells. This is a huge approximation since not only will individuals differ in the numbers of their memories, but it assumes that all the CA1 neurons are storing memories, that the memory bank is fully occupied. Further, some memories—the ones we are continually making use of, or perhaps the most 'vivid' ones—are likely to involve more neurons than others.

There is a further caveat in that 17,200 neurons cannot code for the same 43 memories, otherwise the brain could not distinguish one memory from the other 42. Instead, there must be content variation among the 17,000 neurons, such that only one memory is common to all. Consensus dictates outcome.

The calculated value of approximately 17,000 hippocampal neurons per memory is an average value and is strongly affected by the proportion of responsive concept cells attributed to the hippocampus in a recording session. Further, it is probable that the strongest, most easily recalled memories involve more neurons than those memories we find ourselves searching for. A greater number of cells are likely to code for the face of one's spouse than for that of a distant colleague at work. Similarly, in the case of episodic memories, those for alarming or particularly enjoyable events will be represented by larger populations of hippocampal cells than those for mundane occasions.

The above estimates are very different to those of the Los Angeles group, even though the same experimental data were used. Rather than a few thousand neurons coding for a single memory, Waydo and colleagues estimated that as many as 2–5 million cells may be involved, with each cell representing 50–150 additional items. Intuition can be a poor guide to truth but, even so, the representation of a single memory by several million neurons seems unlikely. However, the main reason for such a high value was that the latter was based on the total number of neurons in the hippocampus and surrounding MTL (medial temporal lobe) structures rather than on the number of pyramidal neurons in CA1.[6] Such a wide inclusion is problematic, for it is unlikely that neurons with different structures and connections are operating in the same way and share the same function. Even if the calculation is based solely on the numbers of neurons in the hippocampus, the pyramidal cells clearly differ from the granule and other cells. Further, Andersen and his Oslo co-workers showed that information flowed from the CA4 pyramids in the dentate nucleus to the CA1 pyramids in the main body of the hippocampus, suggesting that the CA1 cells would be the final repositories of 'memory'. If Waydo et al.'s calculation, like the present one, was based solely on the CA1 cells available and on the number responding, rather than on the whole MTL, then the results would be much closer.

There is one factor, however, that was overlooked in both calculations— the presence of 'silent' cells. Though occasional silent cells were encountered by the Los Angeles group, the great majority of concept cells had been firing spontaneously. If the findings of Henze and colleagues[7] in the rat with their tetrode (four recording surfaces) are applicable,[8] there may have been as many silent cells as spontaneously active ones. Such a situation would not affect the previous calculations appreciably, provided the spontaneous activity was distributed randomly throughout the CA1 cell population. If, on the other hand, *entire* cell populations coding for specific memories were silent, the estimated number of cells per memory would be correspondingly diminished, as would the convergence of different memories on to the same pyramidal neuron.

Regardless of the presence of silent cells, the conclusion from the present calculations, that several different memories must be coded for by the same hippocampal neuron, is borne out by experiment. In their 2015 paper the Los Angeles group reported finding a cell that responded to photographs of two actresses (Jennifer Aniston and Lisa Kudrow), another cell firing to pictures of two buildings (the Eiffel Tower and Leaning Tower of Pisa), and a third to images of two Star Wars characters (Yoda and Luke Skywalker).[9] In a later review Quian Quiroga has taken the issue of linkage further, emphasizing that a hippocampal neuron does not necessarily have to code for items of the same class (i.e. people, buildings, or objects) but rather for any items that are associated in some way. As recounted earlier, his group had been able to show that a concept cell that initially responded only to pictures of the actor, Josh Brolin, could be made to fire to images of the Eiffel Tower as well, once the subject had been shown pictures of Brolin with the Eiffel Tower.[10]

The idea of concept cells coding for 'associations' has added importance in that it could explain episodic memories.[11] As an example, the memory of a car accident might he contained in individual neurons coding respectively for wreckage, for police cars with flashing lights, and for the location of the incident. This idea, that an episodic memory might be the combination of several semantic memories, is not so far from Frederic Bartlett's distant proposal that memories are reconstructions (and therefore open to error).[12]

The tendency of one memory to call up another is something we all experience.

Perhaps the most famous literary example is Proust's evocation of a childhood in Combray, a series of recollections initiated by the taste of a madeleine that had been softened in a cup of tea.

> But, when nothing subsists of an old past, after the death of people, after the destruction of things, alone, frailer but more enduring, more immaterial, more persistent, more faithful, smell and taste still remain for a long time, like souls, remembering....[13]

In my own case, and perhaps for most people, it is usually vision, rather than smell or taste, that triggers memory. For example, if I think of the medical school in Newcastle upon Tyne that I attended more than 60 years ago, it is always the same scene that comes to mind—the front of the red-brick building, the parking spaces beside the two wings on either side, the heraldic shields above the entrance, the silvered bottoms of the pillars, the rotating door, and so on (Figure 42.1). But now that I have this initial picture, others come effortlessly—the physiology lecture theatre with the blackboard at the front, the experimental laboratory where we would record twitches of frog muscles on rotating drums, the anatomy dissecting room with the bodies on the tables, the bicycle racks at the rear of the building. It is as if there is a principal scene (the front of the medical school) and a number of subsidiary ones (the rooms inside). Similarly, if I think of a certain friend, I am immediately aware of his name, and then begin to see

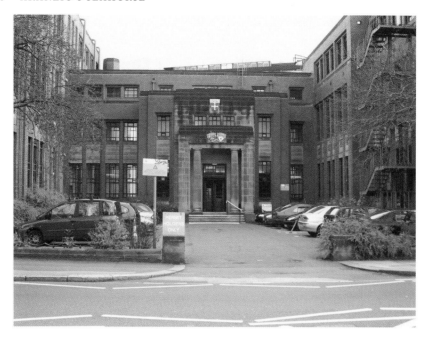

Figure 42.1 The main entrance to the former Medical School in Newcastle upon Tyne.

his house and garden, the interior of his kitchen with the day's newspaper spread on the table, the sunroom where we would have coffee in the summer, and so on.

In *The Organization of Behaviour*, the book that had such a great impact on psychology theory, Donald Hebb envisaged distinct neural assemblies that had formed synaptic connections with each other whenever there had been some linkage in the outside world. For example, in an infant the neural assembly for the sight of a mother would be linked to that for the sound of her voice The concept cell recordings have provided a different explanation for the association of memories, however—rather than by connections between large groups of cells, the different memories are represented on the same neurons.

The recordings from the Los Angeles patients (and subsequently from patients in King's College Hospital in London, following Quian Quiroga's move to the United Kingdom) tell us other important features of the hippocampus. One is that the several thousand neurons comprising a memory/concept are not grouped together in the hippocampus, as might have been anticipated, but are scattered throughout it. Why this should be is not known, but presumably there is some functional advantage and the cellular mechanisms responsible would be an interesting topic for investigation. Also unclear is the function of the concept cells found *outside* the hippocampus—those in the amygdala, entorhinal cortex, and parahippocampal cortex.

A third feature is also surprising—though the hippocampus contains powerful inhibitory neurons (the basket cells investigated by Per Andersen and John Eccles),[14] the multi-unit recordings show little, if any, inhibition of neurons surrounding a discharging concept cell. This is quite unlike the situation in the visual and somatosensory pathways where surround inhibition serves to 'sharpen' the neural signals and enhance discrimination. It may be that the function of the basket cells in the hippocampus is to dampen down excitability throughout the structure, thereby preventing 'spurious' memories from surfacing into consciousness.[15]

Another unknown aspect of hippocampal function concerns the whereabouts of new memory formation. Are new synapses formed on 'naive' neurons that had previously been uncommitted to a memory, or on cells that had already had some association with the new stimulus? And, with the passage of time, is it possible for a pyramidal neuron to 'switch' its memory content, particularly if the latter has been infrequently recalled? Could one set of synapses disappear and another set take their place?

One last but very important deduction from the concept cell recordings is that hippocampal cell activity, by itself, is unlikely to result in consciousness. Even if all the neurons coding for a particular concept were to increase their firing rate substantially (usually severalfold in experiments),[16] the effect would be lost among all the ongoing spontaneous activity in the millions of hippocampal neurons. It can only be the combination of excitation in the hippocampus with that in a sensory pathway that enables a memory to be recalled. The converse is equally important. Impulse activity restricted to the visual pathway might enable faces, animals, and buildings to be fleetingly 'seen' but without the temporal continuity and memory of the hippocampus they cannot be recognized. Clive Wearing provided a dramatic example.

While the calculations reflect the end result of all the complex synaptic activity taking place in the hippocampal complex, they leave untouched some important issues, among them the nature and importance of spatial maps in different species.

Notes

1. S. Waydo, A. Kraskov, R.Q. Quiroga, I. Fried, and C. Koch, 'Sparse Representation in the Human Medial Temporal Lobe' (2006) 26(40) *Journal of Neuroscience* 10232–4. In a later paper Waydo and Koch have taken their 'sparse coding' approach further and shown, in a mathematical model, that an AI system would be capable of learning items (e.g. faces or buildings) without prior instructions. See: S. Waydo and C. Koch, 'Unsupervised Learning of Individuals and Categories from Images' (2008) 20 *Neural Computation* 1165–78.
2. E.T. Rolls, 'A Computational Theory of Episodic Memory Formation in the Hippocampus' (2010) 215 *Behavioural Brain Research* 180–96.
3. P. Andersen, T.V.P. Bliss, and K.K. Skrede, 'Lamellar Organization of Hippocampal Excitatory Pathways' (1971) 13 *Experimental Brain Research* 222–38.
4. A.J. Harding, G.M. Halliday, and J.J. Kril, 'Variation in Hippocampal Neuron Number with Age and Brain Volume' (1998) 8 *Cerebral Cortex* 710–18. The numbers of hippocampal neurons vary considerably and 8 million was chosen for the present calculations, those being the values found for the two youngest subjects by Halliday *et al.* Other estimates for hippocampal cell numbers are given in: J.A. Cobb, J. Simpson, G.J. Mahajan, J.C. Overholser, G.H. Jurjus, L. Dieter, N. Herbst, W. May, G. Rajkowska, and C.A. Stockmeier, 'Hippocampal Volume and Total Cell Numbers in Major Depressive Disorder' (2013) 47(3) *Journal of Psychiatric Research* 299–306.

5. These are the data that Waydo and colleagues used for their calculations of sparseness ('Sparse Representation in the Human Medial Temporal Lobe', see note 1).

6. It is not clear where this estimate came from. Of the three references given in the Waydo *et al.* paper (see note 1), only one—that of Harding and colleagues—includes a reference to actual cell numbers and this was for the hippocampus rather than for 'MTL', the entire medial temporal lobe.

7. D.A. Henze, Z. Borhegyi, J. Csicsvari, A. Mamiya, K.D. Harris, and G. Buzsaki, 'Intracellular Features Predicted by Extracellular Recordings in the Hippocampus *in vivo*' (2000) 84 *Journal of Neurophysiology* 390–400.

8. This is a very big 'if' since the Henze experiments were carried out with a different type of recording electrode and on anaesthetized rats rather than on conscious humans.

9. H.G. Rey, M.J. Ison, C. Pedreira, A. Valentin, G. Alarcon, R. Selway, M.P. Richardson, and R. Quian Quiroga, 'Single-Cell Recordings in the Human Medial Temporal Lobe' (2015) 277 *Journal of Anatomy* 394–408.

10. R. Quian Quiroga, 'No Pattern Separation in the Human Hippocampus' (2020) 24(12) *Trends in Cognitive Sciences* 994–1007. doi:10.1016/j.tics.2020.09.012. Epub 2020 Nov 5. PMID: 33162337.

11. Quian Quiroga makes this novel proposal in 'No Pattern Separation in the Human Hippocampus', see note 10.

12. F.C. Bartlett, *Remembering. A Study in Experimental and Social Psychiatry* (Cambridge, UK: Cambridge University Press, 1932).

13. M. Proust, *The Way by Swann's. In Search of Lost Time*, Vol. 1, translated by Lydia Davis (London: Penguin Books, 2002).. (Original French publication in 1913). A madeleine is a small, rounded biscuit peculiar to France.

14. See Chapter 7.

15. Negative feedback via an inhibitory neuron, itself activated through an axon branch from the primary cell, is found elsewhere in the mammalian central nervous system, viz; cerebellar Purkinje cells via basket cells, neocortical deep pyramids via basket cells, α-motoneurons via Renshaw cells. It is possible that painful muscle cramps, particularly in the elderly, may result from temporary loss of Renshaw inhibition on motoneurons.

16. See: M. Cerf, N. Thirunvengadam, F. Mormann, A. Kraskov, R.Q. Quiroga, and I. Fried, 'On-line, Voluntary Control of Human Temporal Lobe Neurons' (2010) 467(7319) *Nature* 104–8. In this paper Figure 4 shows the average increase in firing rate for a number of concept cells when the patient was concentrating on the subject. In contrast to the modest human values, the firing rate of a *rat* hippocampal 'place cell' (the rat equivalent of the human 'concept cell') can accelerate from a resting value of one impulse per second to 100 impulses a second whenever an animal arrives at a certain position in its neighbourhood (H. Eichenbaum, P. Dudchenko, E. Wood, M. Shapiro, and H. Tarili, 'The hippocampus, memory and place cells: is it spatial memory or a memory space?' (1999) 23 *Neuron* 209–26).

43

Speculations on Spatial Maps and Other Issues

In a rat, once a map of the surroundings is formed in the hippocampus, certain cells will fire whenever the animal is in a particular location, as originally shown by John O'Keefe and Jonathan Dostrovsky.[1] The activity of these 'place cells' informs the rat of its exact position and enables the animal to navigate appropriately. There is now increasing evidence, gathered from single cell recordings in patients with epilepsy, of the existence of place cells in the human hippocampus and allied structures also. Rather than have the subjects move from one location to another, the human experiments have made use of virtual reality. In the study by Andreas Schulze-Bonhage and his colleagues at the University of Freiburg, Germany, the subjects were required to deliver a different virtual object to each of a succession of virtual stores situated at various points in the visual field.[2] When an object was subsequently recalled to mind and its name spoken, increased firing was observed in the 'place' neurons coding for the location of that object. Just as important as the place cells were neurons sensitive to the direction that the virtual traveller was taking in moving from one store to another.

In comparing human and rodent behaviour in relation to their respective spatial maps, however, there are several significant differences between the species. One of them is that a rat, having constructed a map, can use it to navigate successfully in the dark, something most humans are unable to do. In my own case, unexpected power failures leave me, with outstretched arms, colliding with chairs, tables, and other objects on my way to finding a torch, despite familiarity with the previously lighted room. Nor is my spatial mapping very successful in daylight—driving to an address in a city for the first time soon leaves me unaware of the numbers of turns and intervening distances that have been taken.

And yet there is a case to be made that, in the end, most of our conscious activities are based on spatial maps—visual maps, that is. Suppose, for example, that one is walking through a park (Figure 43.1). At first one's glance may be directed to the path leading to a pavilion. Within the next few seconds the rapid saccadic movements of the eyes transfer the gaze to the pavilion itself, first to one corner of the roof then to another, and then down to the pillars on either side of the stage. In this way an image of the front of the building is created and recognized as such by concept cells in the hippocampus. Now, out of the corner of the eye movement is caught and the head turns slightly to observe a child running towards a swing and concept cells for child and swing will now fire. However the activity of the various concept cells—those for path, pavilion, child, and swing—will be associated with impulse activity in hippocampal place cells corresponding to the positions of the objects in the combined visual fields.

Aranzio's Seahorse and the Search for Memory and Consciousness. Alan J. McComas, Oxford University Press.
© Oxford University Press 2023. DOI: 10.1093/oso/9780192868244.003.0045

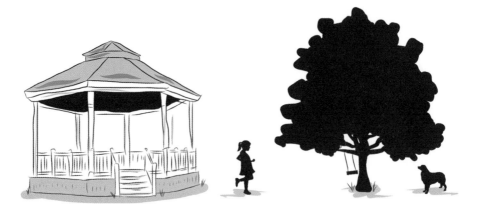

Figure 43.1 Elements in a hypothetical hippocampal spatial map (see text).

We are, in fact, continuously creating object-related spatial maps during out waking hours. Importantly, it is the prolonged discharges in the hippocampal cells (the long-term potentiation discovered by Bliss and Lomø)[3] that provides the time necessary for the objects and parts of objects in different parts of the visual field(s) to be integrated into the unified picture.

The scene in the park, just described, was unremarkable. A tree branch did not fall across the path, the pavilion did not catch fire, and the child was not attacked by a loose dog. Had any of these events occurred there would have been added significance to the scene and some emotion generated in the viewer, enough perhaps for an episodic memory of the occasion to be created and stored in the hippocampus (through the action of the amygdala).

Hippocampal mapping may even be taking place as this book is being read. The two open pages at any instant will fill the visual field. Within the field the margins are noted, together with the presence or absence of an illustration, the positions of the words in relation in relation to each other, and the sequence of alphabetical letters within each word. Combined, the different features give meaning to what is seen.

A person denied the opportunity for visual mapping because of congenital blindness will create other types of spatial map. Objects within reach are touched and a tactile map constructed as the fingers explore the surfaces and estimate sizes and features. Similarly, auditory maps evolve though the reception of sounds from different directions. In all three instances—visual, auditory, and tactile—the maps are laid out in the hippocampus. Common to these maps is the perception of distance; other things being equal, near objects have more significance and evoke the strongest discharges in the hippocampal cells.[4]

An intriguing feature of hippocampal mapping is that it can be consciously employed as a strategy for memorizing substantial numbers of objects, places, words, and people. Sometimes used as a trick at parties, the method allocates each object to a different position within an imagined enclosure—for example, to a different room in a house. During recall, one then works one's way mentally through the house, visualizing the object associated with each of the visited rooms.[5] Something similar occurs on a larger scale, especially in the elderly. A person may forget the reason for entering a room; a return to the previous room restores the purpose and the next sortie is successful.

Returning to the comparison of hippocampal neural activity in humans and rodents, it was mentioned that place cells in the rat only fired when the animal was physically present at a particular location; in humans, by contrast, it was sufficient for the location to be seen. A likely explanation for the difference between the species is that the usefulness of the place cells altered over the course of evolution. In the rat they were needed to guide the animal back to a source of food or to return it to its nest in a wall; the information was essential for the rat's survival. In humans, however, 'what' could become of interest irrespective of 'where." The Grand Canyon or Niagara Falls are memorable regardless of whether the respective images have been seen in a book, during a film or on TV—but the corresponding memories are unlikely to have survival value for the individual retaining them. Since the linkage between 'what' and 'where' is no longer obligatory it became possible for the human hippocampus to store *semantic* information in addition to creating memories for *episodic* events.

There are other differences in hippocampal functioning between rodents and humans. In a rat there is very often a reward, perhaps an item of food, associated with a particular location. Such an association would result in 'pleasure' neurons firing in the reward centre (the nucleus accumbens) whenever the respective place cells were excited. Similarly, an unfortunate visit to a backyard containing a cat could result in synaptic linkage between other place cells and limbic neurons responsible for pain and fear. In humans, however, most of the spatial mapmaking in the human hippocampus, especially that responsible for semantic memories, is devoid of emotional content.

Yet another distinction between humans and rodents is the respective use made of the various senses in creating the spatial maps. In humans vision dominates, as reflected in the large area of cerebral cortex devoted it. Rats, however, have smaller eyes and fewer neurons in the visual pathway, while the closeness of the head to the ground affords a poor vantage point. Although a rat's vision is used to create the boundaries of a spatial map, it is likely that smell is an important identifier for the place cells; the same is probably true for dogs, given their habit of marking out territories with drops of urine. In simpler creatures, particularly those from earlier branches of the evolutionary tree, chemosensation is the primary sense and must therefore be paramount in whatever primitive mapping is possible in their respective nervous systems.[6]

(1) *The origin of the hexagonal grid arrangement in the entorhinal cortex for positional information.* The discovery of place cells in the hippocampus by John O'Keefe and Jonathan Dostrovsky had been unexpected but not difficult to absorb into neural theory. In contrast, the grid cells that Edvard and May-Britt Moser had found in the entorhinal cortex were simply bizarre.[7] How had the hexagonal fields of the cells come about and what was the functional advantage of such an arrangement?

Regarding the latter question, the answer may be that the grid system enabled information to be held and passed on in a way that was much more economical than those found in sensory systems. In the human somatosensory pathway, for example, each of the neurons in the cortical primary receiving area respond to touching a small area of skin on the body surface. The pathway can be traced from the receptors in the skin, through the peripheral nerve fibres in the arm or leg into the spinal cord and then through the dorsal column nuclei and a new set of fibres to neurons in the thalamus, and then through a final set of fibres to the postcentral gyrus in the cerebral hemisphere. The end result is that each cortical cell responds to touching a small area of skin, just as the receptors did in the periphery.[8] Put together, the small areas form a map of the body surface. Similarly, in the visual system, it is easy to see how ganglion cells with concentric receptive fields in the retina are succeeded by cells with similar receptive fields in the lateral geniculate nucleus and then in the primary receiving area within the occipital lobe. Just as in the somatosensory system, when the responses of the visual cells are combined, they form a map, in this case of the visual field. (Through convergence of outputs, the visual cortex then goes on to have higher-order cells with linear receptive fields—lines, bars, slits, and edges—as Hubel and Wiesel had shown in their Nobel Prize-winning experiments in the 1950s and 1960s).[9]

In contrast, each grid cell was found by the Mosers to respond to a large number of positions of a rat within its environment. If the animal's enclosure was small, the points were close together; if the rat's surroundings were more extensive the points were further apart. The recognition of the territorial boundaries depended both on what the rat could see and on how far it travelled in its explorations. If lines were drawn through the points at which a single entorhinal cell fired, they would form a hexagonal grid. The illustrations provided by the Mosers in their publications indicated that a single entorhinal neuron would fire if the rat visited any one of a hundred or so positions (points) in its surroundings. Further, the Mosers showed that any position of the rat could be pinpointed by the overlapping of only eight grids. Thus, rather than a minimum of 100 entorhinal neurons being required to code for 100 positions (in a hypothetical sensory pathway), 13 grid cells (100 ÷ 8) could perform the same function—a very significant economy.

But how had this extraordinary grid cell arrangement evolved? This is a question that the Mosers have attempted to answer.[10] One suggestion is that grids are formed by interference between oscillatory trains of impulses in the theta range, but it transpires that fruit bats have grid cells without theta oscillations while in monkeys, theta activity only occurs intermittently, though grid cells remain present. Other theoretical models are based on 'attractor' circuits or on competitive inhibition.

There is another possibility that deserves consideration, however, and it stems from the work of Richard Axel and Linda Buck on the olfactory system, discussed earlier.[11] Using optogenetics, they showed that there was a spatial representation for odours not only in the olfactory bulb of a mammal but in its insect equivalent, the antennal lobe of a fruit fly. In the mouse they had found that, although the receptors for more than a thousand different odours were scattered among the epithelial cells lining the inside of the nose, the paths of the nerve fibres from the receptor cells were organized so that each odour was represented by two small neuron clusters (glomeruli) at a specific location in the olfactory bulb, the next stage in the olfactory pathway. Axel and Buck had shown that the mouse genome included the instructions for the creation of a spatial map for odours. Since the entorhinal cortex is the next stage in the olfactory pathway, it seems possible that the hexagonal maps of grid cells evolved from the glomerular maps of the olfactory bulb.

(2) *What is the function of the granule cells in the dentate nucleus?* The small granule cells, tightly packed into a single layer in the dentate nucleus, vastly outnumber the pyramidal cells in the adjacent CA4 region of the hippocampus.[12] Comparison with other regions of the brain and spinal cord suggests that the granule cells are unlikely to be interneurons that simply regulate the firing of the pyramidal cells, since relatively few are required for this function, as exemplified by the inhibitory basket cells studied by Andersen and Eccles in Canberra.[13] Nor are the granule cells likely to be shaping the response characteristics of the pyramidal cells, since this has already been done by neurons elsewhere in the temporal lobe—the cells that have been shown to respond to faces and objects, for example. Further, the granule cells are unusual neurons in that they are being constantly turned over, new ones being created as others die[14]—a phenomenon that is difficult to reconcile with the permanence of memories.

One suggestion is that the granule cells act in concert with the pyramidal cells in the final stage of the hippocampal pathway (CA1), serving as non-specific neural amplifiers for messages coded by the concept cells. The analogy of a radio comes to mind, with the volume control represented by granule cells and the wavelength (station) by the concept cells.[15]

(3) *Combination of different modalities in hippocampus to create concept cells.* At some point in the hippocampal complex there is convergence of different sensory modalities, in order to explain the existence of concept cells in CA1 that are responsive to both the image of a person or place and to its spoken or written name. Anatomical studies show that this convergence occurs in the entorhinal cortex, the visual and auditory systems adding to the olfactory pathway that had evolved earlier.

Notes

1. See Chapter 16.
2. J.F. Miller, M. Neufang, A. Solway, A, Brandt, M. Trippel, I. Mader, S. Hefft, M. Merkow, S.M. Polyn, J. Jacobs, M.J. Kahana, and A. Schulze-Bonhage, 'Neural Activity in Human Hippocampal Formation Reveals the Spatial Context of Retrieved Memories' (2013) 342(6162) *Science* 1111–14.

See also: J. Jacobs, C.T. Weiderman, J.F. Miller, A. Solway, J. Burke, X.-X. Wei, N. Suthana, M. Sperling, A.D. Sharan, I. Fried, and M.J. Kahana, 'Direct Recordings of Grid-Like Neuronal Activity in Human Spatial Navigation' (2013) 16(9) *Nature Neuroscience* 1188–90.

3. See Chapter 15.

4. See Jacobs *et al.*, 'Direct Recordings of Grid-Like Neuronal Activity in Human Spatial Navigation', see note 2.

5. It is a very effective method. At a party one usually has to remember multiple objects (e.g. a coin, hairbrush, spoon, playing card, etc.) placed on a tray. I have used the strategy to think affectionately of deceased colleagues, family, and friends, visualizing each of them sitting in different pews within my usual church.

6. As discussed in depth in Chapter 36.

7. See Chapter 21, also: T. Hafting, M. Fyhn, S. Molden, M.-B. Moser, and E.I. Moser, 'Microstructure of a Spatial Map in the Entorhinal Cortex' (2005) 436 *Nature* 801–6.

8. T.P. Powell and V.B. Mountcastle, 'Some Aspects of the Functional Organization of the Cortex of the Postcentral Gyrus of the Monkey: A Correlation of Findings Obtained in a Single Unit Analysis with Cytoarchitecture' (1959) 105 *Bulletin of the Johns Hopkins Hospital* 133–62.

9. For the most readable account of visual neurophysiology, see: D.H. Hubel. *Eye, Brain and Vision* (New York, NY: Freeman, 1988).

10. See Hafting *et al.*, 'Microstructure of a Spatial Map in the Entorhinal Cortex', see note 7.

11. R. Axel, 'Scents and Sensibility. A Molecular Logic of Olfactory Perception' Nobel Lecture, 2004. <http://www.nobelprize.org/uploads/2018/06/axel-lecture.pdf> accessed 24 April 2022.

12. J.A. Cobb, J. Simpson, G.J. Mahajan, J.C. Overholser, G.H. Jurjus, L. Dieter, N. Herbst, W. May, G. Rajkowska, and C.A. Stockmeier, 'Hippocampal Volume and Total Cell Numbers in Major Depressive Disorder' (2013) 47(3) *Journal of Psychiatric Research* 299–306.

13. As shown by Andersen in Oslo; see P. Andersen, *The History of Neuroscience in Autobiography*, L.R. Squire (ed.) (San Diego, CA: Academic Press, 2004) 4: 2–39.

14. See Chapter 25.

15. Another analogy would be a public orator and a crowd. Without an audience the orator (concept cell) can proclaim but no-one takes notice. With a large responsive audience (granule cells), however, the authorities become aware (consciousness) and may need to respond (motor act).

44

Final Note: The Multi-Tasking Hippocampus

The first part of the book presented, in historical form, the body of evidence linking the hippocampal complex to learning and memory. The second part argued that the hippocampus generated consciousness—the latter being short-term memory. Memory and consciousness are surely two of the most important properties of a nervous system but, for reasons already given, it turns out that the hippocampus is involved in other functions as well. As described earlier, Cornelius Vanderwolf detected the onset of rhythmic electrical activity in the hippocampus prior to movement, suggesting that the structure was concerned in the initiation the latter.[1] The same author, using similar technology, had shown the hippocampus to be part of the olfactory system.[2]

Memory, movement, and olfaction are important enough, but other functions have also been attributed to the hippocampus, some set out in the proceedings of a meeting devoted to this issue;[3] they include roles in appetite and hunger, in the response to stress and in regulation of the autonomic nervous system. Through the work of John O'Keefe, presented earlier in the book, the hippocampus had been shown capable of constructing spatial maps by means of 'place' (and other) cells. And long before that, the hippocampus had been identified by James Papez as part of a neural circuit responsible for engendering emotion, and by Paul MacLean as a key element in one of the components in a 'triune brain'.[4]

Given so many functions, it is tempting to compare the hippocampus to a city—both have unique locations and both have important connections to other regions; with births and deaths, both have slowly changing populations. Like the neurons in the hippocampus, the inhabitants of a city have different occupations, some in manufacturing (factories), others in education (schools, colleges, and university), some in food and hospitality (hotels, restaurants), some in health (clinics and hospitals), others in recreation (parks, sports fields, swimming pools), and so on. Extending the analogy further, just as a city may become the seat of government for a region or an entire country, so might the hippocampus have evolved into the chief administrator for the entire nervous system.

Notes

1. C.H. Vanderwolf, 'Limbic-Diencephalic Mechanisms of Voluntary Movement' (1971) 78 *Psychology Review* 83–113.
2. C.H. Vanderwolf, 'The Hippocampus as an Olfacto-Motor Mechanism: Were the Classical Anatomists Right After All?' (2001) 127(1–2) *Behavioural Brain Research* 25–47.

Aranzio's Seahorse and the Search for Memory and Consciousness. Alan J. McComas, Oxford University Press.
© Oxford University Press 2023. DOI: 10.1093/oso/9780192868244.003.0046

3. See: *Psychology Review* 1971, volume 78, for the proceedings of a meeting to discuss non-memory aspects of the hippocampus.
4. See Chapter 31.

E.

RECAPITULATION, SYNTHESIS, AND EPILOGUE

45

Recapitulation and Synthesis

This book has been about memory and its relationship to consciousness. It has been a story about different approaches to understanding the nervous system—evolution, neurophysiology, clinical neurology, and, most recently, optogenetics.

The story began with the discovery of the hippocampus by Aranzio in the 16th century and, after a gap of several hundred years, continued with the descriptions of its internal structure and of its connections to other parts of the brain. As to its possible function, there had been a hint that had not been followed up—the great 19th-century neurologist, Hughlings Jackson, had described a patient with disordered consciousness (a 'dreamy state') associated with a tumour in the hippocampal region. To the anatomists and physiologists, however, the hippocampus remained an enigma. Although it had been relegated to being part of a primitive 'smell' brain (rhinencephalon), even that function had been disputed by Alf Brodal, one of the few anatomists interested in the hippocampus.

And then, in 1957, quite unexpectedly, had come publication of the paper of William Scoville and Brenda Milner with its description of memory loss following bilateral resection of the hippocampus in a young man with epilepsy. The study had been the outcome of a fortunate conjunction of a bold and skilful neurosurgeon, a well-trained and very able psychologist, and an intelligent and compliant patient—Henry Molaison (Patient 'H.M.'). For the first time the hippocampus had been clearly identified as essential for memory in a human subject, but there was a catch, one that may have misdirected much subsequent research. Since Henry Molaison still had short-term memory, the latter had been thought to reside elsewhere than in the hippocampus. It was only when the brain was subjected to careful post-mortem examination a half-century later that appreciable hippocampal tissue was found to have survived surgery.

One of the many to be influenced by Scoville and Milner's paper and its unique findings would be the aspiring psychiatrist Eric Kandel. Forsaking a clinical career, Kandel would embark on a series of electrophysiological and biochemical studies in *Aplysia*, a giant sea slug, that would ultimately reveal the cellular mechanisms involved in creating a memory. However, it was O'Keefe and Dostrovsky's discovery of 'place cells' that had provided the second great advance in understanding the role of the hippocampus and, like so much of science, it had started with a chance observation—in this case, the recording of impulse activity with a misplaced electrode. The impact of O'Keefe's work was heightened by a video showing the building-up of a map in the rat hippocampus as the animal explored its surroundings. It was

Aranzio's Seahorse and the Search for Memory and Consciousness. Alan J. McComas, Oxford University Press.
© Oxford University Press 2023. DOI: 10.1093/oso/9780192868244.003.0047

O'Keefe's work that paved the way for the Moser's discovery of the intriguing 'grid cells' in the neighbouring entorhinal cortex.

Some thirty years after O'Keefe's initial publication (with Jonathan Dostrovsky) the recording of impulse activity in the hippocampal area had led to another great advance, this time by Itzhak Fried, Christof Koch, Rodrigo Quian Quiroga, and others in Los Angeles. Rather than rats, the subjects had been neurological patients undergoing assessment of their temporal lobe epilepsy and it was they who revealed that the hippocampus contained 'concept cells'—neurons that could be excited not only by the visual image of a particular person or building but by their spoken or written names. Different types of information about the subject had been brought together to complete a 'concept' and, when thinking about the subject, the cells had increased their impulse firing. One of the important inferences from this work was that hippocampus housed both semantic and episodic memories, with the latter possibly being derived from the former. Further, the hippocampus did not simply create neural memories and transport them to the neocortex (during sleep, as David Marr had suggested), but was itself a permanent repository. In creating both short-term and long-term memories, the hippocampal neurons were confirming Donald Hebb's postulate ('Cells that fire together, wire together') and behaving in much the same manner as the *Aplysia* neurons studied in such detail by Eric Kandel.

Even in the simple reflex circuitry of the giant sea slug there had been an additional neuron needed to bring about the lingering potentiation of the response (short-term memory). In the same way the hippocampus contains more than one type of neuron; not only are there the large pyramidal cells (the concept cells) but also smaller granule cells (replenished throughout life) and inhibitory neurons (the basket cells), as well as other types. And then, especially crucial for emotional events, there is the influence of the neighbouring amygdala in the conversion of hippocampal short-term memory to long-term. This action of the amygdala illustrates an important point—the hippocampus does not act alone but is dependent on adjacent structures. In addition to the amygdala, there is the entorhinal cortex (supplying sensory information to the hippocampus) and the subiculum (an important source of outgoing fibres). And, of course, many structures further afield also connect to the hippocampus and are affected by it.

The studies summarized above all pointed to the importance of the hippocampus (or, rather, the hippocampal complex) for creating and storing memories. While there would be little argument that such memories are a prominent feature of our consciousness, the second part of the book went further. It attempted to show that, rather than being a feature, memory *is* our consciousness—that we live in a constantly changing and evolving short-term memory, and that the hippocampal complex is where this consciousness is being generated. There were two strong hints that this is the case in the work already referred to. One was the production of abnormal 'dreamy states' by lesions in the hippocampal region, some of them preceded by spontaneous *odours*— of burning, for example. The second hint, equally important, was the observation that thinking about a person or object is associated with increased impulse firing by the corresponding concept cells in the hippocampus.

There was, however, an entirely different argument for the identification of consciousness with memory and this was based on evolution. The core of the argument was that the entire nervous system, a system that includes some 100 billion neurons in the human brain, nevertheless evolved as a system for producing movement. In the simplest, earliest creatures the only guidance for movement was provided by receptors sensitive to specific molecules present in the environment ('chemosensation'). Movement towards the source of these molecules was essential for nutrition and reproduction and was carried out automatically. At some point in evolution, however, the acquisition of food (or successful coupling) was associated a change in the 'state' of the creature that it was able to sense.

Other than it probably involved dopamine release, even in simple organisms, we have no idea of the nature of the reward, the changed 'state' of the creature, that caused it to respond to some chemical cues and not to others. Nevertheless a memory must have developed for those beneficial cues, enabling a creature to seek out sources of food and sex. Rudimentary as it was, this marked the beginning of a consciousness—since rewards were only effective if they could be remembered for future occasions.

The primitive chemosensory systems of the simplest organisms evolved into highly discriminative olfactory ones, with multiple types of receptors and housing systems (antennae, vomeronasal organs, etc.) and ever more complex neural wiring. At the same time other types of receptor would evolve, those for vision, hearing, and touch, with each system developing its own circuitry. These new senses added greatly to the environmental cues that could be used to food and reproduction but, as with chemosensation, were only effective if they could be remembered. Rather than develop independent memory circuits, evolution enabled the new receptors to make use of the system already in place for chemosensation—the nascent hippocampal complex.

The hippocampal complex was but the most conspicuous part of an elaborate array of interconnected neural structures, however. It had been the eminent French neurologist, Paul Broca, who had first recognized an apparent continuity between the hippocampal gyrus and a fold of grey matter immediately above the corpus callosum, regarding them as comprising a 'limbic' lobe. Later workers, tracing neural pathways,[1] would add more and more structures to this limbic 'system', envisaging it as a part of the brain concerned with emotional behaviour, the control of body functions (heart, respiration, appetite, sleep), and with pain and pleasure. That this system, operating with little or no neocortex, could by itself generate consciousness was suggested by observations on children who had suffered strokes *in utero* and by the apparently rational, memory-based behaviour of certain non-mammalian species (particularly amphibians).

As to what kind of consciousness an amphibian or other animal might have, we can only surmise.[2] By their behaviours, birds and mammals appear to experience pleasure and pain, hunger, and satiety, fear and anger, and they obviously see, feel, smell, taste, and hear. There is more to their consciousness than this, however, for animals can plan courses of action and, implicitly, must have created body images—and with the images, a sense of 'self'. A crow, confronted with an otherwise inaccessible source of food, may find a twig or bend a piece of wire to bring the tasty object within reach. A squirrel will contemplate a new birdfeeder before climbing a nearby tree, running along a particular branch and jumping on to the feeder above the baffle intended to keep it at bay. In instances such as these the animal is obviously capable of imagining a future chain of events and is 'thinking' in visual terms, much as a congenitally deaf human may come to think in American Sign Language.

Humans with speech and hearing, however, not only contemplate the future visually but think with an interior voice, one capable of providing a continuous commentary during the course of the day. For obvious reasons this type of thinking is absent at birth and only appears two or more years later, after an elementary grammar and vocabulary have been acquired. This auditory consciousness is most obvious when we are sitting or lying down with the eyes closed and spatial maps are no longer being created (though they may be imagined or remembered). Thinking in sound is unlikely to be limited to humans, however, but a skill acquired by other mammals with large brains. A dolphin, for example, appears to listen to a series of clicks uttered by another dolphin before responding with its own series, just as happens in a conversation between two people.[3] In humans the hippocampus and other parts of the temporal lobe are heavily involved in the auditory consciousness. The evidence comes from the presence of hippocampal concept cells responsive to spoken names, from amygdaloid neurons firing to specific sounds (O'Keefe's early work), and the jumbled speech of patients with damage to the superior temporal lobe (previously termed 'sensory' or 'Wernicke's' dysphasia). As Konorski proposed, there are likely to be gnostic units, presumably in the temporal lobe, that code for ever more elaborate elements of speech—a hierarchy that progresses from sounds and words to phrases and sentences.[4]

The preceding discussion began with the role of memory in the evolution of consciousness in animal species, including the primate *Homo sapiens*. Earlier in the book mention was made of an entirely different, non-evolutionary, kind of argument for considering memory as the essence of consciousness. This approach had to do with the minimum time required for a sensory perception or a thought. To speak a sentence aloud requires a few seconds for the words to be uttered and a similar, perhaps slightly shorter, time, would be needed if the same words comprised an unspoken thought. However, the thought is only complete if the beginning of the sentence is held in memory until the end is reached. When the amnesic Clive Wearing stated that he had never had a thought, it may well have meant that he had never been conscious long enough for anything more than a momentary awareness of something—his short-term memory was too brief for a train of thought to develop. Just as thoughts require time, so do perceptions. The compilation of visual and other sensory information to construct a spatial map is not instantaneous, nor can movements or sounds be appreciated without integration of the respective stimuli over time.

In a person with a fully functioning hippocampal complex the short-term memory is sufficient not only for the construction of thoughts but for the registration of his or her surroundings and of any events taking place. We live in an ever-changing short-term memory. For example, I am presently aware that I am sitting on a chair in front of my desk, my fingers tapping away at the computer keyboard. The fact that two minutes ago

I was in the kitchen, pouring boiling water into a coffee mug, has already gone out of my mind. If I think about what I was doing before resuming work on my laptop, I can come up with an image of the kitchen, the kettle on the countertop, the window looking out over the back garden, and so on. But, unless something unexpected had happened while I was in the kitchen, all of these images were reconstructions from long-term memory rather than 'true' recollections of what actually happened. Coffee-making had been a trivial event, something that had been performed on numerous other days and not associated with any emotional content. What benefit could there be in remembering it? And so, as the day progresses, one short-term memory seamlessly succeeds another, creating consciousness as it does so. We could represent the situation with a figure (Figure 45.1).

The figure assumes that, during waking hours, the amygdala is constantly supplying low-level excitation to the hippocampus, even though it is not critical for short-term memory. However, the amygdaloid input increases dramatically should there be a major, emotive event. As consciousness gives way to sleep the short-term memories will have long since faded but the synaptic strengthening engineered by the amygdala persists and, with it, the (long-term) memory of the major event. Though the duration of Henry Molaison's short-term memory was estimated at around 30 seconds, it is likely that the duration fluctuates, depending on the state of the brain. It is a common experience that, despite considerable mental effort, the names of a small group of people may be almost instantly forgotten after introductions have been made. Since short-term memory is dependent on synaptic potentiation, and since animal experiments have shown the latter to be diminished by stress, this embarrassing behaviour might be expected.

That memory, short-term memory, *is* consciousness seems so obvious, how was it not appreciated as such before? The fault may have been to regard memory as but one

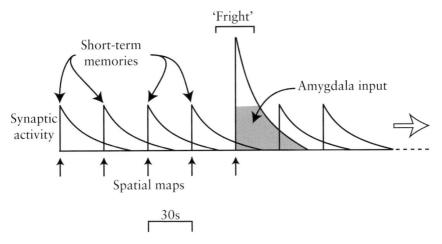

Figure 45.1 Successive short-term memories (simultaneously generating consciousness), of which one becomes long-term due to amygdaloid input. See text.

facet of consciousness, rather than constituting consciousness itself. For example, in describing an elderly relative, we might say:

> 'Aunt Edith is still able to read without glasses. Her memory is fine, too, and she manages to get out for a daily walk through the park.'

In this illustration, memory has been put on a par with reading and walking, rather than as the very essence of the person under discussion. Aunt Edith *is* her memory. Should she be unlucky enough to develop Alzheimer's disease in a few years, and to lose both short- and long-term memory, we might say:

> 'We visited Aunt Edith but she was totally "out of it." She never even knew who we were. She seemed totally confused and unaware of her surroundings.'

Without short-term (and long-term) memory, Aunt Edith's consciousness was diminished. Though still able to respond to immediate stimuli—the switching on and off of lights, the sound of the gong announcing dinner, the presence of another person in her room—she had lost her own identity. The 'Edith-ness' had gone. Were it to be examined post-mortem, Edith's hippocampus would almost certainly exhibit severe degenerative changes, in keeping with the findings in hippocampi of other similarly affected persons.[5]

The equating of consciousness with short-term memory and the attribution of both to the function of the hippocampal complex still leaves the 'hard' problem awaiting a solution. How is it that impulses in nerve cells can be translated into colours, sounds, and tastes, and also into thoughts and the sense of self? In searching for their 'neural correlates of consciousness' (the NCC), Christof Koch and Francis Crick appreciated that, even if they were to succeed in identifying the brain circuitry responsible for generating consciousness, it would leave the hard problem unsolved. And that remains the situation today. Not only does a solution to the hard problem remain evasive but it is impossible to imagine any sort of experiment that might help. There are no bridging steps conceivable between the impulse and the expression of consciousness.

This impasse raises the possibility that we are confronted by a phenomenon of Nature—that consciousness is a necessary consequence of impulse activity in neural circuits shaped by earlier processing of sensory information about an organism and its environment. This is admittedly vague but the intention should be clear. If certain neurons (those in the hippocampal complex in vertebrate brains) have 'learnt' and subsequently become active, consciousness inevitably follows. Rather than regarding the seemingly magical transformation of neural electricity into thoughts and sensations as a supremely difficult problem awaiting solution, it should be accepted as a natural phenomenon. In this view there is no 'in-between'—no hitherto unidentified molecules, no psychic 'force', no quantum mechanics. It just *is*.

Given the extraordinary cognitive abilities of human (and other) brains, together with the range and detail of our sensory perceptions, a phenomenological answer to the hard problem may be difficult to accept. The task is easier, however, if consciousness is seen as a property that evolved over tens of millions of years and that began with a chemically based primordial memory in a primitive creature. And there is a philosophical point to be made. Why should it be any more difficult to accept the equivalence of consciousness and impulse activity in programmed neural circuits than the equivalence, say, of matter and energy in the physical world? Before Einstein, the latter would have been inconceivable to most people and, even now, evokes a sense of wonderment.

If consciousness is indeed short-term memory mediated by hippocampal neurons, what are the consequences for other theories of consciousness? The first obvious casualty is panpsychism, the idea that an elemental consciousness is a feature of all matter. Also untenable is the concept of consciousness as an inevitable consequence of any information processing system with sufficient branching and feedback (computer algorithms, for example). Nor should we be concerned about the possibility of consciousness in automated lawnmowers, vacuum cleaners, and washing machines. However, though it is unlikely, the possibility of consciousness cannot be excluded in a continuously active physical 'learning' system, one that included transducers and circuitry for the acquisition, processing, and storage of information about the state of the system and that of its surroundings. In the end, neurons are themselves aggregates of atomic particles subjected to the laws of quantum mechanics and electromotive forces. Indeed, it is just possible that Alexa, Siri, and Google are more than cleverly engineered gadgets.

The primary importance of the hippocampal complex raises an important question about the remainder of the brain, one that Sir Francis Walshe had been cognizant of. If they are not the immediate source of consciousness, what are the two cerebral hemispheres for?

The answer is that the neocortex is an extremely sophisticated and powerful sensory analyser, one that initially enabled ever more accurate and appropriate movements necessary for life of the individual and procreation of the species. Further, it was the sensory information provided by the neocortex that enabled an infant to acquire its sense of self. At the present stage of evolution the neocortex is employed for much more, however—it is essential for planning the events of the day, it allows world events to be learned from the newspaper, it permits music to be enjoyed from the radio, and, in the case of a physicist, it enables elementary atomic particles to be visualized in the mind. All of this is possible because there is a huge memory in the neocortex (especially the temporal lobe)—memory not just of faces but of cars, trains, trees, houses, drawings, photographs, pieces of music, geometric shapes, mathematical equations, and so on. All of these memories correspond to the 'gnostic units' posited by Jerzy Konorski; they are neurons that have 'learned' to respond selectively to increasingly complex features of the environment.

The consensus among neuroscientists is that the sensory pathways can generate perceptions without reference to the hippocampus. If Clive Wearing had had total destruction of both hippocampi, his ability to see and hear in the acute stage of his illness would have been good evidence for such a proposition. As it is, the full extent of Clive's hippocampal damage is still unknown and it is possible that a residuum is still functioning (and responsible for his few seconds of short-term memory). On the basis of the minimum time argument, it seems possible that the sensory pathways, by themselves, are insufficient and that the very act of seeing (and hearing) is dependent on the hippocampus. As suggested previously, the time-chunking behaviour of the neocortex may render it incapable of creating a perception. While this matter must remain moot, at least for now, there can be little argument that it is the hippocampus that binds the various objects seen into a coherent picture (spatial map), enables objects to be recognized, and links the visual information to that from other sensory pathways.

Normally, the mind's traffic is one-way and dependent on what we are looking at, or listening to, at the moment. The path is from receptors through neocortical analysers (with their gnostic units) to the hippocampus and conscious perception. But how well does the system function in the reverse direction, from hippocampus to neocortex? Suppose we close our eyes and try to imagine a place, a person, or a physical activity such as playing tennis. For most people the construct has poor resolution, the faces and surroundings are not sharply defined nor are the colours bright. The same is true for dreams, for here again the brain is creating imagery in the absence of ongoing sensory information. Presumably the excitation in the sensory neurons recruited by the hippocampus during imagining and dreaming is less than that occurring during a natural sensory experience (Figure 45.2).

Remarkably, in the case of dreams, the brain is able to construct a narrative to give credibility to the images thrown up by spontaneously active groups of hippocampal neurons; so compelling are the stories that we experience fear and joy in their mental enactment, followed by a sense of wonder when we wake. An important feature of our dreams, one indicative of hippocampal involvement, is that we do not see objects, buildings, or people in isolation but as elements in changing scenes ('artificial' spatial maps). The same is true of our visual memory, for if someone is being spoken of or otherwise thought about, the image of the person will come to mind not against a featureless grey background but within an appropriate setting—a certain room in their house, the restaurant where you lunched together, or the footpath followed in a country walk. The various associations suggest that, not only episodic memories but semantic ones too, are held in hippocampal memory as spatial maps.[6]

There is also the matter of 'volition', an important part of consciousness, to be considered. For example, we may decide to leave work early and to call in at a flower shop on the way home. While walking to our home we may consult a mental list as to what to have for dinner. After dinner we will watch a certain programme on TV, but first we have to telephone a friend. All of these intended actions appear to be the result of choice—of volition. But are they?

The decision to leave work early followed a glance at the clock. The decision to buy flowers was prompted by the sight of bunches for sale outside the flower shop. Hunger pangs initiated the thoughts about dinner. And so on. In each case, something seen, heard, or felt ultimately excited memory neurons in the hippocampus and, through existing synaptic connections, excited others. Neurons responsive to the sight of the clock were linked to those for the 'EXIT' sign above the door to the office. 'Flower' neurons

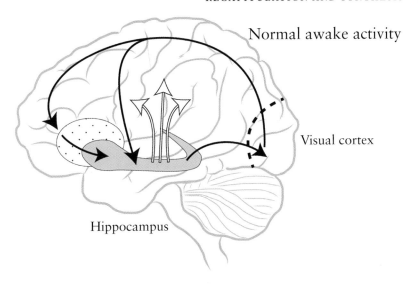

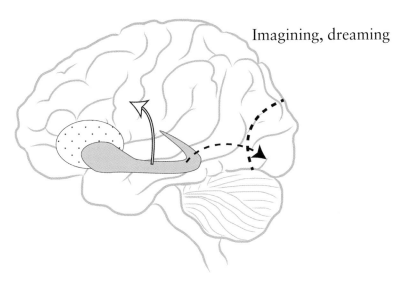

Figure 45.2 Hippocampal inputs and outputs during normal sensory experience (*Upper*) and during imagining or dreaming (*Lower*).

were connected to 'wife' neurons. In each case the excitation of the hippocampal neurons conjured up a picture, a word, or an imagined action.

The idea that what we conceive as 'will' is actually a response is consistent with the results of two very different types of study, by Michael Gazzinaga and Benjamin Libet respectively. Gazzinaga, carrying on with the human 'split-brain' studies pioneered by Roger Sperry, found patients in whom the dominant left hemisphere could fabricate intentions for actions executed by the right hemisphere—actions of which the left hemisphere had previously been unaware.[7] In Libet's study, one of the most famous in experimental psychology, healthy subjects were required to note the moment they became

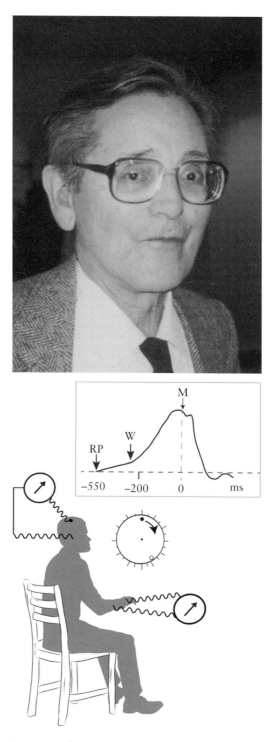

Figure 45.3 *Upper.* Benjamin Libet, attending a conference and appearing much younger than his 80 years (photograph by author). *Lower.* Libet's experiment. The subject noted the position of a spot tracing a circular path on the oscilloscope screen at the time he or she became aware of the 'will'(*W*) to move the hand (*M*, movement). Scalp electrodes recorded a negative readiness potential (*RP*) beginning some 250ms earlier.

aware of the intention to move. This time was found to lag some 250 milliseconds be-hind a surface-negative brain potential (the *bereitschaftspotential* or *readiness potential*) recorded with an electrode on the scalp (Figure 45.3).[8] Though Libet himself did not explore where in the brain the bereitschaftspotential originated, there is evidence from animal studies that the hippocampus, among other limbic structures, may develop elec-trical activity before the cortex, even one to two seconds before a movement takes place.[9] The difference in timing might be further evidence that volition, an important aspect of consciousness like perception and thinking, is also a function of the hippocampus.

If our sense of free-will is an illusion, then the same is likely to be true for 'atten-tion'—our seeming ability to direct our thoughts to this topic or that, to listen to a par-ticular passage in a piece of music or to unexpected news from a colleague, to discern a pattern in a painting or to search for an object dropped on the floor. Although it would be rather difficult to test in the same way that 'voluntary' movements were examined by Libet, it is very likely that the same kind of result would be found—that neural activity preceded a change in attention, and that the latter was not willed at all. A similar argu-ment applies to 'imagination,' the basis for the greatest creativity of which the human brain is capable. Given what is now known about the properties of concept cells in the human hippocampus, is it not likely that 'imagination' is largely due to the different kinds of stimuli that may excite the same cell? Two or more female actresses, perhaps, or similar buildings, snatches of music or mathematical equations? And sights and sounds linking the same object or person?

Precisely how the hippocampal activity is translated into neural activity elsewhere and ultimately into a movement is a matter of conjecture. We do know that the evo-lution of the primary motor cortex (in the precentral gyrus) enabled the fingers and thumbs to perform astonishingly skillful movements. We also know that, if a move-ment has been practiced, the instructions for its execution have been 'learned' by the cerebellum, for the latter is the site of procedural memory. Clive Wearing provided a good illustration. Having lost both short-term and long-term 'declarative' memory as a consequence of the destruction of both hippocampal regions, he had neverthe-less retained a largely intact cerebellum and was still able to play piano pieces from his past. Clive could also cope with the physical activities of daily living—eating, drinking, sitting down, walking—all of them activities that he could perform automatically. His 'procedural' memory had been mostly spared.[10]

There is still much we do not know and this is especially true of the inner workings of the hippocampal complex. However, some boundaries to our ignorance have been es-tablished for we *do* know the numbers of neurons that are involved, as well as the main paths taken by impulses as information flows into and through the hippocampus. And we certainly know a great deal about concept and place cells. It is very likely that major advances will continue to come from recordings of impulse activity in single neurons of conscious human beings, while optogenetic studies (mostly in mice) will prove invalu-able in identifying the locations, types and numbers of neurons performing particular functions.

There may well be surprises along the way, though perhaps none more remarkable than the relatively recent finding linking potentially harmful self-replicating proteins— 'prions'— to memory. Once again it had been Eric Kandel who had been responsible for the advance. With Kausik Si he had identified an intracellular protein (cytoplasmic polyadenlyation element-binding element, CPEB) involved in the formation of long-term memory.[11] On examining its structure, Kandel and Si were surprised to notice a similarity to prions, and they then realized that, as a prion protein, CPEB could quickly assemble and strengthen activated synapses, making long-term memory possible. It was a robust and simple mechanism that did not depend on the transcription of DNA in the neuron nucleus. Who could have imagined that proteins capable of causing fatal neurological disorders were part of the normal memory mechanism?[12]

The present era has been remarkable for its success in the exploration and understanding of the nervous system but there is still much work to be done.

Notes

1. Some idea of the two-way connections of the hippocampus in the human brain has come from the use of tensor diffusion MRI (now the favoured methodology for intact human brains). Unfortunately, the method is not good for fibre paths between the hippocampus and the frontoparietal cortex because of interference from the fluid in the lateral ventricle. Other connections to and from the hippocampus show up well, however, especially with colouring of the fibre bundles. See: J.J. Maller, T. Welton, M. Middione, F.H. Callaghan, J.V. Rosenfeld, and S.M. Grieve, 'Revealing the Hippocampal Connectome through Super-Resolution 1150-Direction Diffusion MRI' (2019) 9 *Nature Scientific Reports* article number 2418.

2. For discussion, with examples of animal intelligence, see Chapter 4 in: A.J. McComas, *Sherrington's Loom. An Introduction to the Science of Consciousness* (New York, NY: Oxford University Press, 2019). A more extensive account of animal behaviours resembling those of humans was provided by Charles Darwin in his great work, *The Descent of Man and Selection in Relation to Sex* (London: John Murray, 1871).

3. V.A. Ryabov, 'The Study of Acoustic Signals and the Supposed Spoken Language of the Dolphin' (2016) 2 *St Petersburg Polytechnical University Journal: Physics & Mathematics* 231–9. Also: <http://dx.doi.org/10.1016/j.spjpm.2016.08.004> accessed 24 April 2022.

4. See: J. Konorski, *The Integrative Activity of the Brain* (Chicago, IL: Chicago University Press, 1967). The concept of a hierarchy of auditory gnostic units is also discussed in: A.J. McComas, *Sherrington's Loom. An Introduction to the Science of Consciousness* (New York, NY: Oxford University Press, 2019).

5. M.J. Ball, M. Fisman, V. Hachinski, W. Blume, A. Fox, V.A. Kral, A.J. Kirshen, H. Fox, and H. Merskey, 'A New Definition of Alzheimer's Disease: A Hippocampal Dementia' (1985) 1(8419) *Lancet* 14–16. In the 1970s Melvin Ball was the only neuropathologist studying Alzheimer's disease in Canada and one of the very few in the world. It took less than two decades for the socioeconomic importance of the disease to become fully appreciated (while determining many future scientific careers and creating a billion dollar industry!).

6. In contrast to the dullish images conjured up in dreaming or imagining, the hallucinations in the Charles Bonnet syndrome (in persons who have lost their sight) may involve brightly coloured solitary objects, people, or animals, suggestive of a non-hippocampal origin.

7. M.S. Gazzinaga, 'Cerebral Specialization and Interhemispheric Communication: Does the Corpus Callosum Enable the Human Condition?' (2000) 123 *Brain* 1293–326. This review surveys the extensive studies on patients with 'split' brains (brains in which the corpus callosum linking the two hemispheres was divided in an attempt to control epilepsy). The review includes a particularly striking 'chicken claw' experimental observation by Gazzinaga and Joseph LeDoux.

8. For discussion of work leading to Libet's critical experiment, and for critique of the latter, see Chapter 13 in: A.J. McComas, *Sherrington's Loom. An Introduction to the Science of Consciousness* (New York, NY: Oxford University Press, 2019).

9. C.H. Vanderwolf, 'Limbic-Diencephalic Mechanisms of Voluntary Movement' (1971) 78 *Psychology Review* 83–113.

10. In addition to the motor cortex and cerebellum, the parietal cortex is involved in the preparation for movement, as are the basal ganglia (caudate nucleus, putamen, globus pallidus, subthalamic nucleus, substantia nigra). Also pertinent is the observation that an amphibian is capable of rational behaviour and yet has no motor cortex—but does possess a limbic system, cerebellum, and basal ganglia.

11. K. Si and E.R. Kandel, 'The Role of Functional Prion-Like Proteins in the Persistence of Memory' (2016) 8 *Cold Spring Harbor Perspectives in Biology* a021774.

12. The discovery of prions and subsequently their role in such neurological disorders as kuru, Alzheimer's disease, amyotrophic lateral sclerosis, and parkinsonism is a book in itself! A brief overview that captures the mystery and excitement of prion research is: M. Brahic, 'The Jekyll and Hyde Proteins' (2021) November 13 *New Scientist* 48–50.

SUMMARY OF PART II

Consciousness evolved from the ability of primitive creatures to retain chemosensory information essential for survival. In mammalian brains the development of the hippocampus resulted in consciousness taking the form of a succession of real or imagined spatial maps that, in humans especially, might be associated with an inner voice.

46

Epilogue

The elderly woman looked back at the young reporter and gave one of her broad smiles before answering.[1] It was her intention, she said, to spend the afternoon of her birthday watching the final of the World Soccer Cup on television. She had favoured France from the beginning of the tournament but anticipated that Croatia would be a tough opponent. She had long been a soccer fan and Manchester City had always been her favourite team. The woman smiled again. In the evening, she said, there would be a party for her.

The reporter would have noted the slight accent in the elderly woman's fluent speech, a relic of her English childhood in Manchester. She would have noted, too, the bright, intelligent eyes and sensed the vitality of the small person sitting in front of her. And the reporter would certainly have admired someone who was continuing to research and teach long after the normal retirement age.

Brenda Milner, revered by her friends and colleagues, and by neuroscientists throughout the world, was about to celebrate her 100th birthday (Figure 46.1)

It had been almost 70 years since she had attended Donald Hebb's seminars in the Psychology Department at McGill and had decided to work for a PhD under the new professor's supervision. Not long after, she had published her paper with Wilder Penfield on the effects of temporal lobectomy in Penfield's patients. Then had come the invitation from William Scoville to examine the memory loss in some of his surgical cases and in one patient in particular, Henry Molaison. It had been Brenda Milner's careful testing of Henry that had demonstrated the importance of the hippocampus for memory and also the fact that there was more than one type of memory.

Henry had died, as had Brenda's former graduate student, the one who had taken over Henry's psychological testing, Suzanne Corkin. Brenda's supervisors had gone too. Donald Hebb had spent the last years of his life in the little town on the Atlantic coast where he had grown up. As for Wilder Penfield, long after his retirement the great surgeon had remained active, using much of his time to continue writing books, the last of which had been the story of his own life. But a far greater legacy than the books and the many scientific papers was the world-famous hospital and investigative centre that he had conceived of and brought into existence, the Montreal Neurological Institute.

Herbert Jasper had also departed, but not before his colleagues at the Université de Montréal had organized an international symposium on consciousness to celebrate the 90th birthday of Canada's greatest neuroscientist. Jasper had given a paper himself and it had been one of the best of the meeting. Brenda had first encountered Jasper at the Neurological Institute when she had been a graduate student and Jasper was in the

Aranzio's Seahorse and the Search for Memory and Consciousness. Alan J. McComas, Oxford University Press.
© Oxford University Press 2023. DOI: 10.1093/oso/9780192868244.003.0048

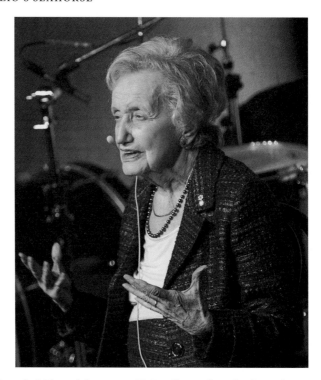

Figure 46.1 Brenda Milner delivering a TED talk, aged 93. (Wikimedia Commons. Photo by Eva Blue: Creative Commons Attribution 2.0 Generic License.)

gallery of the operating theatre making electroencephalogram (EEG) recordings while Penfield operated.

Peter Milner had gone too. He and Brenda had been married for over 60 years, having been brought together by the Second World War. In their different ways both had studied human behaviour and Peter had enjoyed great success too. Had he and James Olds not discovered the presence of a reward centre in the mammalian brain? Peter had died at the age of 99.

Brenda had received many honours in her long life. Her PhD in Hebb's department had been followed by 20 honorary degrees from other universities. She had been made a Companion of the Order of Canada, that country's greatest honour. She had won numerous medals and prizes. Among the latter had been the 2014 Kavli Prize in Neuroscience and before that a Gairdner Award, regarded by many as a stepping-stone towards a Nobel Prize. But the latter, the greatest prize of all, had eluded her. Almost certainly she would have been nominated, perhaps more than once. After all, it had been given to others for their work on the hippocampus and memory—Eric Kandel, John O'Keefe, Edvard and May-Britt Moser. Kandel had even acknowledged that it was Brenda's study of Henry Molaison that had inspired him to begin his own research on memory.

A nomination might have posed difficulties for a Nobel Committee, however. Kandel, O'Keefe, and the Mosers had all spent years toiling away in laboratories, devising new experimental approaches to the study of memory and the hippocampus. In contrast, Brenda's work had come easily. On first meeting Henry, she had asked him to remember a three-digit number; on testing him half an hour later she was surprised to find that although he had remembered the number he had no recollection of having seen her. Brief though it had been, the time had been enough to show the importance of the hippocampus for long-term memory. Then there had been the discovery of procedural memory, a special category of memory quite distinct from the ability to remember people, names, places, and events. Yet that discovery had come easily too—a few minutes spent testing Henry on successive days. Though there would be other examinations and important papers to be written, the two main findings were already apparent.

And what about Scoville's role? Had he still been alive, might he have been considered for a share of a Nobel Prize? It was Scoville who had performed the surgery on Henry Molaison and who had already noted the latter's serious impairment of memory. Moreover Scoville had been the senior author of the 1957 paper in which he and Brenda had described the findings in Henry Molaison and in nine other patients subjected to bilateral temporal lobectomy. But a Nobel Committee would have been obliged to consider the ethics of using an inadequately tested approach to the alleviation of epilepsy. And a Committee would have been aware of an earlier embarrassment. After the Prize had been given to Egaz Moniz in 1949 for treating psychiatric patients with prefrontal leucotomy, that initially popular surgical intervention had been abandoned by the medical profession.

And yet, and yet … If the Nobel Prize were to be awarded solely on the basis of the impact of a scientific discovery in physiology or medicine, then Brenda Milner would be an obvious choice, even at her great age!

Back to Penfield. In his time he had been a giant in his profession and, since his work on mapping the human brain was well known, very much a public figure. He, like Brenda Milner, had won prestigious awards and received numerous honorary degrees, and might well have been considered for a Nobel prize himself. It had been his report of curious symptoms, seemingly evoked from past life by electrical stimulation, that had led him to propose the temporal lobes as keepers of memory—some 20 years before the paper by Scoville and Milner. Indeed, much of Penfield's prestige had come from his thoughts as to how the brain functioned and, in particular, the relationship between the brain and consciousness. Against the conventional wisdom of the time, he had sensed that the massive cerebral hemispheres in the human brain were not responsible for thoughts and voluntary actions, but that the origins of the latter lay deeper.

Though it was a bold proposal, Penfield had made several observations in the course of his work that were in his favour. The problem had been his vagueness as to where, in the base of the brain, the elusive consciousness might reside. Rather than set about the matter in a careful, systematic manner, he had several times shifted his locus. Moreover his language had been more philosophical than scientific, much in the style of his great mentor, Charles Sherrington. It was unfortunate, especially since Penfield had had a man at his side who could have helped him enormously. Herbert Jasper, Penfield's companion in the operating theatre, was one of the most accomplished neuroscientists in the world. He had been a pioneer in both electromyography (EMG) and EEG, had proposed the universally adopted 10–20 electrode EEG recording system, had shown how the EEG could locate tumours, had made some of the first microelectrode studies of the cerebral cortex and thalamus, had helped to identify GABA (γ-Aminobutyric acid) as an inhibitory neurotransmitter in the mammalian nervous system—and done much more. Canada's greatest neuroscientist could have provided the scientific rigour that Penfield needed, forestalling the damaging criticism and embarrassment inflicted on Penfield by Francis Walshe. And Jasper might well have considered the limbic system as a candidate for a 'centrencephalic integrating system', in keeping with Penfield's intuition that his 'centre' was 'to be found in the old brain, not in the new'. How close Penfield had been!

But this is all conjecture. What is not conjecture is the enormous mountain of scientific data available that, somewhere and somehow, contains the key(s) to understanding the neural basis of consciousness. The present book has been an attempt at a soluble problem.

The limbic system, with its amygdala–hippocampal complex, has emerged as the solution.

Note

1. Interview on the occasion of Brenda Milner's 100th birthday (no longer available on the Internet and reference not found).

Acknowledgements

I must begin by stating that there are five books that not only made the present work easier, but provided information and insights that would otherwise have been missed. The first is Wilder Penfield's autobiography, *No Man Alone*, written in the closing years of the great surgeon's life and finished less than a month before his death. Based largely on the letters to his mother, the work is a valuable historical record not only of Penfield's remarkable life (and escape from death in the First World War) but of the development of neurosurgery as a specialty and, of course, of the founding of the Montreal Neurological Institute. Despite Penfield's international renown as a neurosurgeon and clinical neuroscientist the autobiography is free of self-promotion and one can only regret that it concluded in 1934, the year that the Institute opened, for the author must have had much more to tell.

The second of the books is *Patient H.M.* by Luke Dittrich, a grandson of William Scoville, the enterprising neurosurgeon who operated on Henry Molaison (Patient H.M.), inadvertently destroying the young man's long-term memory. Scoville's family background and his professional life are vividly described, though not without criticism, and there is an intriguing account of the fate of Henry Molaison's brain following the latter's death. Thoroughly deserving of its place on the *New York Times* bestseller list, *Patient H.M.* is an excellent read—so much so that several friends received copies shortly after its publication. And I am further indebted to the author, this time for allowing me to reproduce the photo of his grandfather (in surgical gear) and for kindly answering a query about his interview with Suzanne Corkin.

It was the late Suzanne Corkin who authored the third of the very helpful books. Because of some remarks and actions attributed to Corkin in Dittrich's *Patient H.M.*, I had anticipated being critical of her *Permanent Present Tense*. Instead, I found a book that explained the many aspects of memory in a refreshingly direct and simple manner, while recounting her many investigations of Henry Molaison. Towards the end of the book especially, there is a sense not only of gratitude to Henry but of affection for him too. It is therefore unfortunate that, when Corkin's fine career was being brought to a premature end by cancer, her reputation should have been blemished (by her destruction of laboratory records, as stated during her interview with Dittrich).

If asked, those working in the field of memory would probably have had little hesitation in suggesting Erik Kandel's *In Search of Memory: The Emergence of a New Science of Mind* as one of the books so helpful to me. Indeed, how could one write about the history of memory research without drawing on the account given by a Nobel Laureate? In his memoir Kandel succeeded in a difficult task, that of balancing a life story with a description of research, enough to please both a layperson and a neuroscientist interested in memory. The drawings of *Aplysia*, its neural circuitry and its responses to stimulation, were enormously helpful, as was the story of the later biochemical and molecular biological investigations that brought a life's work to a triumphant conclusion.

While Kandel's memoir, like the other books mentioned, provided abundant helpful information, it was the fifth book, *Forever Today: A True Story of Lost Memory and Never-ending Love*, that left the deepest impression. Deborah Wearing's telling of the tragic illness that befell her brilliant husband lingers in the mind. Words like devotion, dedication and determination fall far short in helping to describe Deborah's response to the destruction of Clive's mind. Clive himself, struggling to make sense of every brief snatch of awareness, is surely one of neurology's—and life's—heroes. The debt that neuroscience owes to Deborah and Clive for making their extraordinary story known is very great.

As with *Galvani's Spark* and *Sherrington's Loom*, I have drawn heavily on Larry Squire's superb series, *The History of Neuroscience in Autobiography*. Indeed, I suspect that, other than Dr Squire, I may have read more of these wonderful autobiographies that anyone. What a treasure trove for a medical historian to delve into! None of the many accounts failed to provide information about life and research that would not have been otherwise available. Not surprisingly, the styles of the writings differ as much as the contents, reflecting the personalities of the authors. Were I to be asked which of many I enjoyed most, I would pick the late Patrick Wall's on account of its wit and irreverence. Also of great value have been the Nobel Lectures and Backgrounds of Eric Kandel, John O'Keefe, Edvard and May-Britt Moser, and Richard Axel.

Next, I would like to thank Marie Levesque for once again producing much needed illustrations, just as she had for *Sherrington's Loom*, the present book's predecessor. Marie's drawings display a talent that I lack, and her patience during this difficult COVID-19 time was much appreciated.

I am also grateful to a number of others, all of them distinguished professors but some sadly no longer with us, for discussions and correspondence. They include Arthur Buller concerning John Eccles and the way that experiments were conducted in Canberra. Herbert Jasper became a friend in his later years, following a breakfast conversation at a scientific meeting at Queen's University, Canada. We corresponded over Penfield's reaction to Walshe's article and it was he, Professor Jasper, who kindly invited me to participate in the 1997 symposium on consciousness in Montreal. Sir Andrew Huxley gave me his and others' reaction to a talk at Cambridge University by Francis Crick and I heard Crick myself during a symposium sponsored by the Society for Neuroscience. I was privileged to help host Eric Kandel during a speaking visit to McMaster University (prior to his Nobel Prize) while my own research brought me into contact with two others mentioned in the book— Patrick Wall and Denise Albe-Fessard. I was especially grateful to Denise for allowing me to spend a very instructive month observing her experiments at the Institut Marey in the late 1960s.

Next, I would like to thank those who either gave permission to reproduce photographs or assisted in obtaining it. In no particular order they are Vaina Lucia, Edmund Rolls, Fernando Nottebohm, Jack MacMahon, Shirley Bayer, Elena Novikova, Loma Karklins, Candice Bjur, Scott LaFee, Katherine Fenz, and Kara Sjoblom-Bay. There were some who went further, kindly making suggestions, answering queries, and providing material that I had been unaware of. In this category are Clare Armstrong (regarding her grandfather, Sir Francis Walshe), Jean-Gaël Barbara (regarding Alfred Fessard, Denise Albe-Fessard, and the Institut Marey), György Buzsáki (regarding Case Vanderwolf), Fred Gage (regarding his ancestor, Phineas Gage), Sheena Josselyn (regarding optogenetics), Rodrigo Quian Quiroga (regarding concept cells), Aaron Newman and his Dalhousie colleagues (regarding Graham Goddard) and Terje Lømo (regarding Per Anderson). Thank you all, not least for helping to make the contents of the manuscript more vivid. I must also acknowledge the remarkable person whose research started and concluded the book— Brenda Milner, presently 103 years old and still working(!). I would have asked Dr Milner for a little of her time, gladly taking the train from Hamilton to Montreal and, if it would have helped to gain admission, entering her MNI office on bended knee. Alas, the COVID-19 epidemic made such a quest impossible, but Dr Milner was kind enough to allow me to reproduce an early photograph of her and, just as important, to wish me success with the book.

Next come friends and former colleagues who read the manuscript and who offered encouragement and suggestions. I was surprised and delighted to discover that Norman Jones, a distinguished respirologist but former junior neurologist, had also thought of an evolutionary explanation for consciousness. Jean Delbeke helped greatly over the 'Numbers Game' chapter, preferring neural computations based on a binary code ('fire' or 'not fire') as a means of memory storage. While I did not pursue this direction, Jean's criticisms and wise suggestions led me to reject much of the original draft of the chapter, one that had instead sought explanations in a changing 'signal-to-noise' ratio of hippocampal impulse activity. Erwin Montgomery (the 'philosopher-neuroscientist' in the book's 'Journey' preface) also applied his formidable intellect to the manuscript; while we remain unable to agree upon some scientific reputations and legacies, I am always grateful for his wisdom and insights. David Turner, with admirable patience and considerable skill, dealt with any computer problems, provided one photograph and improved another. Looking further back, there are others, most of them no longer living, who come to mind—Alexander Harper for teaching me physiology in Newcastle, Jack Diamond for the invitation to join McMaster University, Adrian Upton for accompanying me in the Canadian adventure, Roberto Sica for his comradeship in and out of the laboratory, and Moran Campbell for being a supportive departmental Chair. As an aside, how fortunate Adrian Upton and I were to become McMaster faculty in the autumn of 1971! It was a time of optimism and excitement—a new Faculty of Medicine based in a boldly designed building on a beautiful campus, plentiful money and laboratory space for research, freedom to choose topics, and time to do the experiments. One cannot help but regret the economic and social tensions that have since taken away so much of the joy and vigour of university life in the Western world.

Turning now to the actual production of the book, I owe a huge debt to Martin Baum of Oxford University Press for his encouragement, support, and wise counsel (including the choice of title for the book). I had the good fortune to have Jade Dixon as my editor at OUP and no one could have been more pleasant and efficient in getting everything in order and in making helpful suggestions. After Jade's contributions came the arrival of the proofs, the work of Shanmuga Priya, Project Manager for Newgen Knowledge Works––thank you, Priya, for your skill and efficiency. I would have found the checking of the proofs a difficult task without the manuscript skills and keen eye of my long-time friend, Aurelia Shaw, who has kindly helped me before.

Finally, and with profound gratitude, I come to my wife, Marie Ambruz, who continues to make her husband's life a pleasant and comfortable one, to offer inspiration and encouragement, and who kindly accompanied him in a quest to locate the venue of the 1953 Laurentian symposium on consciousness. Because of Marie the past decade has given me a happiness that I could never have anticipated and for which I cannot thank her enough. Had it not been for her love and care, the book would never have been written.

Index

For the benefit of digital users, indexed terms that span two pages (e.g., 52–53) may, on occasion, appear on only one of those pages.